PRAISE FOR

Toxic Superfoods

"One conversation with Sally Norton transformed my health. Thankfully, she has shared her life's work about the dangers of oxalates in this book. Everyone needs to hear her message."

—Dr. Bill Schindler, author of *Eat Like a Human*

"Sally Norton does a super job of revealing the many ways oxalates can promote the health of plants and undermine the health of people. You'll be shocked by the many foods and drinks that contain oxalates and you'll be alarmed to learn of the potentially harmful effects. This book is a must-read for people who eat plant-based superfoods."

—Fred Provenza, PhD, author of *Nourishment*

"An invaluable book that tells the story of the deleterious health effects of oxalate in our food."

—Miki Ben-Dor, PhD

"This book has the power to change the course of your health, happiness, and longevity for the better."

—James L. Oschman, PhD, author of *Energy Medicine*

"Juicing, raw food, and vegan trends have come and gone over my 30 years in the integrative oncology world and are currently all the rage again. This trend has created an illusion of health, and yet, clinically, I have seen the opposite. Sally has done an excellent job confirming what I have been seeing clini-cally."

—Dr. Nasha Winters, ND, FABNO

"Sally Norton has made a major breakthrough in our understanding of plant toxins. For believers in the health benefits of plant-based diets, this will be an unsettling yet actionable book."

—Kaayla T. Daniel, PhD, author of *The Whole Soy Story* and coauthor of *Nourishing Broth*

TOXIC
SUPERFOODS

HOW OXALATE OVERLOAD
IS MAKING YOU SICK—AND
HOW TO GET BETTER

SALLY K. NORTON, MPH

RODALE
NEW YORK

Published in the United States by Rodale Books, an imprint of Random House, a division of Penguin Random House LLC, New York.
RodaleBooks.com
RandomHouseBooks.com

RODALE and the Plant colophon are registered trademarks of Penguin Random House LLC.

Library of Congress Cataloging-in-Publication Data
Names: Norton, Sally K., author.
Title: Toxic superfoods : how oxalate overload is making you sick—and how to get better / Sally K. Norton, MPH.
Description: First edition. | New York : Rodale, [2022] | Includes bibliographical references and index.
Identifiers: LCCN 2022013492 (print) | LCCN 2022013493 (ebook) | ISBN 9780593139585 (trade paperback) | ISBN 9780593139592 (ebook)
Subjects: LCSH: Low-oxalate diet—Popular works. | Oxalic acid in the body—Popular works. | Oxalic acid—Toxicology—Popular works.
Classification: LCC RC918.O9 N67 2022 (print) | LCC RC918.O9 (ebook) | DDC 613.2/6—dc23/eng/20220716
LC record available at https://lccn.loc.gov/2022013492
LC ebook record available at https://lccn.loc.gov/2022013493

ISBN 978-0-593-13958-5
Ebook ISBN 978-0-593-13959-2

Printed in the United States of America

Book design by Andrea Lau
Art by Forrest Alexannder Higgins
Reference art for Raphide tips: photograph from C. J. Prychid et al. (2008), *Annals of Botany*
Reference art for Raspberry seeds: photograph from Franceschi and Nakata, 2005
Cover design by *the*BookDesigners
Cover photo illustration based on images from © Shutterstock

10 9 8 7 6 5

First Edition

In memory of Golding Bird and Clive Solomons and with gratitude to Joanne Yount, Susan Owens, and others whose suffering and caring led them to discover something new and make a gift of it to the world.

[W]e often let many things slip away from us,
which deserve to be retained; . . . either in tract of time obliterated,
or at best so overwhelmed and buried under more frothy notions,
that when there is need of them, they are in vain sought for.

—ROBERT HOOKE, MICROGRAPHIA, 1664

Contents

Part 2: The Low-Oxalate Program

Acknowledgments

First and foremost, my deepest gratitude to the founder and executive director of The Vulvar Pain Foundation, Joanne Yount; researcher and advocate Susan Costen Owens; and her champion and cheerleader, Edythe Pumfey Steffens. These pioneers clued me in to a solution to my pain when no one else could. Their work essentially saved my productive life.

Joanne Yount and Susan Owens not only rediscovered the healing power of low-oxalate eating, but their fresh insights and the resources they created made it possible for me and many others to find our way back to health. Joanne Yount's foundation (VPF) has pioneered systematic and extensive food oxalate content testing, and since 1993, VPF's newsletters provided a treasure trove of information on oxalate illness and the use of low-oxalate eating to reclaim health.

Thanks to crucial support from Pumfey Steffens, Susan Owens's Autism Oxalate Project (AOP), and the Trying Low Oxalates (TLO) community that formed around it, which have created a worldwide opportunity for sharing knowledge, experience, and practical wisdom about oxalates.

This book is my contribution back to both those communities: I hope it helps many more people see the value of oxalate awareness. If readers find value in this book, I encourage them to support those organizations.

In practice, low-oxalate eating would be nowhere without the hundreds of food oxalate content tests performed and reported by Dr. Michael Liebman and his colleagues on behalf of VPF and AOP. Joanne Yount's and Susan Owens's work was launched with the research and educational support of the late Clive Solomons, Ph.D., who recognized that oxalate was a concern after helping one woman. He went on to conduct thousands of urine tests, which provided the initial evidentiary basis for the emerging modern understanding of oxalates and health, and developed support therapies such as the use of calcium citrate in an effort he called the Pain Project.

Thanks also to Dr. Susan Marengo and Dr. Tanecia Mitchell for talking with me about their research on oxalates. Their work helps to explain the mechanisms of acute and chronic oxalate toxicity.

Hundreds of people have shared their stories of suffering and healing with me over the past nine years, propelling me to understand the nature of this disease by relating their experiences of oxalate overload and recovery. They have taught me just how widespread oxalate overload is and how much it can mean to find a path to recovery. I love you all. You too helped make this book possible. I hope our collective years of suffering and healing can also help others avoid needless pain.

Many special folks quickly saw the wisdom in what I shared with them and supported and encouraged me to continue to get the message out and create tools for their friends and family. My thanks to Kathleen Rose, Judy Hart, Cheryl Dingman, Jackie Dean, Rick Medley, Mary Ann Boyd, Jeannie DeAngelis, and many others who have passed this message forward and cheered me on.

A special shout-out to my low-oxalate support groups—the loyal in-person Richmond, Virginia, crowd who so believed in this work and showed up every month for five years, and the global community that formed when I took the support group online. Thank you to everyone who corresponded with me or who participated in interviews.

Thank you to the many readers who peeked at my drafts at every stage and were willing, patient, and encouraging (if not adequately critical!), but especially to Diane York and Tom Keeler.

Karin Wiberg kept me moving forward, taught me valuable new writers' tricks, sharpened my eye for punctuation and clarity, and helped with the book title. Many thanks to Donna Loffredo and the Harmony/Rodale Books team for helping to bring this book to the world.

To John Looseman, the middle school science teacher who inspired my choice of profession. To the memory of my loving father, Malcolm, who never doubted that my health problems were real. And to my husband, Jeremy Raw, who helped me discover the VP Foundation and its message—without his unfailing support, this book would not exist.

List of Tables

Introduction

When Healthy Isn't

Despite the fact that oxalate-containing plants are used in cooking, their ingestion may nonetheless lead to poisoning.

—Pedro Sanz, MD, and R. Reig, MD,
American Journal of Forensic Medicine and Pathology, 1992

I f you've joined the ranks of conscientious eaters by loading up on almonds, spinach, turmeric, tea, or chocolate, this book is for you. If you know anyone with a diet featuring "wholesome" foods like blackberries and quinoa who is *not* the picture of vitality and sturdiness, this book can help them. If you're suffering from gut problems, joint pain, inflammation, or a host of other symptoms that are stumping your doctors, it is very possible this book will point you toward relief.

What is the invisible culprit hiding within your favorite "superfoods"? Oxalates: chemical toxins that are produced by many plants.

I am an oxalate overload survivor. I ignorantly consumed excessive amounts of oxalates for most of my life—despite receiving a bachelor's degree in nutrition from Cornell University and a master's degree in public health leadership from the University of North Carolina at Chapel Hill. I had to learn about oxalates the hard way: through personal experience. My eventual enlightenment came after decades of striving for good health and painfully missing the mark.

I did not know that many of today's beloved "health foods" can *cause* health problems. And the culprits are so deeply trusted, it seems no one dare make the connection between our "best" foods and our most common maladies, including digestive problems, aches and pains, low energy, poor sleep, and worse. This book asks you to take a fresh look at an all-too-common problem: the failure of healthful eating to help us feel truly well.

Many of our most popular foods, such as potatoes, peanuts, and even today's "superfood" darlings like spinach, naturally contain tremendous amounts of overlooked (but long-known) natural toxins called oxalic acid, oxalate salts, and oxalate crystals (collectively known as "oxalates"). Oxalates are poisonous. Consuming a lot of them is destructive to your health. This simple fact remains controversial, despite 200 years of science and human experience to back it up. It's time to look past unquestioned beliefs and overpowering trends that are, in fact, leading us into serious trouble.

If you want to maintain the best possible well-being and long-term health, or if you are seeking optimal performance, then learning to avoid oxalates is a sensible move. If you're ailing and can't figure out why, you owe it to yourself to give this a try.

Many people have finally found some relief from—or have even reversed—a variety of conditions and syndromes, such as hypothyroidism, osteopenia, chronic pain, and chronic fatigue, simply by swapping their high-oxalate foods for low-oxalate alternatives. Low-oxalate eating has improved their sleep, energy, concentration, and mood. In the long term, avoiding oxalates can potentially prevent injury, arthritis, and osteoporosis, and can slow age-related degeneration. Such a choice may even calm a hyper-reactive immune system. Given the modern explosion of all these problems, oxalate-aware eating is critically important for everyone today. Undertaken correctly, it can dramatically improve quality of life and health.

Toxic Superfoods presents the existing science to explain the surprising healing responses and gradual recovery that a properly conducted low-oxalate diet can bring about. In developing this book, I've done a lot of heavy lifting for you—literally. I've lugged countless heavy volumes of medical journals up and down stairs to the library scanner, so you don't have to. Here's some of what I've learned, and what I share with you in Part 1 of this book:

- What oxalate is and where it occurs in nature, in our foods, and in our bodies
- Facts about oxalate that will help you navigate the thicket of oxalate-related misinformation on the internet
- Trends that have caused oxalate intake and related health issues to increase in recent decades
- Why it is risky to be "trendy" in your food choices
- How oxalates cause health problems—and, yes, we're going to dig a bit into the science because you need to understand it
- Why we don't see the connections between oxalate consumption and our health troubles
- The vast array of symptoms of oxalate overload and the diseases it can lead to

In Part 2, you'll learn how to adopt a low-oxalate eating pattern. You'll also find these practical resources:

- How to adopt a healthful low-oxalate diet
- Supportive strategies for healing from oxalate overload, including supplement suggestions for minerals and B vitamins that are easy to obtain and adapt to individual needs

❖ A Risks, Symptoms, and Exposure Self-Quiz (page 277) to see if you're headed for oxalate trouble

❖ Tables identifying high-oxalate foods and low-oxalate alternatives

❖ Recommended readings and additional online resources (page 298). Please visit toxicsuperfoods.com or sallyknorton .com for recipes, additional oxalate data resources, and an alphabetical bibliography of the source materials.

This book will guide you through the process of recognizing your risk factors and symptoms, altering your diet, and aiding your recovery with clear, simple steps. Armed with the information you'll find here, you can be confident in your new dietary choices, even when your health-care providers don't get it.

An Effective Path to Better Health

Oxalate-aware eating is completely within your reach. Armed with just the basic information in this book, you'll find a simple and inexpensive way to switch for a few months and see what it does for you. You, too, may be convinced.

"Low-oxalate" is not "no-oxalate," and many people experience prompt relief just by breaking their daily habits of eating handfuls of high-oxalate foods. *The key is to know what you're eating and how much, and to choose your daily staples from nourishing foods with less potential to create chronic problems*. The benefits of eating to reduce the oxalate loads in your body are rewarding and meaningful, often showing up within the first two weeks.

The foods you will be eating in place of your high-oxalate "frene-mies" are widely available (though sometimes not as well-known). It's simple to select turnips and cauliflower in place of potatoes, to try pumpkin seeds or cheese in place of almonds and peanuts, or to use romaine lettuce or arugula instead of spinach or mixed baby greens in your salads and smoothies. These changes are a good place for anyone to start.

Reducing your oxalate intake is simply the first step, though. If you're experiencing oxalate-related health problems, undoing the chronic damage of oxalate overload is not an instantaneous process. Initial improvements may be followed by intermittent symptoms as the oxalates, which have accumulated in the body over years or decades, make an often harrowing exit. Symptom flare-ups may continue over an extended period, as I discuss in Chapters 11, 12, and 13.

> **TESTIMONIAL**
>
> "I will admit I had been skeptical of the dangers of oxalate . . . until yesterday. I had a very high oxalate day with spinach. All I had to do was pay attention, and I noticed I had almost every symptom people are describing here. My worst symptom was a very bad shift in mood." —Joe

Fortunately, many people have been through the low-oxalate transition, sharing their experiences and learning from each other. We know a good deal about what to expect as we heal from oxalate overload. One thing is that everyone's case is unique. Here is how one of my clients described his experience:

"Since consulting with you last summer my health has improved more in five months than in the last three years. My quality of life has improved 90 percent, I no longer get nocturnal feet and leg cramps, my brain fog is gone, and I don't have kidney pain anymore. My 'incurable' hyperthyroidism was declared by my Kaiser endocrinologist to be officially cured without radioactive iodine

or medication. My thyroid panel levels are all back within the standard ranges. . . . I think adding your supportive protocols sped up the recovery process."

            —*Chris Knobbe*, MD

I fervently hope this book will inspire you to avoid, or recognize and recover from, the damage wrought by our oxalate-overloaded diets. I also hope *Toxic Superfoods* inspires a new generation of scientists to look deeply into the role of oxalates as a source of ill health. That important work is long overdue.

  Hang on, dear reader. We're about to adventure into a hidden world that will challenge you to reconsider everything you thought you knew about healthy eating.

PART 1

HOW OXALATES HARM

1

Health Food or Health Disaster?

*The greatest obstacle to discovering the shape
of the earth, the continents, and the ocean
was not ignorance but the illusion of knowledge.*

—Daniel J. Boorstin, *The Discoverers*, 1983

Actor Liam Hemsworth publicly blamed spinach smoothies for a 2019 kidney stone episode that required surgery. At age 29 he had to miss a movie premiere and an awards banquet because of it. In 2020, *Men's Health* magazine quoted Mr. Hemsworth as saying: "February last year, I was feeling really low and lethargic and wasn't feeling good generally. And then I got a kidney stone." He added: "Every morning I was having five handfuls of spinach and then almond milk, almond butter, and also some vegan protein in a smoothie. And that was what I considered super healthy. So, I had to completely rethink what I was putting into my body."

This book invites you to do just that: Rethink your "health" food.

Even moderate, relatively common levels of oxalate in a habitual diet can fuel the customary aches and pains of life: digestive distress, inflamed joints, chronic skin issues, brain fog or mood problems, as well as health declines associated with "normal" aging. And then there are those painful kidney stones. Eighty percent of them are formed from oxalate, much of which comes from the foods we eat.

Mr. Hemsworth was one of the lucky ones. Three weeks after completing a 10-day "green smoothie cleanse" for weight loss, a New York City woman with a history of gastric bypass surgery went to the Nassau University Medical Center on Long Island, complaining of persistent nausea, weakness, and poor appetite. She was immediately put on a low-oxalate diet, but it was too late, her kidneys did not recover, and she remained dialysis-dependent.

Similar examples of kidney failure due to consumption of "health foods" include a man, also attempting to lose weight, who juiced celery, carrots, parsley, beets with their greens, and spinach. The man's kidneys were seriously damaged. His doctors at the Mayo Clinic prescribed dialysis and a low-oxalate diet. He stopped juicing. It took more than four months for his kidney function to improve.

And it's not just kidney failure. Damage from dietary oxalate can hit any—or every—bodily system and cause serious chronic health problems. It's no accident that Mr. Hemsworth's kidney stones were preceded by malaise, depression, and lethargy. However, most medical journals reporting health crises from overzealous oxalate consumption fail to mention the non-kidney problems that likely also occurred.

Because it is so easy to overeat oxalates, chances are you may already be experiencing occasional oxalate-related aches and pains somewhere in your body. Do you tend to get a stiff neck? In those of us with dietary oxalate overload, pain, knots, or stiffness in the top of the shoulders or in the upper or lower back are typical. Some people experience chronic or intermittent joint inflammation, gout, arthritis, carpal tunnel syndrome, or a more generalized stiffness, often accompanied by a lack of pep.

Or perhaps you have long-standing injuries or chronic itching, tingling, or pain that never fully resolves. Your doctors can't help you figure
out what is going on; they seem to think you're "just fine" and should
just live with life's little miseries. If any of this rings true for you—if you
don't feel "just fine"—this book may be your golden opportunity to turn
things around.

Other seemingly small things can be indicators of oxalate overload,
including itchy or dry eyes, eye floaters, excessive tartar on the teeth,
tooth sensitivity, sensitive or frail skin, and odd things like pressure or
pain in the loins, irritable bladder, urinary tract infections, frequent
urination, or cloudy urine. Liver stress from oxalate overload can aggravate chemical sensitivity. Digestive problems like indigestion, reflux, bloating, excessive belching, constipation, and irritable bowel
syndrome are especially common. Additional symptoms can include
shortness of breath, sinus problems, yeast infections, and even cold
hands and feet.

Do you ever feel especially clumsy or occasionally have poor coordination? Do you get muscle spasms or eye twitches, or have memory or
word-finding difficulties, headaches, or anxiety and panic disorder?
Being neurotoxic, oxalates can get in—and on—your nerves. Oxalic
acid chemically bonds to calcium and other minerals and interferes
with cell energy production. Relentless oxalate consumption can cause
oxalate to build up inside the body *without* obvious symptoms and may
culminate years later as "old-age problems" such as bad bones, chronic
pain, and vision and hearing loss. Oxalate deposits are also associated
with brain cell damage that leads to Parkinson's disease and dementia
disorders.

You don't have to have symptoms to have a disease, and oxalate toxicity is no exception. But a wide spectrum of potential symptoms can
occur in the wake of oxalate overload, and each of us will (eventually)
suffer from our own unique subset of them if we persist with high-oxalate
eating. To make it easier to consider your own situation, you can take the

Risks, Symptoms, and Exposure Self-Quiz (in the Resources section, page 277) or look over **Table 10.1,** which lists body systems and oxalate-associated symptoms. Keep reading to get the interesting details.

There are several factors that increase the likelihood that your high-oxalate diet may be leading to oxalate overload and symptoms, including:

- ♦ A diet low in calcium and other minerals (dairy-free and vegan diets are two examples)
- ♦ Frequent use of gut-irritating foods, including beans, bran, whole grains, quinoa
- ♦ A history of repeated use of antibiotic or antifungal medications
- ♦ Long-term use of nonsteroidal anti-inflammatory pain medications (NSAIDs)
- ♦ Obesity or diabetes
- ♦ Crohn's disease, irritable bowel syndrome (IBS), leaky gut, food sensitivities, bariatric surgery, or gut dysbiosis
- ♦ Frailty or other chronic non-oxalate illness
- ♦ Poor kidney health, history of kidney stones, family history of kidney disease.

As you will see in Part 2 of the book, simply trying a low-oxalate diet for a few months is another way to assess your situation.

The Hard Road to Enlightenment

Maybe, like me, you have always considered yourself a healthy eater. It was healthy eating that led to my ill health. I was beyond exhausted—unable to read with comprehension, unable to work. A high-tech sleep study showed that I was waking up 29 times every hour. Medications did nothing to improve the situation. I was stuck, and no one could help me. I had problems with joint pain and symptoms of genital burning, but I did not connect them to my exhaustion and sleep issues. It was my genital burning that, in 2009, led me to The Vulvar Pain (VP) Foundation, and under the fog of my heavy brain fatigue I decided to try the low-oxalate diet they recommended, hoping for relief from genital pain, not understanding the potential scope of effects or the long period needed for full recovery from oxalate damage.

In my ignorance, I drifted back to my beloved sweet potatoes and celery, and in 2013, I added kiwifruit to my diet in a desperate attempt to resolve my chronic constipation. After three months of a daily kiwi (sometimes two), my arthritis and stiffness became severe (all over again). This led to the brain-twisting recognition that dietary oxalate was related to my decades of joint pain. Grudgingly, I finally got serious about maintaining a low-oxalate diet.

Once I consistently shunned my go-to high-oxalate foods (for me, mainly sweet potatoes and chard), multiple personal miracles unfolded. The debilitating sleep disorder vanished, *decades* of pain and joint problems receded, and I started to feel younger. I never imagined anything like that was possible. The contrast between the years of intractable problems and then dramatic, lasting, and wholly unexpected benefits in the wake of the diet change was eye-opening.

While doing the research that led to this book, I started giving free talks in my community about what I was learning. Those talks quickly blossomed into a monthly educational support group that continued for five years and later went online. Because so many people wanted and needed ongoing support and personalized attention, my nutrition consulting grew into an oxalate-education specialty practice. I was perplexed by (and slightly skeptical of) the wide array of healing responses my "students" were reporting. Take, for example, the disappearance of Barry's unsolvable itching and Amy's chronic muscle pain:

"Many things have really gotten better since I started eliminating oxalates. Most importantly for me, itching has been reduced significantly. I have been suffering with itching for years and no one could help me. I feel I have control over it now. This has been truly amazing. My stomach feels a lot better also. So, I feel that I have a great future. Thanks mainly, to you. You are amazing."

—*Barry*

"I just wanted to let you know how blown away I am by the complete pain relief in my psoas. Blown AWAY. It was so debilitating for so long. BLESS YOU, WOMAN!"

—*Amy*

My astonishment felt somewhat disorienting yet thrilling. Of all the things I've learned from the stories shared by oxalate-injured people, the most important and unexpected was this: we are not alone, we are not oddities. My research in the medical literature confirmed the connection between oxalate and many health problems. Oxalates are messing with a lot of us in a wide variety of ways. It's time we take notice.

My Cautionary Tale of Healthy Eating

Over the years I had tried every diet imaginable—for my general health, for my irritable bowel and bloat, for my fatigue, for my arthritis and muscle pains, for my injured feet that wouldn't recover, for my osteopenia, for my allergies.

I never imagined any reason for limiting the oxalates in my diet. Nor did the countless medical doctors and alternative health providers I turned to for help, with whom I found only frustration and expense. As far as I knew, the little-used low-oxalate diet was for kidney patients, not me. I had no obvious kidney impairments. However, the kidney indicators on my standard blood tests tended to be a bit "off," and for 30 years my urine was frequently cloudy. Chronically cloudy urine is a visible sign of high levels of oxalate crystals, a condition called *crystalluria*. Crystal-laden urine is a risk factor for kidney disease, yet it gets little attention, and no doctor ever commented on mine.*

Like so many others, prior to learning about oxalates, I was following the prevailing health advice of our times. I cut out salt, wheat, gluten, and sugar, and I added more salads, sweet potatoes, and occasional smoothies. My eating style had shifted to embrace plant-based whole foods. Careful to limit red meats and fats, I shopped the produce department where "food is medicine." Despite all this wholesome organic goodness, as months and eventually years went by, I didn't get the results I hoped for. Instead, my health got worse. Does this sound familiar?

Health problems from excessive oxalates in our bodies may begin with no symptoms at all—not a one. Worse still, oxalate overload doesn't have to be silent to be overlooked. When I was a 20-year-old vegetarian, a Cornell University doctor told me that I had gout, a type of diet-related joint pain. That seemed odd to me because gout is generally associated with meat and alcohol consumption, neither of which were in my diet. Neither the doctor nor I was aware that the oxalates in our diet promote the two hallmarks of gout: generalized oxidative stress and crystals collecting in the joints. Unsurprisingly, my doctor did not mention the possibility of "oxalate gout," a known sub-type of gout, and showed no curiosity as to why a trim, young female vegetarian would have gout. At that time, oxalate gout was inexplicably being dropped from diagnostic consideration and is now called "pseudo-gout" (or non–uric acid gout).†

---

* I did tend to have high BUN and sometimes elevated creatinine revealed by standard blood tests, but this was shrugged off or ignored.

† More updated and comprehensive understanding of gout is that it is an expression of a generalized inflammatory and metabolic disorder, and is not confined to the joints. (See Georgiana Cabău, Tania O. Crişan, Viola Klück, Radu A. Popp, and Leo A. B. Joosten, "Urate-Induced Immune Programming: Consequences for Gouty Arthritis and Hyperuricemia," *Immunological Reviews* 294, no. 1 (March 2020): 92–105.)

In an ideal world, gout would be a red flag to inquire about dietary habits, including oxalate intake.

My episodes of gout were a relatively minor element in a deeper, decades-long puzzle of "bad feet." Over a year earlier, at age 19, I was diagnosed with a painful broken foot bone and a stiff big toe. Instead of healing, my foot pain turned into a saga involving both feet and years of crutches, wheelchairs, and doctors issuing injections, prescription-strength Motrin, expensive orthotics, surgery, and rehab, none of which fixed my feet. For years, there was never even a fleeting thought (on my part), or any hint from any health-care professional, that diet could be a factor in either the initial onset or the lack of resolution. Around the age of 27, I eventually got off the crutches, orthotics, and pain medication. I'd always credited my swimming a mile every day for this progress and I failed to notice (until now) that I also moved away from vegetable gardening, stopped eating chard, and ate fewer vegetables generally.

Despite moving past the need for crutches or meds, my subpar feet lingered. For the next 20 years, I could not run or tolerate the jumping and dodging required to play most sports. Dancing? Heels? Both were out of the question. I could not even stand bare-footed at the kitchen sink. Yet, suddenly, at age 50, just months after fully adopting the low-oxalate approach to my diet, everything changed. For a nephew's wedding, I hiked from parking lots, across city streets, up and down stairs, posed for photos, and mingled for seven hours wearing three-inch-plus heels without pain. I was stunned. Soon I was running on pavement in bare feet—no pain, no problem.

Not only are doctors unaware of the connection between health problems and oxalate, but also their dismissal of the symptoms and off-the-mark diagnoses leave many of us accused of imaginary illnesses or psychological problems. That dismissive attitude may be compounded by the fact that oxalate is documented to have neurological effects, which include emotional brittleness, despondency, heightened irritability, and anxiety.

In 1998, at the student clinic at the University of North Carolina, I was harshly told I didn't have "real" problems, but that I clearly needed "psych services" because surely anyone wondering if there was a dietary or environmental element to my aches, fatigue, and food sensitivities was verging on mental health collapse. Even at Cornell University in 1986, it was not my orthopedic doctor who recommended a leave of absence for foot surgery but, rather, the mental health services office. Lack of awareness of oxalates and their toxic effects leaves folks like the younger me damaged, stuck, and in decline.

Countless recovery stories like my own or those of Chris, Barry, and Amy demonstrate relief from perplexing problems just by putting less oxalate into our shopping carts and blenders. None of us suspected a connection nor did we expect the dietary shift would be so broadly helpful—yet it was.

Getting Our Heads Around Oxalate Overload

If medical reports about oxalate poisoning caused by spinach smoothies or stories of significant health revival are shocking, it's because we're getting a skewed, incomplete story about high-oxalate plant foods that ignores their potential to do harm. In today's world, blaming produce and nuts for health problems sounds like blasphemy. But maybe a little rebellion is needed in an era of universally declining health, escalating autoimmune problems, and epidemic issues with overuse, abuse, and addiction to pain medications.

Health is not preserved by wishfully thinking that plants are always benign. In fact, plants make toxins that can damage us, even the plants we consider "edible" and "beneficial." Because this fact doesn't align with currently favored nutrition theories promoting phytonutrients and fiber, and demonizing animal fats, we ignore plants' toxic effects, hoping they won't matter much.

I myself was an ignorant skeptic. I had a lifetime of "healthy food" programming from professors, alternative-health experts, the whole-foods movement, magazines, and numerous veggie-diet advocates and their books, not to mention cultural "truisms" illustrated by iconic figures like Popeye and his spinach. . . . None of that deep-seated indoctrination was easily set aside. So, let's take a closer look at the science of oxalates so that we can understand how our beloved plant foods can wreak such havoc on our bodies. First, let's consider why plants contain oxalates.

2

Oxalates Are Weapons for Plants

*Feed a man pulverized glass and he will die: permit him
to chew the leaves of the* Dieffenbachia seguine
*quickly his tongue is pierced by a million oxalate
raphides and he suffers untold agony.*

—B. G. R. Williams, MD, and E. M. Williams, MD,
The Archives of Diagnosis, 1912

For a great majority of plants, oxalic acid and oxalate crystals are essential to their growth, survival, and reproduction, and they are also secret weapons in the defensive warfare plants wage to keep from being eaten. Plants use oxalic acid's toxic powers to shun a variety of predators, including infectious fungi, other microorganisms, insects, and other plant-eating animals—including humans.

Humans use the natural biocide powers of oxalates in several ways. For example, oxalic acid is a registered pesticide and drug used in bee-keeping to kill mites that infect bees. Its use at recommended levels seems to be safe for adult bees. However, because oxalic acid is very toxic to honeybee larvae, its use may be a factor contributing to the very colony collapse problems that the treatment is intended to contain.

If you're wondering about oxalate in honey, know that the oxalic acid content in plants is much higher than in honey, and the oxalate content of honey from treated colonies is only slightly increased over that of untreated colonies.

In an ancient technique, central and southern African hunters harnessed the power of oxalic acid by driving wooden arrowheads into banana tree trunks about 24 hours before the hunt. The oxalic acid in the tree sap is powerful enough to paralyze prey. It's a nerve toxin.

When oxalic acid molecules bind to minerals (such as calcium), the resulting *oxalates* tend to form *crystals*. Plants deliberately construct a variety of shapes of calcium oxalate crystals by first erecting scaffolding made from proteins that have a strong affinity for calcium. The shapes of these creations include rough sand, diamonds or pyramids, rectangular blocks, spiky "disco balls," and long fine needles with barbed tips. The needle shapes are called *raphides* (see **Figures 2.1** and **2.2**). Raphides are designed to carry poisons as they puncture cells in the mouth, throat, and gastrointestinal (GI) tract. The toxins they deliver include oxalic acid, enzymes, glucosides (poisons bound to sugar molecules), and neurotoxic peptides, which can wound, stun, and paralyze those who dare eat them. One study used raphide crystals from kiwifruit to demonstrate that even natural vegetarians like caterpillars can die from the one-two punch of the raphide crystal arrows "dipped" in natural toxins.

The inedible houseplant *Dieffenbachia* is famous for its ability to propel raphide crystals into the cells of the mouth and throat of pets and people. The irritating effects escalate and persist owing to immune reactions. Even a momentary taste of *Dieffenbachia* sap can cause a massive release of histamine and temporary paralysis of the vocal cords, rendering the victim unable to speak for days. That is why *Dieffenbachia*'s common name is "dumb cane."

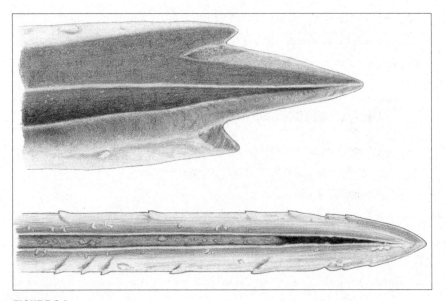

FIGURE 2.1
Raphide tips specifically designed by plants to serve as weaponry.

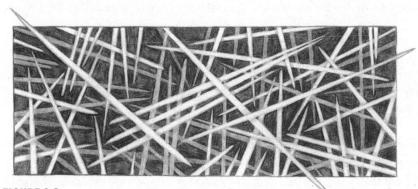

FIGURE 2.2
Raphides from kiwi have a simpler toothpick shape that can damage us.

Oxalate crystals are abrasive and resist cooking and digestion. Other forms of oxalate in foods include caustic oxalic acid ions that enter our bloodstream following meals, exposing all our tissues (and cells) to harm. We'll see that such damage, though invisible, can eventually escalate into degenerative illness.

Being aware that oxalate is a health risk, researchers have tried to develop spinach cultivars that are lower in oxalate, so far to no avail. While *plants* may need oxalates for survival, *we* absolutely do not.

THE FUNCTIONS OF OXALATES IN PLANTS

✦ Protecting from infections and predators
✦ Managing (storing and discarding) calcium
✦ Saving carbon
✦ Capturing sunlight

Oxalate crystals in foods are harder than teeth and cause tooth wear in humans. It's no wonder that they may also cause irritation to the mouth and digestive tract. Typically, we don't experience sensations in our mouth from the crystals in foods because we don't grind up the plant cells enough while chewing. It is possible to unleash these nasties, however. One eater described the reactions she and her fellow diners had from eating pulverized kiwifruit:

> "For my final course of dinner, I had a super healthy salad with a kiwi/macadamia nut dressing. The kiwi was blended in a Vitamix, causing the seeds to also be blended. WOW! I believe that the seeds REALLY irritated my mouth. My lips got chapped, and my mouth really hurt. I couldn't finish the salad due to such strong irritation."
>
> —Online post to the Rawtarian Community Forum

The raphides in the kiwifruit that caused her mouth irritation are located adjacent to the seeds, embedded in an envelope of pectin mucilage. This coating was disrupted by the high-power blender, releasing the crystals to do their damage. Regardless of the presence of oxalate crystals, though, liquefying foods with blenders and juicers breaks open the hard-to-digest plant structures that might otherwise partially limit the oxalates' irritating effects. When we pulverize our foods—turning them into nut milks, for example—we not only free crystals to abrade the digestive tract but we're also setting oxalic acid free and enhancing its ability to do us harm. Almond milk, being a dilute solution of pureed and filtered almonds, contains a lot of *bioavailable* oxalate that readily moves into the bloodstream.

Regularly consuming almond beverages can lead to health problems, as it did for three young children identified at the Pittsburgh School of Medicine, who sustained serious kidney injury from the oxalate in almond beverages. That result was unexpected, as earlier research suggested that calcium added to the beverages might bind to the oxalate and lower the amount that gets into the bloodstream. So much for that theory. Rat studies long ago found that oxalate bound to calcium enters the blood intact. Much older research suggests that the more dilute the oxalate, the more toxic it is.

We don't need to use blenders for sharp oxalate crystals to cause irritation and abrasion. Skin irritation from oxalate crystals is a well-known problem for workers on agave plantations and in tequila distilleries.

Other oxalate crystal shapes in leaves, stems, bark, and seeds are also invaluable tools for plant self-defense. A single large tree produces hundreds of pounds of blocky oxalate crystals every year to discard excess calcium while also keeping burrowing insects at bay. Cinnamon—which is a tree bark—is very high in oxalate crystals (but low in oxalic acid). The oxalate crystals in tree bark are a chief component of smoke, soot, and ash released when trees burn.

As with tree bark, some fruits defend their seeds with rings of oxalate crystals in their outer layers—see, for example, the cross-sectional drawing of a raspberry seed in **Figure 2.3**. Calcium oxalate crystals help seeds be durable and survive many threats (including predators' digestion) during dormancy. When the seeds germinate, they break down the protective oxalate crystals into a source of calcium (which is required for building proteins), while releasing free oxalic acid. Soaking nuts and grains kicks off germination, converting some of the oxalate crystals into free oxalic acid, which is the form most able to enter our circulating blood.

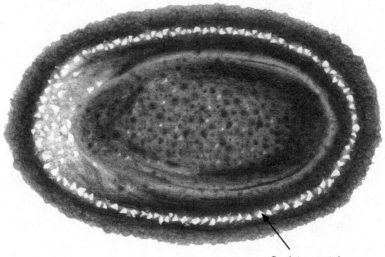

Oxalate crystals

FIGURE 2.3
In this cross-section view of a single raspberry seed, oxalate crystals can be seen as a ring of white specks just under the outer layer.

In food testing, the current practice is to distinguish oxalate as either *soluble* (free oxalic acid) or *insoluble* (crystals and calcium-oxalate molecules). Only a small fraction of insoluble oxalate (~1 percent) is believed to enter the bloodstream, but how much stomach acids and food combinations alter the oxalate molecules and crystals is hard to know.

In some plants, oxalate crystals may act like "bones" by helping them stay upright, as well as by serving as a mineral reservoir. The bone analogy fits here because in animals and humans, our actual bones not only hold us up but also are reservoirs of calcium that can be tapped when calcium levels drop in the bloodstream. Calcium is essential for plant and animal life, but it must be carefully managed because too much or too little at any moment can cause serious problems.

Sometimes plants create calcium oxalate crystals as a "discard pile," allowing them to manage and excrete calcium to prevent the amount of free calcium from reaching toxic levels in their cells. For that reason, oxalate levels tend to be higher in plants grown in soils that are high in calcium. Interestingly, in tomatoes, the combination of too much calcium and too much humidity promotes oxalate crystal formation in the fruits, visible as gold specks on the fruits' shoulders. The gold-speckled tomatoes are less attractive and spoil quickly because the crystals can damage cell structures.

Cleverly, desert plants use oxalate crystals as if they were air. During the day, while the sun shines in impossibly dry air, cacti and other desert plants must close their air holes to hold on to moisture, but that cuts off the supply of carbon dioxide required for photosynthesis. These plants build oxalate crystals during the night, amassing carbon they can then use for photosynthesis during the day. Not surprisingly, cactus leaves (nopal) are high in oxalates.

Food Oxalate Levels Vary

The varying levels of oxalates in plants and the relative lack of good information on those levels make estimating our oxalate intake an imprecise art. Plants are living things and their oxalate content (and oxalate type) can vary substantially depending on their growth environment, metabolism, varietal genetics, and other factors. Even the stage of maturity can be important. For example, a very ripe Hass avocado has only about 7 mg of oxalate, yet a firm one that is barely ripe contains about 50 mg—seven times as much.

The black and white peppercorns used in everyday cooking are the fruit of the same pepper vine, but their oxalate content is quite dissimilar. The black peppercorn is picked when unripe and is high in oxalate

(~13 mg/teaspoon). In contrast, the white peppercorn is picked when fully mature and is very low in oxalate (<2 mg/teaspoon). By weight, immature black peppercorns are 10 to 20 times higher than white peppercorns. In soybeans, a similar pattern is observed: oxalate levels are highest when the beans are immature. Soybean varieties (there are over 100) vary widely in oxalate content, even when fully mature.

An additional degree of fuzziness to oxalate content numbers comes from vague serving sizes (amounts are often underestimated) and variable food densities (how finely chopped, for example). Keeping in mind that numbers indicating the total oxalate content of foods are not precise (nor are your portions), the honest thing to do is to use rounded-off numbers when estimating oxalate intake, as I have throughout this book.

The reliability of published numbers is also a common source of error and confusion, partly because accurate analysis of oxalate content in biological materials is a very tricky thing. Together, analytical challenges and the failure of researchers to specify variety, maturity, and other distinguishing characteristics increase the fuzziness of the oxalate data. The abundance of poor-quality and poorly documented data is a major impediment to the recognition of oxalate overload. Unreliable and fragmentary data prevents us from accurately estimating our consumption of oxalate and obscures dietary oxalates' powers to harm.

AN OBJECT LESSON IN SNIFFING OUT POOR DATA

Like cauliflower, turnip and rutabaga are members of the brassica family. They are low in oxalate and can easily substitute for potatoes. Peeled baking potatoes—Russet and Idaho—have 25 to 50 mg oxalate per 100 grams; boiled red-skinned new potatoes are lower in oxalate; a small number of tests suggest they have about 20 mg per 100 grams.

Cooked turnip contains only 2 mg of oxalate per ½ cup,

according to testing done at the University of Wyoming. But if you didn't know turnips are *brassicas,* you'd be fooled by some sloppy data available online. In a list hosted by the Harvard School of Public Health Nutrition Department, and widely circulated online, their data claim that turnips have 15 times that amount of oxalate (30 mg). That's probably a decimal point error, but it illustrates a key reason as to how using online data can be confusing. Evaluate your source of information and check it carefully for accuracy.

Indeed, you *can* trust the brassicas to provide bioavailable minerals. They are a flexible culinary family that can not only fill in for potatoes but also be a substitute for chard and spinach as a side dish or be added to enrich soups, stews, and casseroles. Just use the brassicas in moderation and make sure they are cooked well; they are harder to digest when raw or undercooked.

Relative Levels of Oxalate in Various Plant Families

Worse still are inaccurate beliefs about oxalates in foods. The categorical idea that *all* "leafy greens" must be avoided is false. And, although some foods like spinach have been tested over and over, many other foods have not been tested at all with accurate techniques, let alone thoroughly tested for variations across or within specific varieties, growing conditions, or ripeness and maturity. Because some foods either haven't been tested adequately or may naturally vary so widely in oxalate content, we rarely (if ever) know the precise oxalate content of a specific serving we are about to eat. That is why it's important to plan your menus around reliable food-content data and to limit your use of untested foods or foods that are highly variable. The data and general tips provided in this book can help keep your guessing to a minimum.

Here's one helpful tip: sometimes knowing the plant family to which a food belongs can suggest whether that food is likely to be very high or very low in oxalates (or relatively unpredictable). Plant foods that are *reliably low* in oxalates come from these two families:

- The cabbage family (Brassicaceae or Cruciferae), which includes broccoli, cauliflower, arugula, collards, mustard, kale, watercress, radish, turnips, rutabaga, and other common vegetables
- True lettuces (Asteraceae family), including butterhead, romaine, iceberg, and leaf varieties

Foods that are *consistently high in oxalates*:

- Tend to be seeds. High-oxalate seeds include chia, poppy, and hemp seeds, for example, as well as most tree nuts, beans, teff, whole grains, and several spices including caraway.

- Or come from these two families:
  1. Amaranth family (Amaranthaceae), including beets and their leafy green tops, chard, spinach, lamb's quarters, amaranth, quinoa
  2. Buckwheat family (Polygonaceae), including buckwheat and rhubarb

Nightshades (Solanaceae family), including potatoes, tomatoes, and eggplant, tend toward higher oxalate content, but they vary considerably. Ripe red peppers (bell and hot) are often low in oxalate, yet green, yellow, and orange bell peppers are inexplicably two or three times higher. Hot peppers vary, too. They are generally higher in oxalate compared with bell peppers but are used in smaller amounts. According to a limited number of tests, habanero peppers are one of the lowest and Anaheim the highest. Baking potatoes (including chips and fries) are high, but new potatoes are lower. Fresh tomatoes tend to be "medium-high" depending on variety (and portion size). While having a few to-mato wedges on a salad is fine on a low-oxalate diet, tomato sauce and other concentrated forms of tomatoes are considered high-oxalate foods and need attention to portion sizes. Concentrating the foods by cooking or drying them typically increases their density and the amount of oxa-late they contain. A ½ cup of boiled spinach has a lot more spinach (and oxalate) than a ½ cup of raw spinach.

Another potential source of the variability of oxalate content of many foods is contamination by oxalate-producing molds, specifically *Asper-gillus* and *Penicillium*. These oxalate "generators" are the most common fungal contaminants in wheat flours and the products made from flour. Likewise, fresh and dried fruits (including figs, grapes and raisins, ap-ples, apple juice and apple products), almonds, sesame seeds, hazelnuts, and pistachios are examples of foods prone to contamination from oxalic-acid–producing molds. The variable oxalate content in breads and pastas may be influenced by varying levels of mold contamination, which is impacted by changing conditions and practices used in harvest-ing, milling, packing, and storing of flours. When mold-contaminated products such as bread flour dominate our diets, they, too, contribute to the oxalate load of modern diets.

Yet another possible source of variability of oxalate content in pro-duce is the use of oxalic acid to slow yellowing in leafy greens during postharvest storage.

Oxalate is a toxic compound that has been effectively harnessed by plants (and fungi) for their defense and survival. In the next chapter, we'll look at how much oxalate we can tolerate without toxic conse-quences.

3

How Much Is Too Much?

"No, I'll look first," she said,
"and see whether it's marked 'poison' or not,"
for she had . . . never forgotten that,
if you drink much from a bottle marked "poison,"
it is almost certain to disagree with you, sooner or later.

—Lewis Carroll, *Alice's Adventures in Wonderland*, 1865

It's remarkably easy to overeat oxalate and get sick from doing so. Even natural herbivores like insects, sheep, and cattle get sick from eating oxalate-loaded plants. When Cornell University researchers in 1949 fed beet greens (a high-oxalate green) to baby chicks, the oxalate killed all of them within two weeks. When horses consume high-oxalate forages, they develop a stiff and stilted gait owing to calcium depletion and problems with the function of their muscles and nerves. This oxalate-induced disease is called "big head" because the lame animals eventually develop distorted, swollen faces. As their facial bone cells gradually die and the connective tissue structures fall apart, disorganized scar tissue takes over and cannot successfully revert to normal bone. Similarly, high-oxalate foods can create mineral deficiencies that are deadly for sheep, even though sheep, unlike horses, are ruminants with bacterial digestion that gives them better tolerance for oxalates.

For a flock of Egyptian sheep in 2006, it took only a few days of eating beet greens—a by-product of the sugar beet industry*—to cause tremors, teeth grinding, dry mouth, stumbling, anorexia, weight loss, and even depression. The medical team used intravenous calcium and magnesium to save 46 ewes, but 2 died despite treatment. In humans, oxalates also disturb calcium metabolism and create deficiencies that harm bones, muscle, nerves, the brain, and other organs.

The amount of oxalates humans can consume without ill effect, while variable, is surprisingly low. Kidney researchers tell us that **a "normal" and safe intake level is within the range of 150 to 200 mg a day. "High-oxalate" eating—with great potential to get healthy people into trouble over time—is typically defined as 250 mg or more per day. Diets over 600 mg a day are considered "extremely high."** (Note: As we saw in the previous chapter, estimates of oxalate content of foods tend to have a "ballpark" specificity because actual content in foods depends on many variables.)

Even if these intake thresholds were well known—and they are not—we still would be clueless about how much we eat and what it's doing to us, because nutrition labeling does not require testing and reporting of the oxalate content of foods. Like sheep and cattle stumbling into a dangerous thicket of weedy high-oxalate forages, we can easily blunder into astoundingly high—and dangerous—levels of oxalate consumption, yet never know it. **Table 3.1** is a list of typical servings of

---

* Sugar beet tops, like other leftovers from industrial agriculture, are sometimes added to animal feed—despite the risk of illness or death to the animals.

high-oxalate foods contributing to the high levels of oxalate consumption you may be inadvertently consuming daily.

Table 3.1: Worst Offenders

Note: Oxalate content data presented in this table (and throughout the book) are summarized from test results reported by trustworthy laboratories and research reports. Where multiple test results are available, the numbers have been combined into a practical estimate for making dietary selections. A table of oxalate content data listing the values and published sources for all the foods mentioned in this book is available on my website, sallyknorton.com.

Item / Preparation	Serving Size	Mg Oxalate per Serving (total)
Beverages		
Beet juice	⅔ cup (160 ml)	95
Black tea, brewed	1 teabag (~1.7 g)	20
Green tea, brewed	1 teabag (~1.25 g)	15
Milk with 2 Tbs. chocolate syrup	1 cup (240 ml)	18
Hot cocoa, made with 1 Tbs. cocoa powder	6 g cocoa powder	40
Starbucks Latte Dark Chocolate Mocha, tall	1½ cups (360 ml)	75
Desserts		
Carob powder	2 Tbs. (12 g)	55
Chocolate, 70% dark	1.75 oz. (50 g)	110
Chocolate, 85% dark	1.75 oz. (50 g)	140
Cocoa powder	2 Tbs. (11 g)	80

Item / Preparation	Serving Size	Mg Oxalate per Serving (total)
Fruits and Berries		
Apricots, dried	¼ cup (35 g)	30
Blackberries, fresh	4 oz (113 g)	60
Clementine, peeled	1 (75 g)	20
Figs, mission, small, dried	6 (60 g)	50
Kiwifruit, fresh	1 (75 g)	30
Pomegranate, seeds and juice	½ cup (85 g)	30
Star fruit	1 (90 g)	270
Grains and Pseudo-Grains		
All-Bran cereal	½ cup (30 g)	75
Amaranth, raw	¼ cup (50 g)	75
Brown rice, cooked	1 cup (195 g)	24
Buckwheat, cooked	1 cup (180 g)	230
Quinoa, boiled 30 minutes	1 cup (180 g)	110
Shredded wheat cereal	2 biscuits (50 g)	40
Soba noodles (buckwheat)	1 cup (110 g)	30
Teff (flour)	⅓ cup (45 g)	100
Wheat germ	½ cup (55 g)	25
Whole-grain bread	2 slices (75 g)	30

(table continues)

Item / Preparation	Serving Size	Mg Oxalate per Serving (total)
Green Vegetables		
Beet greens *or* red-stemmed chard, raw	1 cup (40 g)	380
Beet greens *or* red-stemmed chard, boiled 6 minutes	½ cup (90 g)	400
Cactus (nopal), boiled 30 minutes	½ cup (75 g)	260
Chard, white-stemmed, boiled 6 minutes	½ cup (90 g)	270
Mixed salad greens/mesclun, raw (typical)	1½ cups (45g)	75
Rhubarb, cooked	½ cup (120 g)	370
Sorrel, boiled 15 minutes	½ cup (90 g)	520
Spinach, raw	1½ cups (45g)	450
Spinach, boiled	½ cup (90 g)	450
Herbs and Spices		
Black pepper	½ tsp. (1 g)	8
Slippery elm	½ tsp. (0.75 g)	18
Turmeric	½ tsp. (1.1 g)	25
Legumes		
Black beans, boiled	½ cup (90 g)	65
Great Northern beans, boiled	½ cup (90 g)	70
Navy beans, boiled	½ cup (90 g)	50
Peanuts, roasted	28 nuts (28 g)	45
Pinto beans, boiled	½ cup (90 g)	40
Soybeans, boiled	½ cup (90 g)	50

Item / Preparation	Serving Size	Mg Oxalate per Serving (total)
Nuts		
Almonds, whole, with skins	24 nuts (28 g)	120
Cashews	24 nuts (28 g)	75
Pecans, halved	17 halves (28 g)	18
Pine nuts (pignoli), raw	3 Tbs. (28 g)	60
Walnuts, halved	14 halves (28 g)	16
Root Vegetables and Starches		
Beets, boiled	½ cup (85 g)	45
Plantain, fresh, cooked in oil	½ cup (85 g)	95
Potatoes, russet, baked, flesh only	1 medium (170 g)	85
Sweet potatoes, baked, flesh only	½ cup (110 g)	120
Seeds		
Chia seeds	¼ cup (40 g)	260
Hemp hearts	¼ cup (40 g)	22
Poppy seeds	1 Tbs. (8 g)	180
Sesame seeds, hulled	¼ cup (30 g)	45

It is easy to exceed the 250 mg daily intake defining a high-oxalate diet, especially if you're trying to eat well by current standards. Liam Hemsworth's morning spinach smoothies, mentioned in Chapter 1, which led to his kidney-stone surgery, clocked in at more than 1,000 mg. Given his high-calorie needs (owing to his athleticism) and his vegan diet (at the time), his daily intake could easily have added up to at least twice that amount, perhaps over 2,000 mg. That is a high-oxalate diet times 8! Clearly, it's possible to eat way more oxalates than we can handle, and the toxic effects are not recognized as a medical problem.

Human deaths have occurred from meals containing as little as 3,500 to 4,000 mg of oxalate. In most healthy people, the lethal acute dose is surely higher. Death, of course, is a crummy standard for defining harm.

It's hard to avoid eating too much oxalate. Take, for example, the impulse-buy area at a typical retail store checkout. It's usually loaded with chocolate, nuts, and other high-oxalate treats like plantain chips. Trader Joe's, for example, even offers plantain chips sprinkled with dark chocolate. Based on tests of similar products, this snack probably has 45 mg oxalate per ounce. But who eats just 1 ounce of chips?* Worse still, a 2-ounce peanut butter Clif bar has 70 mg of oxalate, and a small 1.4-ounce dark chocolate bar has about 100 mg. A scant ¼ cup of almonds—just 26 nuts—has nearly 150 mg oxalate.

Even if you resist those temptations, other uninformed choices can add up to big but invisible differences. See how this might play out with two very similar menus, shown in **Table 3.2.**

Notice that the oxalate content of Menu 1 in **Table 3.2** is 10 times as much as that of Menu 2. But they look very similar because we are not oxalate aware, and the importance of this difference is lost in our oxalate-oblivious world. Based on current health precepts, we tend to favor the menu containing 1,000 mg of oxalate over the 100 mg menu because it includes "healthy" fiber and dark leafy greens.

Sadder still, professional training and academic degrees make little difference. Even licensed dietitians typically have only a vague and limited idea about which foods are high in oxalates, and like most other nutrition professionals, they would not see the oxalate content difference between the two menus. Nearly everyone blithely ignores the toxicity of oxalates when recommending foods.

Our standard way of evaluating food safety is to read labels and to focus on fat, salt, and carb content. Through this lens, similar foods can

---

* The amount of oxalate in the chocolate-sprinkled plantain chips is less than TJ's banana chips and Terra brand sweet potato chips, which have ~60 mg oxalate per ounce, but more than Lay's potato chips with 25 mg per ounce.

vary widely in oxalate content—for example, "leafy greens." A 2-cup serving of raw arugula has only 3 mg of oxalate, and a 2-cup serving of romaine lettuce has even less: 2 mg. Raw spinach, however, has over *two to three hundred times* the oxalate of lettuce and arugula, with a whopping 600 mg of oxalate (or more) in a 2-cup serving. Packaged salad greens, especially the "baby" mixes, typically contain spinach, chard, and beet leaves mixed with lettuce. The content of these mixes varies, but they may contain over 80 mg of total oxalate per 2-cup serving. You don't have to eat spinach and beet greens to get into oxalate trouble, but it's a popular way of doing so.

The smoothie, relentlessly promoted on TV and websites, in social media, and in books, is today's best-selling answer to improved energy, weight loss, fitness, and longevity. When we met, my colleague May proudly told me about her healthy diet of the very best fresh foods—not knowing that her diet was way overloaded with oxalates. Her daily menu featured a green smoothie that contained 2 cups of chopped raw spinach, 1 cup of berries, 1 cup of almond milk, and frequently half a raw beet.

The rest of her day was also overloaded. Her standard lunch was a spinach and kale salad with avocado and chopped almonds. Her afternoon snack was black tea and crackers with peanut butter and honey. For dinner, she frequently had steamed spinach or chard, potatoes, some sort of fish, and a bit of dark chocolate for dessert.

Table 3.2: Which Menu Is "Normal"?

Numbers are provided as an educational tool and are rounded in the oxalate content columns to the nearest 5 mg, because exact precision with oxalate content estimates is impossible (and misleading).

	Menu 1: 1,000 mg Total Oxalate		
Meal	Food Items (mg oxalate)	Meal Total Mg Oxalate	
Breakfast	½ cup All-Bran cereal (73) ½ cup fresh raspberries (12) ½ cup whole milk (0.5)	85	

Lunch	Black bean burrito
	[white flour tortilla, large (10),
	    ⅔ cup black beans (85),
	    cheese (0) seasoned with
	    ⅛ tsp. each cumin (3)
	    and black pepper (2)]
	¼ cup picante salsa (10)
	8 corn chips (5)
	½ cup mandarin orange sections (20)
	small iced tea (10)
		145	

Dinner	1½ cups Hormel bean chili (75) 1½ cups baby spinach salad (465) 7 oz. baked Idaho potato with skin (140) and butter (0) 1 oz. dark chocolate with almonds (87) 12 oz. Budweiser beer (3)	770	
~ Day Total		1,000	

Menu 2: 100 mg Total Oxalate	
Food Items Mg Oxalate	Meal Total Mg Oxalate
1 cup Rice Chex (5) ½ cup fresh blueberries (4) ½ cup whole milk (0.5) Black coffee (2)	12
Cheese (0) quesadilla with mushrooms, canned (¼ cup) (0.3), and baby shrimp (0), white flour tortilla (10) Corn salsa [½ cup corn (2) with 2 Tbs. each: red onion (0.5), red bell pepper (0.25), ½ clove garlic (0.1), 2 tsp. each lime juice (0.2), olive oil (0), ¼ tsp. chili powder (2), cayenne (1.5)] Apple and banana fruit bar (3) Club soda with lime (0)	20
Baked chicken seasoned with Shake 'N Bake (4) 1½ cups Caesar salad, romaine (1.5), croutons (3.5), dressing (1.5) 1 cup steamed broccoli (9) ½ cup white rice (3) Chocolate ice cream with chocolate sauce (45) 5 oz. red or white wine (0)	68
	100

BOX 3.1: A SUMMARY OF DIETARY DESIGNATIONS

Daily Oxalate-Intake Categories

✧ "Normal" diet: 130–220 mg/day

✧ Low-oxalate diet: under 60 mg/day

✧ High-oxalate diet: over 250 mg/day

✧ Extremely high-oxalate diet: over 600 mg/day

Food Designations

✧ Low-oxalate food: under 4 mg/serving

✧ Moderate-oxalate food: 4 mg to 9.9 mg/serving

✧ High-oxalate food: over 10 mg/serving

✧ Very high-oxalate food: over 15 mg/serving

From the spinach alone, May was easily consuming over 1,000 mg of oxalate a day. Add in the oxalates from her almonds, almond milk, peanuts, berries, potatoes, chard, black tea, and chocolate, and her total daily ingestion of oxalate was at least 2,500 mg. That's roughly two-thirds of a potentially lethal dose in someone with underlying health problems—and she was consuming this *every day.* No wonder that since starting this supposedly healthy diet, she had been experiencing back pain, brain fog, and severe afternoon energy crashes! But the connection to her diet didn't dawn on her until a mutual friend introduced her to my work.

"Normal" and Safe

In healthy people, a diet under 200 mg a day is probably low enough to avoid oxalate problems (60 mg oxalate per meal). This intake level offers recovery potential for mild kidney problems and even symptom relief for the oxalate poisoned. Moving to this target range is Phase One in adopting an oxalate-aware lifestyle. Relief from oxalate-related symptoms may be just 5 to 10 days away when oxalate intake is consistently lowered. All you need is a bit of sustained attention, and you'll see that it's doable.

Therapeutic Low Oxalate

Oxalate researchers suggest that an oxalate intake under 100 mg per day is the goal for anyone with a history of kidney stones, and that 75 mg daily is feasible. The typical clinical definition of a truly low-oxalate diet is under 60 mg per day* (20 mg or less per meal). That is the target used for reversing the chronic disease caused by oxalate deposits. Before you rush to adopt a low-oxalate diet, however, be aware that getting to this level is Phase Two in a process of undoing oxalate overload, *not* job number 1. We'll discuss later how to get there safely, but as a preview, look again at Menu 2 listed in **Table 3.2.** To transform that 100 mg oxalate, "low-normal" menu into a diet that encourages the body to remove oxalate deposits from the tissues, the simple fix is just to choose vanilla ice cream instead of chocolate ice cream with chocolate sauce. With oxalate awareness, the taste of vanilla is delightfully satisfying, empowering, and rewarding.

My spinach-loving associate May took my advice to heart and stopped drinking smoothies altogether. She also replaced spinach with

---

* Often expressed as 40 to 60 mg daily.

arugula, bok choy, and romaine, and quit the nuts, almond milk, potatoes, black tea, and chocolate. Within 10 days of changing her diet, her brain fog lifted and she stopped having afternoon energy crashes. Within two months, her chronic low-back pain also went away.

Why "Too Much" Is Too Much

Overloading with oxalate will eventually establish the two essential roots of all disease: toxicity and deficiency. Oxalate itself is toxic. Be it in your GI tract or blood vessels, your bones or your brain, an excessive amount of oxalate can scramble the cell structures and energy systems and disrupt basic cell function. Over time, routinely eating oxalates in excess causes oxalate accumulations and creates chronic inflammatory toxicity. To make matters worse, oxalates can enable and amplify the effects of other toxins and yet escape blame.

Overloading your diet with oxalate creates or worsens a variety of nutrient deficiencies and starves your cells of the nutrients they need to do their work.

Long-term toxin exposure (of many types) plays a central role in the development and progression of neurodegenerative diseases and gut dysfunction. Exposure to lead, thallium, or mercury early in life and over a lifetime causes a significant proportion of what is often considered to be "normal" age-related cognitive decline. Even among such commonly recognized poisons, there has been little attention to *subclinical* effects (meaning symptoms that do not draw clinical attention or lead to treatment).

Lower-level exposures to hazards may not have obvious and immediate effects on your health. Persistent metabolic stress and chronic low-level inflammation resulting from toxicity eventually can tip you into illness. Toxicity can take years to reveal itself, and the effects are easily overlooked. Part of the problem in recognizing toxicity is that we associate it only with life-threatening crises (acute poisoning, cancer, or sudden kidney failure).

Many of the dietary shifts steering us toward greater oxalate consumption also make it more likely that we will become deficient in key nutrients. If toxicity and deficiency remain unnoticed and uncorrected, disease and accelerated aging are inevitable. Toxicity in tandem with deficiency assures human suffering.

How and what we eat today has led to unimagined troubles as we eat more oxalate than at any time in human history.

4

Toxic Delusions and Troubling Trends

*Salad gluttons, defined as people who eat salad more
than twice a week in winter or four times a week in summer,
are insidiously programmed with three related beliefs:
first, that all foods are either poisons, which make you fat and
feeble, or medicines, which make you sleek and lovely;
second, that raw vegetables, including salad and crudités,
fall into the medicine category; and third, that the plant kingdom
has been put there by some benign force for man's pleasure and
well-being. All three are toxic delusions.*

—Jeffrey Steingarten, *The Man Who Ate Everything*, 1997

Today, thanks to industrial-scale processing, refrigerated trucks, and intercontinental shipping, a phenomenal conveyor belt relentlessly pushes oxalate at us 365 days a year. High-oxalate foods are increasingly used as daily staples. U.S. agricultural statistics show that sweet potatoes and spinach—two very high-oxalate foods—

were the crops with the highest increases in acreage from 2012 to 2017. Sweet potatoes saw a 38 percent increase and spinach increased 51 percent. Popular high-oxalate foods are often recent additions to the human diet; most edible vegetables were invented through human horticultural practices.

The list of popular high-oxalate foods is not long (see **Table 3.1**, Worst Offenders), yet remarkably, we consider most of these foods "wholesome." Many are marketed as nature's nutritional "gifts"—even by researchers.

There was a time, not that long ago, when winter in northern climates necessitated a meat- or seafood-centered diet—especially so in our deeper hunter-gatherer past, when the few edible plant foods available were a last resort during times of scarcity. With the spread of agricultural technologies, scarcity of plant foods in advanced economies is no longer the human condition. Now, blackberries and spinach are available no matter the time of year. Marketing, global shipping, and ideology determine our food choices. Mother Nature has no say.

Even as increased year-round availability has made high-oxalate foods more plentiful and affordable, other cultural shifts have rendered them more universally popular—making oxalate overconsumption almost inevitable. Let's look at how we are putting so many people in harm's way with present-day dietary fashions, a plant-centric food culture, and flawed nutritional theories—all ignoring the nutritional shortcomings and toxic secrets of high-oxalate foods.

Snacking Too Much

Snacking is a distinctively modern eating pattern of eating convenience foods in between full-sized meals. According to a study conducted at the University of North Carolina, the percentage of adults who snack on any given day increased from 71 percent in 1977 to 97 percent from 2003 to

2006. Three big influences fueling this trend are low-fat, high-carb dietary recommendations; weight-loss food products; and more meals eaten on the go with fewer sit-down meals.

Whereas one protein-rich fatty meal might last us hours (or even all day), carbohydrate-rich meals create greater blood sugar highs and lows, and the lows predispose us to perpetual hunger. To address these problems, dietary professionals have promoted the practice of *grazing* — eating frequent small meals (including convenience snack foods). Yet nutritionists and researchers worry that high meal frequency is a potential cause of dental caries, obesity, and cancer. If we were eating full-sized meals with more fat and protein, we would dramatically lessen the physical drive to snack.

Popular snacks include packaged nuts, chips, pretzels, and obviously processed "foods" like Cheetos. Snacks are increasingly sold as snack-meal hybrids, often in the form of bars featuring high-oxalate nuts, seeds, and chocolate. New arrivals such as chips made from plantains, bananas, sweet potatoes, purple potatoes, and beets are even higher in oxalate than white potato chips. **Figure 4.1** shows oxalate levels per ounce in six popular snack chips. These are concentrated dehydrated foods and are easy to overeat. We've grown accustomed to the "crunch" and carbs that make chips not only palatable but also addictive. Overeating would be less an issue if we were snacking on cheese, hard-boiled eggs, or plain full-fat yogurt, but these foods have been demonized for containing cholesterol and fat. Instead, retailers offer huge selections of convenient "trail mixes" containing tree nuts, peanuts, chocolate, and dried fruit—all marketed as "healthy whole foods."

Substitute Foods

Modern eating is rife with substitutes for traditional foods. Over time we've settled for inferior flavor and inferior nutrition, *and* we are unaware of the greater toxicity. A well-established example is the mistake of

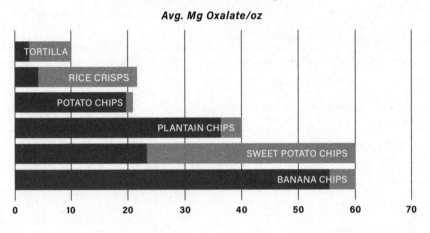

FIGURE 4.1: Oxalate per Ounce in Selected Snack Chips

Avg. Mg Oxalate/oz

displacing butter and lard (which contain essential vitamins and minerals) with nutrient-devoid and toxic margarine and shortening. At least there is some progress on this issue, as the trans fatty acids in these synthetic fats are now essentially illegal. Remember that for over five decades, these toxic fats were pushed on us as healthier.

Perhaps the most obvious example of nutritionally inferior high-oxalate foods displacing traditional low-oxalate foods is the mainstreaming of milk look-alike beverages fabricated from the seeds of legumes, grasses, and trees. In recent years, plant beverages have become big business. In 2016, U.S. soymilk sales alone generated about $881 million. U.S. almond milk sales soared to $1.3 billion in 2019.

Table 4.1: Oxalate Content of Alternative Milks

Beverage Type	Oxalate per cup (mg)
New Types	
Almond milk, homemade (80 g nuts per cup)	160
Almond milk, commercial types	14–35
Soy milk, chocolate flavor, commercial product (Silk)	20
Soy milk, unflavored commercial types (Silk and others)	4–20
Hemp milk, unflavored	11
Rice milk, vanilla flavor	2–10[*]
Cow's milk, chocolate flavor	9
Oat milk, Pacific organic brand	8
Coconut milk	3
Flax milk	0.5
Classic Milks	
Cow's milk	2
Goat's milk	0

[*] *25 mg, as reported by the VP Foundation in* The Low Oxalate Cookbook II, *is likely a data entry error.*

Today, every food store offers some variety of nondairy formulations made from hydrolyzed and homogenized extracts of soybeans, rice, almonds, cashews, oats, hemp seeds, coconut, and flax seeds. Manufacturing "veggie milks" involves blanching, grinding, chemical extractions, treating with high heat—which makes the delicate oils and proteins toxic—and adding water, flavors, colors, stabilizers, thickeners, preservatives, vitamins, and minerals.

Many (though not all) of these products have very high oxalate content (see **Table 4.1**). For example, 1 cup of Almond Breeze contains between 18 and 30 mg of oxalate. Homemade almond milk, which includes more almonds, can be dramatically higher. Note that cow's milk and coconut or flax beverages are low in oxalate.

The recent trend toward nondairy milk substitutes is often motivated by lactose intolerance and milk allergy—often signs of poor gut health, a modern epidemic in itself. Without better answers to explain our lost tolerance for milk, consumers find it comforting and convenient to adopt the new plant-based beverages. People use plant-based milk substitutes as if they were equivalent to real milks, but nutritionally they're very different. More of their calories come from carbohydrates, and they lack the complete protein, vitamins, and bioavailable calcium and minerals found in cow's milk. While packages claim that fortified plant beverages have calcium levels equivalent to cow's milk, settling and poor solubility of the added calcium carbonate (chalk) means that much of that calcium is not even consumed, let alone absorbed. Bioaccess to the added calcium may be further reduced by oxalate present in the drink.

It's interesting to note that for several of my clients, apparent milk (and gluten) intolerances seem to subside with low-oxalate eating.

Highly processed plant protein isolates are widely used as food additives, and in vegetarian protein powders, soy baby formula, faux cheese, and plant-based "meats." The standard method used to manufacture them severely damages protein molecule structures and creates additional toxins, including a kidney-toxic substance called *lysinoalanine*. The problematic results include reduced protein digestibility and lower nutritional utility. Despite the health implications, especially for children and older adults, attention from public health officials is lacking.

Consumers perceive these highly processed products as a healthful and ethical alternative to animal-sourced foods, and they are unaware of the potential toxicity and poor nutritional value. Eating nutritionally inferior and toxin-containing foods can eventually result in a wide range of frustrating symptoms. The initial damage doesn't typically create symptoms, and when it does, we don't recognize that our diet is working against us.

Deficiency and Toxicity

According to the National Research Council, more than 80 percent of Americans consume a diet deficient in vitamins and minerals. Even a slightly suboptimal level of nutrients inside the cells can add up to poor health—although the connection may not ever be apparent. Mineral and vitamin shortfalls can result in neurological impairment, such as mood and behavioral problems, learning deficits, poor manual dexterity, weakness, and muscle atrophy. Nutrient deficiency can predispose us to injury, poor recovery, and diseases of all kinds, and it directly contributes to human death. The contribution of oxalates to deficiencies is a key factor in their toxicity.

Maternal malnutrition impairs fetal and early life organ development, which puts children at high risk for adult diseases later in life. Adult outcomes include "mystery" ailments, premature aging, and inflammatory conditions, such as arthritis or digestive problems.

We know junk foods promote our nutrient-deficient state because processing removes and destroys nutrients. Today even whole foods are less nutritious than they once were because of the soil-depleting industrial farming methods used to grow them.

Less obvious still are the bioaccessibility problems inherent in all plant-based nutrients, even in organic, locally grown, fresh "whole foods." The essential nutrients they do contain (such as calcium, iron, zinc, and some vitamins) may be in forms that are either hard to digest or are rendered partially unavailable due to oxalate, fiber, and other naturally occurring compounds that impede their absorption.

Oxalate ions are mineral snatchers robbing us of the minerals in foods. As a result, a high-oxalate diet is inherently mineral deficient—especially in calcium and magnesium. Dietary oxalate has accomplices that magnify this effect. Two key examples are *phytic acid* and *polyphenols* (a broad category of over 8,000 plant compounds). The polyphenols tannic acid and gallic acid interfere with the digestion of carbohydrates, proteins, and fats (the *macronutrients*). Indigestible phytic acid (or phytate) also interferes with macronutrient digestion and, like oxalate, prevents the absorption of calcium, magnesium, zinc, and iron.

Although we can measure how much calcium is in foods, that measurement often does not tell us if our bodies can use the calcium. Here is an explanation from oxalate experts P. M. Zarembski and A. Hodgkinson, writing in 1962:

> It is well recognized . . . that the calcium [and magnesium] content of food is of little nutritional significance unless considered in conjunction with the oxalic and phytic acid contents. . . . The avoidance of a high-oxalate diet would appear to be particularly important for elderly persons, who . . . can ill afford wastage of calcium from combination with oxalate. A diet high in oxalate is also undesirable in . . . malabsorption syndrome and in vitamin D deficiency.

Worse still, compounds in foods that bind nutrients and obstruct digestion alter our nutrient requirements. The higher the proportion of plant foods in our diets, the greater the volume of food we need to eat to get adequate nutrients. Ironically, these plant foods are considered "low calorie," but their low nutrient content makes that a fallacy in practice.

Plant-centric eating predisposes us to eating too many calories while remaining malnourished. Obesity is a malnutrition disease and a world epidemic.

The Triple Threat of Oxalate

Oxalate has multiple ways to create malnourished bodies. Not only does it block us from accessing minerals in food, but when oxalic acid enters our bloodstream, it also steals minerals from body fluids and cells. If that wasn't bad enough, oxalic-acid ions and the crystals they form directly interfere with the proper functioning and integrity of our cells and tissues, which further leaches nutrients from cells and increases our nutrient needs.

We've known for nearly 75 years about the potential for dietary oxalate to cause malnutrition. In 1939, the *Journal of Nutrition* published the results of an experiment in which 5 out of 12 rats who were fed spinach died. The surviving rats developed weak, thin bones, had low body weight, and could not successfully reproduce. The researcher, Dr. E. F. Kohman, who worked for the Research Laboratory of the National Canners Association, in Washington, D.C., tried to use spinach to assure adequate calcium in the context of a canned-food diet. But to his surprise, the spinach did not deliver the expected calcium, based on mineral analysis of the food. Instead of *providing* calcium, the spinach starved the rats of needed calcium. Dr. Kohman might have known better than to use spinach, given that by 1937, several studies had demonstrated that feeding spinach to human infants depletes them of calcium and iron. Yet some researchers were dismissive of the need to call out this toxic property of spinach, and it remained hidden. Subsequent research (using high-oxalate foods) has confirmed this early research, including a 1968 study using rhubarb, a 1988 study feeding spinach to humans, and a 1989 study in humans showing that "spinach not only has poorly bioavailable calcium, but spinach appeared to decrease the bioavailability of calcium from non-fat dry milk if consumed at the same time."

Dr. Kohman explained that because of its oxalate content, "spinach . . . decidedly interferes with both growth and bone formation. . . . On the other hand, greens with negligible oxalate content, such as turnip greens, kale, mustard greens and collards, markedly improve growth and bone formation under similar conditions."

Growing children have a harder time excreting oxalate and are more susceptible to the effects of nutrient deficiencies and toxic exposures.

The oxalate in today's baby foods featuring high-oxalate grains and pureed vegetables, including sweet potatoes, carrots, and beets, should concern us.

Inattention to poor *bioavailability* in plant foods is a tremendous shortcoming in modern nutrition. Nutritional analyses of high-oxalate foods still do not account for the fact that minerals may be bound to oxalic acid. The lack of usable information about the quantities and implications of compounds that obstruct access to nutrients in foods is a hidden and unacknowledged source of confusion about healthy eating. Today, spinach is widely praised for its high calcium content, even though the calcium is useless (and toxic, because it is calcium oxalate). Yet there has been little effort to educate nutrition professionals about the bioavailability and toxicity problems inherent in high-oxalate foods.

In addition to depriving us of calcium and other essential minerals, oxalate overload creates extra demands for vitamin B_6 and B_1, contributing to functional deficiencies of those nutrients.

Deficiency is only half the story of oxalates' interference with good health. While it's easy to give lip service to the truism that a well-nourished body grows properly and is protected from life-threatening illness, we have largely neglected the complementary axiom: a poisoned body is fundamentally compromised and can't get well, no matter how many nutrients, supplements, or drugs one takes.

"Better Eating" Ideas

Since one of the principal objections to low-oxalate eating is that we won't "get enough plants," let's take a closer look at some of the ideas that keep us wedded to eating high-oxalate plants, even as our bodies cry out for something better.

For decades, the American Heart Association, public health agencies, and many diet books have been telling us to lower fat and calorie intake by replacing high-fat cheese, eggs, meats, and milk with reduced-fat versions and to consume lots of fresh fruits and vegetables, especially "dark leafy greens." As consumption of butter, eggs, and meat has dropped in the last 30 years, obesity and diabetes have exploded. To fix this, we're told to eat more low-fat "whole" foods like beans, whole grains, or "high-protein" pseudo-grains like quinoa and buckwheat.

Replacing meats with tofu and black beans, drinking almond water instead of dairy milk, and sating hunger with trail mix and chocolate — what could possibly be wrong with that? Grains, legumes, fruits, and many vegetables lack vitamin B_{12}, complete protein, and other nutrients supplied by animal-sourced foods. To the modern person, the resulting reduction in protein and other essential nutrients is not obvious. The additional toxic load is even less so.

Over time, the emphasis from health gurus and in diet books has shifted from just weight loss to broader health gains. Many people feel energetically underpowered or downright sick, and they are looking for relief. Along with the pressure to keep pace with our high-activity world, the hope for even a modicum of relief makes us ready converts to new dietary philosophies that promise abundant energy and health.

Increasingly, "health diets," using the substitution method for "bad" foods, unknowingly favor the consumption of high-oxalate foods. One author claims that eating 9 cups of vegetables a day will reverse serious progressive neurological degeneration, recommending high-oxalate foods like spinach and chard, which themselves can aggravate neurological degeneration!

Food Intolerance

Many recent diet programs attempt to address the issue of food intolerance or claim that eating at least one wrong ingredient (wheat or gluten, for example), or maybe several (including dairy, soy, eggs, corn, peanuts, and additives), will slow you down and make you fat because they trigger inflammation. Avoiding allergenic foods purportedly lowers inflammation and improves metabolism, thus liberating energy. The concept is basically good, but it lacks awareness of the natural toxins in plants. Thus, the solutions aren't good—especially when our superfood-colored lenses lead us to select pro-inflammatory and toxic high-oxalate foods that contribute to food intolerance and inflammation.

My own efforts to avoid increasingly numerous food allergies motivated my heavy reliance on sweet potatoes for over 10 years. Sweet potatoes made it easy for me to avoid wheat, soy, and other legumes that I thought were fueling my extreme fatigue and hormonal issues. It didn't work. Despite careful avoidance of allergens, I went on to need a total hysterectomy, and my fatigue progressed to a devastating collapse that ended my working life and my ability to exercise.

A popular allergy-avoiding food-intolerance diet that recommends green drinks and shakes made from vegan protein powder and chia seeds is the Virgin Diet, a trademark of J. J. Virgin. For good "poops," Virgin advises a high-fiber diet featuring high-oxalate raspberries, nuts, chia seeds, and quinoa, with 1 to 5 grams of supplemental vitamin C daily. Unfortunately, excess vitamin C is a potentially significant source of oxalate, and high-oxalate foods are major instigators of chronic inflammation.

Another noteworthy feature of modern eating is that so many of us are studiously following some named nutrition protocol that promises weight loss, better health, avoidance of major diseases, and longevity. Examples include the DASH diet (said to lower blood pressure without medication), Paleo, autoimmune Paleo, pescatarian, and "keto."

A *Paleo* diet excludes all beans, grains, and most dairy foods, based on the observation that Paleolithic (Stone Age) humans did not eat those foods and, based on analysis of skeletal remains, they were hearty and robust. It makes sense that we base our diet on species-appropriate foods available to humans during the millions of years preceding the industrial and agricultural eras of technology. Today's "Paleo" dieters favor nuts, salads, smoothies, low-fat meats, and piles of vegetables. They are rewarded with veggie chips and chocolate, while continuing to eat breads, cookies, muffins, and desserts constructed from modern ingredients such as nut flours and sugar substitutes like xylitol. More honest renditions of Stone Age diets would, no doubt, be less fraught with oxalate.

Autoimmune Paleo (AIP) is a stricter version of the Paleo diet that also avoids foods frequently identified as inflammation triggers (eggs, tomatoes, peppers, white potatoes, grains, and legumes), in hopes of calming autoimmune inflammation. Unfortunately, high-oxalate vegetables including spinach, beets, chard, and sweet potatoes are popular among AIP proponents and followers.

Keto—which is short for "ketogenic"—is a popular version of very low-carbohydrate dieting (20 grams of carbs or less daily) intended to create a healthy metabolic shift to burning fat (ketones) for energy. Indeed, sharply reducing our use of empty, high-carb foods is invaluable for correcting today's epidemic health problems. But, in practice—like Paleo dieters and food-intolerant eaters—keto dieters are encouraged to use nuts and nut flours to imitate baked goods. Using almond flour turns our daily breads, muffins, pizzas, and pancakes into "oxalate bombs."

Other dietary protocols include *pescatarian* (fish, but no other meat), *vegetarian* (no animal flesh), and *vegan* (no animal products at all). Each of those approaches emphasizes plant foods and readily embraces fashionable high-oxalate foods. It is possible to maintain a plant-based diet that is low-oxalate, but without sufficient awareness, any of these modern trends will steer us rapidly toward oxalate overload and related problems with nutrient deficiencies. We forget that shunning foods sourced from ruminant animals is an untested diversion from millions of years of humans relying on them for our development, survival, and heartiness. Not a choice to be taken lightly.

To illustrate how oxalate can add up, see **Table 4.2,** which shows a set of contemporary daily menus representing three popular approaches to "healthy" eating. The calculated oxalate content of these menus adds up to about 800 mg per day, roughly five times higher than the 150 to 200 mg per day that researchers consider to be "typical" and safe. (I'll show you later how to stay low-oxalate within the bounds of these diet strategies.)

The Plant-Based Mindset

Oxalate toxicity is a symptom of the love affair with eating plants that pervades our contemporary food culture. Though we treat them as facts, many of the plant-loving myths that reinforce our needless attachment to high-oxalate foods are highly debatable. For example, as Nina Teicholz describes in her book *The Big Fat Surprise*, the Mediterranean diet has mistakenly been characterized as a plant-heavy diet featuring olive oil with little saturated fat or red meat. That portrayal was formulated on very limited, heavily biased, and possibly even fraudulent data, and was funded heavily by the olive oil industry. The "real world" Mediterranean diet (to the extent that there even is such a thing) is quite divergent from the popular description. And there is less evidence that any of the features attributed to it have distinctive health benefits. The saturated fat we once thought was toxic turns out to be benign and even beneficial. As with so much of modern nutritional advice, today's Mediterranean prescription diet is driven by what we *want* to believe, not what has been shown to work.

Phytonutrients

Having failed to adequately consider inherent toxins and anti-nutrient problems, many health claims for plant foods are undeserved. The risk of deficiency and toxicity from oxalate is often downplayed or excused, because plants contain allegedly beneficial compounds known as *phytonutrients* (phyto- means "from plants"). A long list of fruits, vegetables, nuts, seeds, and herbs are called "superfoods" because natural

Table 4.2: Three Modern Diet Styles

Sample menus provided here include multiple options in some cases to illustrate additional examples. Numbers in the oxalate-content column are rounded to the nearest 5 mg.

	Mixed Diet Based on Whole Foods		Pescatarian Diet
	Foods	Oxalate Content (mg)	Foods
Breakfast	1 cup oatmeal (20 mg), 1 Tbs. raisins (1 mg), 1 Tbs. cashews (23 mg), and dash of ground cinnamon (0) 1 cup coffee (2 mg)	45	Chia pudding: ¼ cup chia (265 mg), 1 cup almond milk (30 mg), and 1 Tbs. strawberry jam (3 mg) Starbucks White Chocolate Latte (8 oz.), made with skim milk (10 mg) OR 4 Boca breakfast patties (120 mg) 2 slices multigrain toast (32 mg) and 2 Tbs. almond butter (120 mg) 1 kiwi (30 mg) Small coffee with ⅛ tsp. turmeric (7 mg)
Lunch	Tuna salad (10 mg) on multigrain bread (32 mg), 1 celery stalk (8 mg) 1 oz. potato chips (20 mg) 1 cup V-8 juice (20 mg) OR Applebee's Paradise Chicken Salad (55 mg) 3-inch brownie (37 mg)	90	1½ cups black bean soup (45 mg) 1 bagel (15 mg) 1 cup green tea (15 mg) 3 oz. carrot sticks (40 mg) OR Chickpea mint and green pea tabbouleh (43 mg) 1 clementine (20 mg) 3 oz. carrot sticks (40 mg) 1 cup green tea (15 mg)
Snack	1 clementine (20 mg)	20	1 oz. dark 86% Ghirardelli chocolate (90 mg)
Dinner	Small romaine salad (5 mg) with pickled beets (20 mg), 1 Tbs. pine nuts (17 mg) Chicken thighs (0), with 6 oz. roasted potato wedges (85 mg) ½ cup cooked chard (500 mg)* or spinach (500 mg)	625	Indian-spiced salmon (10 mg), with cumin-spiced carrots (30 mg) and pear chutney (5 mg) 1 cup quinoa (100 mg) 1½ cups mesclun salad (70 mg) Decaf tea (10 mg)
Dessert	2 small chocolate chip cookies (20 mg)	20	10 vanilla wafer cookies (10 mg) 2 Tbs. peanut butter (50 mg)
~Total		800+*	

* The oxalate content for chard could be as high as 900 mg.

	Oxalate Content (mg)	Paleo Diet	Oxalate Content (mg)
		Foods	
	310	Shake (150 mg total): 1½ cups almond milk (46 mg), 1 cup mixed fresh berries (25 mg), 4 Tbs. hemp powder (50 mg), ½ banana (5 mg), ½ tsp. ground turmeric (24 mg) 5 Tbs. Paleo granola (60 mg)	210
	115	Kale salad: 1 cup chopped kale (5 mg), ¾ cup roasted sweet potato (140 mg), dressing (3 mg), 1 Tbs. sunflower seeds (5 mg), and 7 black olives (9 mg) OR 1½ cups Paleo clam chowder with cashews (80 mg) 1¼ cups mesclun baby greens salad (60 mg), 2.8 oz. marinated artichoke hearts (20 mg)	160
	90	Trail-mix nut bar (65 mg)	65
	225	Zucchini parmigiana made with nut "cheese," sausage and a hint of spinach (250 mg) 1½ oz. raw fennel sticks (10 mg) 2 small tapioca-flour garlic rolls (20 mg)	280
	60	3 homemade chocolate macaroons (85 mg)	85
	800		800

compounds in them are said to have extraordinary powers. The super-food idea makes for great marketing by giving products a heroic, healthy glow. But the effects that power the reputations of superfoods are never as clear-cut as they seem.

The term "phytonutrient" is a misnomer. In everyday language, we misuse the word "nutrient" simply to mean "something that is good for us." *Essential nutrients* are something we must ingest for the body to function, including carbohydrates, proteins, and fats (the *macronutrients* that supply energy and structural materials), as well as vitamins and minerals (the *micronutrients* that keep the chemical reactions going to maintain life).

Phytonutrients are not essential nutrients. Not having them will not lead to deficiency. In fact, their mode of action is more like a toxin that, when consumed occasionally, stimulates metabolic defenses and modifies metabolic processes, which can be beneficial under occasional use, though often with undesirable side effects.

In research studies, phytonutrients have often shown no evidence of benefit and sometimes show explicit evidence of harm.

Tea, for example, has been studied extensively for its health-promoting potential, but the research has not conclusively demonstrated any benefits beyond the alertness boost from tea's caffeine. Concentrating green tea into supplements amplifies the power of certain flavonoids (catechins) to impair thyroid function and cause liver damage.

Quercetin (a plant pigment flavonoid found in onions, green tea, and other foods) is a popular health supplement that disrupts cell membranes yet falsely shows up as beneficial, owing to inaccurate research methods. Similarly, a review of research on turmeric and its extract curcumin emphatically observed, "No double-blinded, placebo controlled clinical trial of curcumin has been successful [found beneficial effects]." The authors point out that curcumin is "unstable in a biological setting" and are highly critical of the volume of inconclusive research, explaining that "cautionary [research] reports [of toxic effects and ineffectiveness] appear to have been swept away in the torrent of papers, reviews, patents, and Web sites touting the use of curcumin." One of those cautionary reports observed, "The fact that curcumin is a common dietary constituent is not enough to prove its safety, as other common dietary constituents [such as beta-carotene] have shown toxicity when used as dietary supplements." The body limits curcumin absorption and the liver quickly degrades it, treating curcumin like a toxin. It's a good thing that our digestive tract and liver detoxify curcumin—unless taken with black pepper, as is now recommended—because curcumin otherwise would likely cause DNA damage and (reversible) infertility.

Constant exposure to these compounds leads to constant metabolic stress. In a direct experimental study, researchers found that *avoiding* plant flavonoids and polyphenols *lowers* cellular stress. They fed volunteers a diet of only eggs, meats, fish, shellfish, grain products, potatoes, carrots, freeze-dried coffee, and mineral water. As they reported, "The overall effect of the 10-week period without dietary fruits and vegetables was a *decrease* [emphasis mine] in oxidative damage to DNA, blood proteins, and plasma lipids. . . ." This finding may not compute: no fruits and fewer vegetables improved cell health! (In case you're wondering about the daily oxalate consumption of the study volunteers, based on the menus given, the total oxalate content of this diet was probably 130 to 200 mg daily, with lunches providing between 85 and 125 mg oxalate from rye bread, carrot salad, and sometimes potatoes.)

In another study of healthy nonsmoking adults, the daily consumption of 600 grams of low-oxalate fruit and vegetables for 24 days had *no beneficial effects* on oxidative DNA damage in immune cells or urine compared with complete removal of fruits and vegetables, or daily ingestion of the corresponding amount of vitamin and mineral supplements. The researchers concluded that consuming fruits and vegetables does *not* protect cells. It's important to note that the researchers (perhaps accidentally) selected low-oxalate foods (including orange juice, apples, broccoli, and onions), altogether containing between 50 and

100 mg oxalate daily, and probably less. So, even in the context of a low-oxalate diet, increasing vegetable consumption was not beneficial. Large human trials using antioxidant supplements have found harmful effects, including digestive problems, cancer, cardiovascular disease, and overall increased mortality.

Other researchers agree. One put it this way: "There is no good evidence in human populations 'overall' that in the absence of deficiency, consuming high levels of nutritional antioxidants [polyphenols, carotenoids, ascorbate, or vitamin E] will protect against disease development." Likewise, an extensive review of polyphenols in human health concludes: "[I]t is premature to use polyphenolic compounds as therapeutic agents." On the other hand, getting enough of the essential nutrients is critically health protective. Vitamin B_1, for example, in addition to being essential to energy production and brain function, directly protects cells from oxidation. Pork, by the way, is the best source of B_1, while consuming tea, coffee, and berries destroys B_1.

Despite the "5-a-Day" recommendations, we don't really know how much or which plant foods can support a long, healthy, productive life. It's impossible to resolve the question of how much of the phytonutrients are needed to produce the claimed benefits—and at what cost, given the unacknowledged effects of oxalate and other plant toxins. My intention is to give you some confidence that if you need to lower your plant food intake to avoid oxalate or heal your gut, harm is unlikely. Still, it is possible to eat a lot of plant foods and avoid oxalate. But, as the clinical study using apples, onions, and other low-oxalate foods showed, there may be few benefits of a high fruit and vegetable intake in terms of protecting our cells. What you gain is culinary pleasure.

Overlooking Harms

Importantly, these seemingly unlikely findings have a higher-than-average likelihood of approximating reality because, as one prominent researcher put it: claimed research findings may often be "accurate measures of the prevailing bias." The prevailing bias is that plant foods and the compounds they contain are appropriate, beneficial, and even necessary for health—and so they can't possibly be bad for us. Our simplistic adoration of plants systematically ignores a vast amount of contrary evidence.

Proponents hawking the nutritional value of plants frequently overstate the benefits of phytonutrients as having antioxidant powers, and they downplay the risks of *phytotoxins* such as oxalate. They make it easy to believe that eating organic plant foods loaded with the so-called antioxidants allows us magically to withstand and disregard the oxalate damage. We need not go into all the ubiquitous and often exaggerated theories of the benefits of these compounds. From a practical point of view, during my years of "perfect" vegetarianism, I should have been experiencing benefits, not just believing in them.

Antioxidant chemicals in foods are mostly powerless over oxalates' toxic and malnourishing effects. Your body has to compensate, eventually becoming depleted and somewhat "deranged" from the effort and sacrifices required to avoid the worst short-term symptoms of oxalate overload. There is no magic in your chocolate or beet greens (or any other high-oxalate food) that will compensate for oxalate poisoning.

People who insist high-oxalate foods are beneficial without making an effort to examine the downsides are indulging in a dangerous form of cherry-picking. Focusing only on the theoretical benefits of plants can be deadly. Starfruit and its juice retain popular "health food" status (especially in Asia), despite very high levels of oxalate. There are hundreds of documented cases of people getting ill (hiccups, vomiting, and back pain) and even dying from as little as 10 ounces of juice (300 ml). As a team of nephrologists and pathologists wrote, "[the] neurotoxicity provoked by the ingestion of the fruit or juice, sometimes fatal, is far more frequent than reported." Being aware of that danger does not stop others from praising starfruit, and dismissing the harm and deaths it has caused, even calling it "an important gift from nature to mankind."

Plants Are Toxin Cocktails with Mixed Effects

Plants have plenty of other risky compounds that become active toxins owing to todays' favored amounts and current preparation strategies. Tannins, for example, are made by plants for microbial self-defense. These bitter-tasting polyphenols are abundant in tea and coffee; cocoa and carob; fruits—including berries and red wine; beans and peas; and sorghum and millet.* Tannins are known to be carcinogenic, and can cause metabolic problems and liver damage. A team of food scientists explains it this way:

> *Tannins are considered nutritionally undesirable because they precipitate proteins, inhibit digestive enzymes [and pancreatic function] and affect the utilization of vitamins and minerals [including iron]. . . . It is not advisable to ingest large quantities of tannins, since they may possess carcinogenic and antinutritional activities, thereby posing a risk of adverse health effects. However, the intake of a small quantity of the right kind of tannins may be beneficial to human health. Thus, it is important to determine the right dose of the right kind of tannins to promote optimal health.*

Their message is this: we should eat fewer tannin-containing plant foods and know exactly which kinds are okay and how much we can tolerate, and maybe even benefit from—but we don't have this knowledge yet. The take-home message is to eat limited amounts of foods high in tannins.

Thankfully, human saliva has proteins that disarm tannins taken in excess, offering some degree of self-defense against their toxic effects.

---

* Tannins got their name from their use in tanning, the process of converting animal hides into leather.

But when we don't chew tannin-containing foods because we've included them in smoothies, juices, teas, and whole-food supplements, we bypass our initial defenses. Although juices and smoothies are promoted for their ability to concentrate and expedite nutrient access from plant foods, they may also expedite their toxicity. Thankfully, the intestines and liver also work to disarm tannins and prevent their absoption.

Overall, the research suggests potential benefits from many plant compounds, such as flavonoids and phenols (formerly thought of as antioxidants), provided you have the "right" gut bacteria and the "right" genetics. Determining which compounds and in what amounts is hard enough; and even if we could identify the right combinations of bacteria and genetics that make plant compounds especially beneficial, hopes of achieving these benefits through plant-heavy eating are impossible dreams. The state of the science gives just enough promise to promote plant foods and supplements, and zero assurance that any individual person will necessarily gain meaningful benefits from using them.

Our cultural attachment to the idea of phytonutrients, and the belief that plants are benign and essential, keeps us from recognizing the dangers of oxalates. Although a low-oxalate diet works, some kidney specialists explicitly oppose or only reluctantly recommend it, out of fear that as people restrict their vegetable intake, they will stop getting important nutrients. A well-informed response is simple: oxalates and other phytotoxins are not good for us, and the theoretical benefits of phytonutrients and phantom minerals do not warrant indiscriminate consumption of dangerous high-oxalate plants.

Fiber: An Example of Going Astray

Fiber is another example of how our focus on theoretical benefits seduces us into consuming high amounts of oxalate. We are told that we simply must have fiber! That is another myth. Fiber has highly vaunted but poorly supported associations with gut health, weight control, cancer risk, and reduction of heart disease. And we rarely hear about fiber's documented malnourishing effects and its ability to promote inflammation, bacterial overgrowth, and constipation.

Back in the 1980s, before everyone was afraid of gluten, the bran muffin and cold bran cereals were kings of healthy high-fiber eating. But even then, there were concerns that fiber's glowing reputation was undeserved. As Jane Brody, health columnist and cookbook author, wrote in 1985, "A . . . serious drawback of increasing the fiber content of your diet concerns its possible interference with the absorption of essential minerals, especially calcium and iron, which are already in short supply in the diets of many Americans. Other nutrients that may be partly blocked by dietary fiber include zinc, magnesium, copper, and vitamin B_6. There is no question that more minerals are excreted on a high fiber diet. . . . Problems arise primarily if an individual's diet starts out with inadequate amounts of the nutrients that are inhibited by fiber."

Long considered inedible, and historically removed with the husk as "chaff," bran is the outer seed covering left over from milling grains and seeds. The idiom "to separate the wheat from the chaff" means to distinguish what is valuable from what is inferior.

Because bran is the major form of protection for the plant embryo, it should not be surprising that bran is high in oxalate. Just 2 tablespoons of any kind of bran delivers a significant amount of oxalate: rice bran has 25 mg, wheat bran 20 mg, and oat bran has as much as 10 mg. A cup of bran flakes (or Raisin Bran) cereal contains nearly 60 mg of total oxalate. That's halfway to a "normal" daily total in just 1 cup of cereal.

If you must have a source of fiber, oat bran, oatmeal, and psyllium (Metamucil) are relatively lower in oxalate. Coconut flesh and flour are better sources of insoluble fiber because they have almost no oxalate; they also taste good. The deeper issue is that keeping fiber in our diet is unnecessary and need not be a high priority.

Ubiquitous messages also claim that a high-fiber diet is required to tend and feed the *microbiome,* the diverse community of health-supporting microorganisms (or flora) living in the gut. That may be the reverse of the truth! The gut actively manages the bacteria it harbors. Gut cells make mucus (with protein-sugar molecules called glycoproteins) as "food" for healthy bacteria. When bacterial populations get too high, they ignite inflammation in the gut (and elsewhere), as the immune system attacks the gut bacteria with antimicrobials to cut back on their numbers. The body's own efforts to manage gut flora are obstructed by dietary fiber. Fiber indiscriminately feeds both beneficial bacteria and pathogenic microorganisms, potentially causing an imbalance, overgrowth, or *dysbiosis.* Chronic inflammation is more likely when bacterial populations (even beneficial ones) stay high owing to excessive fiber.

When you're feeling challenged to keep your fiber intake high, keep in mind that a low-fiber diet (including low-carb, high-fat diets) may support a balanced and healthy state of microbial life (and inflammation) in the colon.

You may also have heard that fiber helps prevent kidney stones. But, in a trial with 99 volunteers, researchers at the Kaiser Permanente Medical Center, in Walnut Creek, California, found that a high-fiber, low-purine, low animal-protein diet *increased* the likelihood of getting another kidney stone — by six times!

The classic delivery mechanism for fiber was once the bran muffin. Today, the muffin remains a popular food, but nutritionally it closely resembles a cake. Most diet books, be they keto, Paleo, or other protocol, offer muffin recipes, often still fiber enhanced. See **Table 4.3** for a comparison of the oxalate content of a "standard" muffin from *The Joy of Cooking* (high at 21 mg of oxalate per muffin) and the Virgin Diet "power" muffin, which has more than 3 times that amount of oxalate, or 68 mg. It is possible to make a muffin that is low in oxalate (only 2 mg), yet with similar fiber content (from coconut flour). Eating less bran fiber on a low-oxalate diet is probably nutritionally advantageous and better for digestion and our microbiome.

Table 4.3: The Muffin: A Comparison

A standard banana nut muffin contains about 20 mg oxalate (and 3 g fiber).

The Virgin Diet Muffin contains 68 mg oxalate, or three and a half times that of the standard banana nut muffin.

Two small gluten-free and low-oxalate muffins made with coconut flour contain only 2 mg of oxalate (and 3 g fiber).

Standard Banana Nut Muffin (*Joy of Cooking*)		Today's Fat-Fighting Low-Allergy "Power Muffin" *Virgin Diet Book*
Ingredients (12 muffins)	Mg Oxalate (Alternative Ingredient)	Ingredients (12 muffins)
all-purpose unbleached wheat flour (1½ cups)	50	Bob's GF biscuit and baking mix (1⅓ cups)
wheat bran [or whole wheat flour] (½ cup)	70 (40)	ground raw almonds (4 oz.)
cinnamon (1 tsp.)	40	chia seeds (4 Tbs.)
nutmeg (½ tsp.)	5	ground flax seeds (¼ cup)
chopped walnuts (⅔ cup)	50	monk fruit extract
light brown sugar (¾ cup)	18	ground cinnamon (1 tsp.)
mashed banana (2 to 3 bananas)	21	SO Delicious coconut milk (1½ cups)
baking powder, baking soda, salt, vegetable oil, egg, vanilla extract	negligible	blueberries (½ cup) baking powder, salt, macadamia oil, vanilla extract
Oxalate Total Recipe	**255 (225)**	
Per Muffin	**21 (19) Calories: 215 Fiber: 3 g**	

Note: Alternative ingredients are in brackets and total oxalate, if using the alternative ingredients, are in parentheses.

Don't Ignore the Downsides of Plant Foods

Even if you have trouble letting go of faith in the benefits of phytonutrients or fiber, the takeaway is that our favorable opinion of them was formed through a lopsided, "benefits only" mindset: embracing tenuous evidence of benefits while ignoring the risk of real harm from plant

Mg Oxalate	Low-Oxalate Muffin	Mg Oxalate
	Ingredients (10 muffins)	
35	coconut flour (½ cup)	4.4
	potato starch (¼ cup)	1.3
460	shredded coconut (¼ cup plus 1 Tbs.)	1
260	organic sugar (⅓ cup)	2.5
2	water (coconut water)	0
0	mashed banana (½ cup)	7
55	nutmeg (2 mg) [or allspice (5 mg) (¼ tsp.)]	2 (5)
4	butter, eggs, salt, baking soda, vanilla extract, almond extract, ghee, or coconut oil	negligible
5		
negligible		
821		**18 (21)**
68		**2**
Calories: 175		**Calories: 167**
Fiber: 4 g		**Fiber: 3 g**

compounds. I'm inviting you to relax the white-knuckled grip on the supposed need for a vegetable-heavy diet. Remember, many plants are assessed on perceived benefits and the risks are ignored.

The contemporary tsunami of propaganda touting the presumed

health benefits of plant-, nut-, and seed-based "natural" foods is not easily resisted. Plant-centric eating is a faith we're loath to give up, and it complicates the effort to avoid or reverse oxalate poisoning.

As my client Liz put it, "I was trying to figure out how I could spin this for myself to make my life philosophy still fit. Oxalates could not be the problem because these foods are the foods of the Bible. These foods are intrinsic to our lives, you know; there are whole cultures that use them, [so] they can't be toxic." Liz wanted to remain a vegetarian, but her body disagreed. Who was right? In the end, her body won her over.

The downsides of plant-based eating extend far beyond oxalates. Vegetarian foods don't supply adequate total protein or the complete spectrum of essential amino acids, and they lack an array of other essential nutrients. A fully plant-based vegetarian diet is nutritionally incomplete, requiring fortification with essential vitamins and minerals. Key vegetarian protein sources—beans and nuts—are minefields of oxalate, as well as other toxic "anti-nutrients" that contribute to digestive problems and reduce their nutrient value. Nutritional supplements alone do not prevent or correct the toxic effects of oxalate.

Still, it is feasible to maintain a plant-based diet and not poison yourself with oxalates. However, you'll have to work harder at it, and you may not fully regain your vitality.

But Doesn't Eating Plants Make Us Feel Better?

I used to be convinced that, for me, a twice-daily romaine lettuce salad was critical to normal bowel function. (Now I see my salads were a tasty and workable crutch for my gut, so damaged by ibuprofen, lectins, and oxalates.) Likewise, many people say they feel good when they increase their vegetable consumption. Even my oxalate-sickened clients often felt good for a time on the plant-heavy diets that ultimately poisoned them. The initial "wellness" response they were experiencing is created by a strong elixir: the combined powers of biology, psychology, and culture.

Let's first consider the role of our biology. The plant-centric diet starts with the power of subtraction. Healthy diet changes almost always include cooking at home and the subtraction of many harmful ingredients. Home cooking reduces the use of soybean oil, fried foods, excessive sugar, processed grains, and other low-quality ingredients used by restaurants. Healthy home menus also limit convenience junk foods loaded with addictive artificial flavors and preservatives, and they may include substantial changes in the routine use of alcohol. Not only may we rightly feel proud of ourselves for wrestling free from the addictive pull of these foods, but our bodies will also likely thank us for relief from man-made toxins with better sleep, mood, and alertness.

Also, veggie-heavy meals (such as smoothies, stir-fries, and rice bowls) tend to be low in protein and calories. Protein and calorie restriction, when undertaken for a short duration, may stimulate a healthy process of cleaning up damaged tissues, which can create some of the "revitalizing" benefits of fasting. But it is unsustainable in the long term. Similarly, there are medicinal effects of several plant compounds which can stimulate the body's defenses and may bring on healthy reactions in the short run. Whatever the therapeutic effects of high levels of plant consumption, the rewards are temporary and may mask the hidden price tag: longer-term toxicity.

In the case of oxalate overload, the body can hold on to oxalate in ways that may hide what is going on: an increasing load of oxalate crystals, constant metabolic stress, and a deferment of the ultimate costs. The time gap between cause and effect keeps the negative effects invisible to us. That seems to have been the case for Liam Hemsworth, who told *Men's Health*, "The first two years [of my vegan diet] I felt great. I felt that my energy was high. I felt like my body was strong, cardio was high, everything felt really good." Yet his veggie diet landed him in the hospital operating room.

Then, of course, we buy into the promising story of plants, and blenders, and "superfoods." We invest time, money, and effort—and our hopes and aspirations. All this buy-in colors our interpretation of the results. To make it worse, a strongly ritualized experience (such as a morning smoothie) is known to be the basis of the placebo effect. When we're convinced that juicing spinach is healthy and feeling good about doing the right thing, it will take longer to notice that what we're doing isn't working—or we'll credit the negative signs as "detox" effects. As a result, many people will stick with it even after the negative health consequences have become seemingly impossible to ignore. Again, Mr. Hemsworth in the *Men's Health* article illustrates this attitude, telling the reader they ought to "keep doing it" (a vegan diet) until "you're not feeling great, then you've got to reassess it and then figure it out."

Eating a veggie-heavy diet is also massively reinforced by today's cultural norms and people's anxiety over sustainability. With everyone in lockstep on eating in a plant-centric fashion, we misattribute the source of our failure to thrive on it. We "know" this stuff is healthy and should be working, so when we're sick and getting sicker, it's a personal failure of our individual body. And often the response to feeling worse is to eat even more of the "good stuff." For many people who suffer in that way, it is a huge revelation to discover that they are not alone. The problem is not an individual failing; the problem is the advice we've gotten, and the general ignorance about how toxic superfoods are actually wrecking us. This knowledge is liberating.

None of that means you can't eat plants and vegetables (or use herbal remedies for specific ailments). It does mean you can relax about "getting enough" vegetables. Learn to select them carefully rather than lean on them as staples or as the ultimate saviors; and recognize that it *is* possible to eat too many. Vegetables add aromas, textures, and color to our meals, which has value for sure. Use them as (seasonal) pleasure foods, but don't force yourself to eat them. Remember our core beliefs about healthy foods are at best incomplete and, in certain dangerous ways, completely wrong. (It is still excellent advice to avoid restaurants and much of what is sold in grocery stores.)

See the "Safe Bets" in **Table 4.4** for your pleasure veggies and other low-oxalate foods.

I can't assure you that you can maintain all your old beliefs in the face of what the story of oxalate toxicity reveals. Our incomplete and misguided opinions about healthy foods have put us on a fast track to oxalate overload. Think about which is more important: giving your body a chance to heal by trying low-oxalate eating, or holding on to foods that are, in all likelihood, not nearly as good for you as their reputations suggest.

The paradoxical and challenging story of oxalates ruining our health should not be news; yet it is because we've forgotten so much. Next, let's take a quick look at how we first learned of oxalate's noxious (and useful) qualities.

Table 4.4: Low-Oxalate "Safe Bets"

Very Low (< 4 mg/serving)	Moderately Low (4–10 mg/serving)
Animal Products	
Meats, dairy, butter, eggs, animal fats	Tuna (most seafoods have not been tested)
Beverages (8–12 oz servings)	
Apple cider, typical beer, coffee, coconut milk, fruit juices (apple, cherry, cranberry, lemon, lime, orange), ginger ale, herbal teas, dairy milk, kefir, sparkling water, wine	Some beers
Desserts, Snacks, and Treats	
Flax crackers, pickles, pork rinds, toasted coconut flakes, blueberry jam, candied ginger (4 tsp.), dates (6), ice cream (vanilla or coconut), whipped cream, white chocolate	

(table continues)

Very Low (< 4 mg/serving)	Moderately Low (4–10 mg/serving)
Fruits and Berries (serving size: ½ cup whole fruits, 1 cup juice)	
Apples, blueberries, cherries, coconut, cranberries (fresh), dates, grapes (seedless), Hass avocado (ripe), melon (cantaloupe, honeydew, watermelon), kumquat, peaches, pear (Bartlett only), fruit juices (apple, orange, lemon, lime, pineapple)	Banana, mango (fresh), papaya, plums (fresh)
Grains and Grain Substitutes, Grain Products (serving size: dry ¼ cup, cooked ½ cup)	
Coconut flour, cornstarch, potato starch (not flour), rice starch; cooked white rice, Uncle Ben's Rice; cellophane (mung bean) noodles, shirataki "rice" or noodles, white rice spaghetti, corn on the cob, coconut wraps	kelp noodles, pearl barley
Greens and Other Vegetables (½ cup servings)	
Alfalfa sprouts, arugula, bok choy, chives, red bell pepper, cabbage, capers, cauliflower, celery root (celeriac), cilantro, cucumber, escarole, kale (lacinato or purple boiled), kim chee, kohlrabi, lettuce (romaine, Bibb, butter, and iceberg), mizuna, mushrooms, mustard greens, onions, radishes, rutabaga, turnips, winter squash, watercress, water chestnuts, zucchini	Asparagus, broccoli (boiled), Brussels sprouts (boiled), collards, endive, green peas (boiled), green bell pepper, kale (raw), pumpkin
Herbs and Seasonings (serving size: ¼ tsp. dried, 2 Tbs. fresh or sauce)	
Salt, white pepper; Frank's RedHot sauce, Tabasco; horseradish; garlic (fresh or dried); sweeteners (honey, stevia, sugar); dried herbs (bay leaf, dill, marjoram, onion powder, poultry seasoning, rosemary, sage, savory, tarragon, thyme); spices (cayenne, mace, mustard seeds); extracts (chocolate, lemon, peppermint, vanilla)	Ground cardamom, Italian seasoning, oregano (dried)

Very Low (< 4 mg/serving)	Moderately Low (4–10 mg/serving)
Legumes / Beans (½ cup servings)	
Black-eyed peas, butter beans Use in modest portions. Always soak legumes prior to cooking them with high heat to disarm lectins.	Green peas (fresh or frozen), mung beans, split peas (yellow or green), No-Nut Butter made from yellow split peas
Nuts and Seeds (1 ounce serving)	
Seeds: flax, pumpkin, watermelon Oils: Although they are low in oxalate, avoid oils from soy, corn, cottonseed, sunflower, and safflower as much as possible owing to inflammatory breakdown products and the unstable/rancid nature of these oils.	Sunflower seeds, chestnuts

5

The Many Faces of a Poison

"Salts of lemons" . . . is much used by servants for taking out ink stains and cleaning harness, and by dyers . . . on a large scale in the preparation of cottons. But the worst feature in its character is its treacherous resemblance to . . . Epsom salts [which] might easily be mistaken for oxalic acid, as might oxalic acid conversely for it.

—J. Clendinning, MD, *London Medical and Surgical Journal*, 1833

A bottle containing Oxalic Acid should be marked poison, and kept on a high shelf.

—Fannie Merritt Farmer,
The Original 1896 Boston Cooking-School Cook Book

My own unexpected outbreak of good health after changing my diet drove me to the medical libraries at Virginia Commonwealth University and the National Institutes of Health, hunting for an explanation. Why did this low-oxalate dietary approach work so well? What is going on with the oxalates we eat and their effects on our cells, organs, bones, and tissues? How much of the damage is reversible? And how did we miss this oxalate problem so completely that hardly anyone is paying attention to it?

At the library, I was intrigued by the curious and often indirect way the connections between oxalates and common health problems reveal themselves. What emerged from countless hours of poring over the medical literature was fruitful, yet disturbing. Scattered across centuries of science and medicine, in thousands of articles, the pieces of information came together to tell a big story about oxalates' consequences for our health. For *nearly two hundred years*, highly respected authors— toxicologists, medical researchers, authors of case reports, and other clinicians—have pleaded for awareness of the dangers of high-oxalate foods.

The subject of oxalates appears repeatedly in the medical papers of many subspecialties, where it is identified as a factor in a wide range of health concerns. New studies and warnings continue to appear in scientific publications. The fascinating history of oxalate as a cleaning chemical and a glance at its chemistry help us begin to understand why this tiny molecule is bad for us.

Culinary sorrel (genus *Rumex*)—a classic leafy green vegetable beloved by Europeans and upmarket American chefs—and a woodland plant called wood sorrel were principal sources of oxalic acid for the early chemists. Sorrel plants share a strong sour flavor owing to their high oxalic acid content. The name "sorrel" comes from the Old French term *surele*, meaning "sour."

The term "oxalic acid" comes from the wood sorrel plant, a type of shamrock in the genus *Oxalis*, but it did not get this name until 1787.

When first described by chemists in 1632, oxalic acid was fittingly referred to as "tartar" (a generic term for "any solid concretion of biological material"). When dried, the oxalic acid extract from sorrel juice forms an odorless white granular powder. Oxalate *microcrystals* can appear as a saltlike residue in the chemists' labs as very fine, dusty grit visible under a microscope and as crusty deposits elsewhere.

"Salts of sorrel" or "sorrel salts" (now called oxalic acid or potassium oxalate) has been used industrially since the 1780s—for example, as a bleach and dye fixative in textile manufacturing, as an electrolytic etching solution and polish in engraving, and as a developing solution in photographic printing. Oxalic acid has *chelating* power (the ability to bind with minerals), which makes it a good cleaning agent. With impressive versatility, sorrel salts remove tarnish from copper, brass, and aluminum; pull rust from concrete and radiators; lift ink, paint, and varnish; and bleach wood and fabric. By the early 1800s, oxalic acid was used commercially under the name "liquid blue" as a disinfecting bleach in laundries and sold as a versatile household cleaning powder marketed with the friendly name Essential Salts of Lemon.

Despite being marketed as a cleaning product, pinches of "salts of lemon" were even used in the 1820s and '30s to impart a lemony taste to food and drink. (Lemon juice itself is very low in oxalates.) Using oxalic acid for its sour taste was an unfortunate practice, since it can have serious toxic effects, including mineral malnutrition; thin, soft, or brittle bones; hemolytic anemia; or even death. The same properties that make oxalic acid a powerful cleaner also make it a powerful poison.

Easy access to sorrel salts in the early 1800s led to a rash of accidental fatalities in England—typically when oxalic acid was mistaken for Epsom salts and taken to treat a stomach complaint (making this mistake is like consuming eight spinach smoothies in one single gulp!). This emergent public health problem inspired the 1823 Scottish publication of a major experimental toxicology study—the first of its kind—showing that ingestion of diluted oxalic acid leads to systemic poisoning.

Ten years later, the day-to-day dangers of oxalic acid cleaners continued to be a public health issue. Speaking in 1833 before the Royal Medico-Botanical Society of London,* toxicologist J. Clendinning, MD, opened his remarks with this lament: "Since 1814, [oxalic acid] has fully vindicated its dignity as an active poison and has occasioned more accidental deaths than perhaps any other." He called out oxalates' "noxious qualities" with concern that it was being commonly used, was easy to obtain, and had the "alarming name, 'salts of lemons.'"

Oxalic acid is still used in the twenty-first century for many industrial applications and in household products such as Bar Keepers Friend cleaning powder and Zud cleanser. If you must use cleaners containing oxalate, it's important to use gloves because prolonged skin contact can cause serious damage. A 1979 toxicology text described the problems arising from skin absorption: "prolonged contact with solutions of oxalic acid has resulted in paresthesia [tingling and numbness], cyanosis of the fingers [bluish discoloration due to low oxygen in the blood], pale yellow discoloration of the fingernails and even gangrene."

Even foods containing oxalate have potential industrial uses because of oxalic acid's power to grab minerals. A modern lab experiment demonstrated the power of the oxalic acid in dried and ground banana peels to snatch toxic heavy metals (lead, copper, nickel, zinc) from contaminated water. The university researchers hope that their banana peel "bio-sorbant" process might scale to water-treatment facilities and create additional income for poor Malaysian farmers.

Given oxalic acid's industrial cleaning prowess, it's reasonable to wonder how the oxalates we eat impact our bodies. To do so, we need to know a bit more about the various forms that oxalates take.

---

* The Royal Medico-Botanical Society of London was an institution devoted to the investigation of the medicinal properties of plants.

Names for Various Oxalate Forms

Today's official and unambiguous chemical names for oxalic acid are a bit tedious: 2-hydroxy-2-oxoacetate or *ethanedioic acid*, and in practical terms a bit overly specific. Instead, the terms *oxalic acid*, *oxalate*, and *oxalates* are still used interchangeably in the scientific literature (and in this book), because the various forms they take in any given situation are generally mixed, indefinite, and changeable. That is also why we often refer to "oxalates" in the plural. The differing forms they take (depending on their biochemical surroundings) each have different effects.

In the watery environment of foods and in the body, soluble oxalate salts (potassium or sodium oxalate and oxalic acid) dissolve into very tiny ions that move and react freely within their surroundings. Even *free oxalic acid* ions can take two different forms (with either a single or double electrical charge), adding to the complexity of the various biological consequences.* For hours following high-oxalate meals, an influx of these ions enters the bloodstream. They travel around the body, damaging cell structures, creating oxidative stress, causing inflammation, and entering cells, where they disrupt cell function and interfere with cell energy production.

Oxalate ions readily attract minerals from the blood plasma, body fluids, or cells. They are especially drawn to calcium and magnesium, and the resulting *insoluble* oxalates do *not* easily come apart (at least not at typical body acidity and temperature). When insoluble oxalate molecules form, essential minerals are lost and are converted into toxins that can damage cells. For example, calcium oxalate is especially prone to becoming nanocrystals with electrostatic charges that can destroy the very machinery of life—cell membranes. When they hook up to healthy

---

* Sorrel salt is potassium oxalate—a soluble oxalate that easily dissolves in water into reactive charged particles (oxalic acid ions).

red blood cells, oxalate crystals produce enough membrane damage to cause the cells to spill their contents. The cells lose not only small molecules such as potassium ions but also large hemoglobin molecules, which carry oxygen to tissues.

Oxalates' ability to damage cell metabolism even has clinical applications! Potassium oxalate is placed in the collection tubes used when testing blood glucose levels. Oxalate ions quickly grab magnesium ions in the blood cells and prevent the cells' enzymes from using the glucose to produce cell energy. The lab then gets an accurate measure of the amount of glucose in the blood many hours after it was drawn. If this mineral binding happens frequently in the body, turning food into cell energy becomes harder.

Nanocrystals have the potential to accumulate within tissues and grow into larger glass-like microcrystals anywhere in the body. This gritty trash creates arduous housekeeping challenges for tissues and the immune system.

In the wake of high-oxalate meals, oxalic acid's calcium "poaching" reduces calcium levels in the blood—especially if meals themselves do not contain ample calcium. The resulting electrolyte imbalance and calcium shortage in the blood and in other bodily fluids require the body to leach calcium and other minerals from the bones to compensate. Even temporary low blood calcium may interfere with the electrical activity of the heart, muscles, and nerves, sometimes leading to visible symptoms in the form of tremor, twitches, hiccups, seizures, coma, palpations, or heart failure. Other, more common signs of nerve damage associated with oxalate toxicity include poor sleep, sensitivity to noise and light, moodiness, lack of motivation, anxiety, and depression. In the digestive tract, transient shortages of calcium and electrolytes in the muscles and nerves create gut-function problems such as reflux, belching, colic, intestinal cramping and pain, diarrhea, and fecal incontinence. In the inner ear, low magnesium can cause dizziness, tinnitus, and hearing loss.

In one published case, the oxalic acid from a soup prepared with culinary sorrel "cleaned up" the minerals in a man's blood, disrupted his heartbeat, and triggered fatal heart failure. In this case, the lethal dose of oxalic acid was about 3,900 mg—consumed in just one meal (which is rarely done).* The report in the *Lancet* medical journal begins:

> A *fifty-three-year-old man, with a four-year history of insulin-dependent diabetes, who was a heavy smoker and drinker, was admitted to hospital because of vomiting, diarrhea, and progressive impairment of consciousness soon after the ingestion of a vegetable soup containing about 500 g[rams] of sorrel. . . .*

The doctors, nurses, and technicians at Barcelona's finest hospital used every measure to save their delirious patient. They began fluid replacement and placed him on a mechanical ventilator and dialysis. Despite the life-saving machinery, he quickly lapsed into a coma. Two hours later, he was dead. The authors warned: "Plants containing oxalic acid are used in cooking and for medicine purposes, and awareness of their hazardous potential is important."

Metabolically Extra Vulnerable to Healthy Foods

Today, sorrel is considered a health food and is used as a medicinal tea, even though the word "sorrel" has been associated with poisoning since

---

* The doctors who wrote the *Lancet* report estimated that his 500-gram portion of boiled sorrel contained 6 to 8 grams (6,000–8,000 mg) of oxalate. But according to an analysis of sorrel conducted at the University of Wyoming, and reported by the VP Foundation in 2010, raw sorrel contains about 779 mg per 100 grams. This suggests that a more accurate estimate of his acute oxalate load was barely 4 grams (3,900 mg) of oxalate. It's important to acknowledge that accurate data on oxalate content are scarce, and this creates a lot of confusion, misunderstandings, and frank ignorance about how much oxalate we are eating and how little it takes to harm us.

1814—a fact long since discarded as trivia. It is likely that the man described in the *Lancet* report elected to gorge on sorrel soup in an attempt to "get healthy" or to compensate for his drinking. People with chronic health challenges often feel desperate for a better life, and they think superfoods like sorrel might rescue them. Sadly, oxalate-heavy foods, including sorrel and spinach, make poor nutritional choices for any metabolically stressed person.

Although it is impossible to know how long and to what degree that sorrel soup victim had been ingesting oxalate-loaded plant foods before his final and fatal dose, even minuscule amounts of oxalate in the wrong place at the wrong time can have potent negative effects. The higher the frequency and amount consumed, the more likely dietary oxalate will cause problems and trigger fresh sites of crystal accumulation and metabolic stress—or even, as in this unusual case, death—just not necessarily in such an acute and recognizable fashion.

When you spread a lethal dose of high-oxalate foods over several days, the mineral depletion and other damaging effects are much more subtle and no longer acutely fatal, but that doesn't mean you are not being harmed.

6

Why Don't We Know About Oxalate Overload?

Prevention of dietary hyperoxaluria
[high levels of oxalate in the urine],
by avoiding excessive intake of foods high in
oxalate or its precursors, should be a part of
the dietary education of the public.

—Y. Sun, MD, et al., *Cureus*, 2017

The story of oxalate overload gets even more surprising when we look at how it vanished as a topic of inquiry from medicine and nutrition, even as the body of scientific evidence about the diversity and severity of oxalate's effects on our health continues to grow.

In 1842, the nascent *oxalic diathesis* emerged as a medical condition associated with diet and involving elevated oxalate in urine. (*Diathesis* refers to a constitutional tendency to a disorder or set of disorders.) Affected patients suffer from digestive problems; arthritis; back pain; anxiety, nervousness, despondency, or other mental distress; fatigue; soft bones; boils; rough and scaly skin; cardiac symptoms; pain or heaviness in the loins; urinary tract stones or distress, semen in the urine, and cloudy urine. Urinary expert Golding Bird and a handful of his colleagues from the tea-drinking British Isles believed that excessive oxalate in the body was bad for the "general health."

Bird was a gifted teacher, careful researcher, experienced doctor, and world-renowned authority on kidney diseases. He wrote a famous and comprehensive textbook, *Urinary Deposits: Their Diagnosis, Pathology, and Therapeutical Indications,* in which he insists that "oxalate of lime . . . merits special attention . . . [pointing to the] importance of carefully studying the relations of [oxalate deposits] to certain states of health." He and his colleagues were able to recognize the connection between diet and the symptoms of oxalate illness, thanks to the seasonality of a novel high-oxalate food—rhubarb. At the dawn of the nineteenth century in England, rhubarb was wildly popular and was strictly a seasonal treat featured in delicate tarts and posh desserts enjoyed by those who could afford sugar.

By 1933, the disease was called the *oxalic acid syndrome,* and the list of symptoms included (1) dyspeptic and intestinal troubles, (2) weakness or low energy, (3) anxiety and depression, (4) migraine, (5) rheumatic pains, (6) kidney stones, (7) irritable bladder, (8) hypotension, (9) colon microbe imbalance or overgrowth, and (10) erratic behavior.

Kidney stones are often accompanied by other problems. Urologist Carl Burkland noted in 1941 that "many patients suffering from oxalate stones are nervous, neurasthenic, pessimistic individuals, often suffering from chronic intestinal disturbances." *Neurasthenic* means they are depressed, anxious, or fatigued and prone to headaches, heart palpitations, and nerve pain. At the time, neurasthenia was (wisely) thought to be the result of the exhaustion of the central nervous system's energy reserves, but it was later categorized as a "neurotic disorder" (and still is) by the World Health Organization (WHO).

Oxalate toxicity can indeed manifest as neurasthenia. The depression, low energy, and kidney stones experienced by Liam Hemsworth as a result of his daily high-oxalate smoothies and vegan diet might, in 1933, readily have led to a diagnosis of oxalic acid syndrome.

Golding Bird feared that the establishment would ignore oxalate toxicity as a medical problem, and he expressed his personal frustration at getting the wider medical world to recognize the seriously detrimental effects of oxalate on one's quality of life, stating that oxalate "seems now to run some risk of being tossed aside as a thing of no consequence." Bird's insights into oxalate toxicity were cemented by his personal experience with joint pain, cloudy urine, kidney stones, and ill health. Tragically (in an era when accurate tests of oxalate levels in foods were not available), he died at age 39 from complications of kidney stones.

The oxalic acid syndrome remained a puzzling and debated condition, not always easy to identify, partly because we have never had good diagnostic tests and have always lacked precise knowledge of oxalate in foods. Bird's apt prediction came true: the diagnosis fell out of favor in the mid-twentieth century, and we stopped recognizing it.

Medicine Gives Up on Oxalate

By the late 1930s, while foundations funded by the Rockefellers were pouring millions of dollars into medical research, medicine was gradually moving away from recognizing diet's power to generate acute symptoms and chronic problems. This shift began in earnest in 1910, when the American Medical Association and the Carnegie Foundation for the Advancement of Teaching published a critique of American and Canadian medical education. The so-called Flexner Report laid out a program that would make medicine more "scientific," establish professional solidarity and orthodoxy based on standardized educational requirements, and guide the medical profession's future. In the aftermath, doctors were trained to use "objective" standardized laboratory testing as the foundation for medical diagnosis. The "art" of diagnosis (which emphasized patients' accounts of symptoms and physicians' observations) took a back seat to test-based diagnosis. Dr. Abraham Flexner, lead author of the 1910 report, later lamented the stifling uniformity and lack of creativity it had encouraged.

Test-based diagnosis led to improvements in handling certain health conditions, but there was also wisdom lost in this push toward standardization. Concern for preventive care was narrowed and gradually handed over to high-tech screening tests, and medicine became more focused on symptom abatement and preserving life, especially in the later, deadlier stages of disease.

The clinical course of oxalate toxicity is an especially poor fit for our modern test-based and compartmentalized medical system. As we will see, urine and blood testing cannot tell us whether we are or might be sick with oxalate, or how sick we might be. Even if urine tests could reliably detect post-meal surges in the body, they have no power to detect subtle toxic effects, be they immediate or delayed.

Today, oxalate research is essentially owned by the urology profession. Scientific conferences on oxalate held since 1986 focus solely on kidney stones and chronic kidney disease, having been organized and co-chaired by a kidney stone pathologist. The "kidney-centric" approach to the study of oxalate-related problems makes no room for recognition of toxic effects elsewhere, or a debilitating oxalate toxicity syndrome.

Importantly, the shift to the kidney-centric view of oxalate illness was solidified in the years following the 1972 expansion of Medicare coverage to include individuals with end-stage renal disease. By the late 1970s, about a decade after Medicare was established, community-based charitable hospital care was displaced by corporate ownership and control of an increasingly high-tech and profit-oriented medical enterprise.

Diet-related illness and dietary solutions offer little hope of bolstering profits. Diet as a form of medical therapy (or even prevention), once standard, became tangential to conventional health care. Dietary consultations are typically not paid for by health insurance, and most doctors are unlikely to "order" them, being under the impression that the potential benefits are mild and slow and that patients are unlikely to "comply" and consistently change their behavior. And even though a low-oxalate diet is used for treating kidney stones (and works), it is treated with skepticism even by leading nephrologists.

As a result, oxalate has become a matter principally of academic interest, and there are wide gaps in the understanding of oxalate's deleterious effects over time. The extensive evidence of oxalate's toxicity—found in cell biology studies, experiments using lab animals, and in human and animal case reports—is scattered across diverse fields of study. When taken together, though, they show that oxalate is clearly a serious problem. Yet, this evidence has led to few human intervention studies of the acute effects of dietary oxalates, and none look at their painful, disabling, and potentially deadly long-term consequences.

Not Seeing Oxalate Toxicity

No field of science is charged with (or even interested in) developing a "whole body" theory of what excessive dietary oxalate does to us, so it is especially difficult to recognize dietary oxalate overload as a unified problem with a common cause. The early signs and symptoms of oxalate poisoning are not well known, can be quite common and diverse, can appear gradually and intermittently, and are dissimilar from person to person. Most important, we don't notice the gradual erosion of tissues and their lost function until metabolic reserves are depleted and the disease process interrupts our lives.

Focusing on symptoms independently and expecting different causes for each also makes it difficult to see the common root.

Not recognizing that health foods lead to health problems is certainly understandable. Medical doctors have no idea that "healthy" foods contain toxins that can provoke specific symptoms in the near term and cause delayed and indirect effects that lead to chronic illness. Like the rest of us, doctors are steeped in conventional dietary advice to eat more plant foods (and to avoid high-fat foods and salt). They see that their patients are anxious and stressed out, and they counsel them to stop worrying about their "imagined" ailments, which don't stand out in diagnostic testing.

Even if physicians were to concede that some of their patients might be suffering from oxalate-induced problems, they don't have effective tools for making the diagnosis—not even an accurate list of high-oxalate foods or a list of oxalate-related symptoms. (See the Resources section of this book.)

Oxalates' effects on our biology are not getting enough attention, yet evidence of oxalate toxicity keeps growing in the literature. As researchers wrote in 2008, "For many years, oxalate has been viewed as a metabolic waste product, a counter ion in transport studies, or an experimentally useful chelator of calcium, and it has not been considered worthy of detailed study. However, neither the excretion of oxalate nor the regulation of its transport are as investigators had expected, and evidence is mounting that oxalate affects normal physiology."

The Nutrition Profession Overlooks Oxalate

Sadly, the field of nutrition has paid no more attention to the risks of dietary oxalate than medicine has, despite statements in their own journals, such as this one from the *American Journal of Clinical Nutrition* in 1972: "Excessive consumption of oxalic acid by human beings deserves serious attention because it has been implicated in several clinical disorders."

The initial focus in the field of science-based nutrition was not food safety or therapeutic diets. Instead, science-based recommendations grew from the early food chemistry of the mid-1890s, when a U.S. agricultural chemist developed a system to calculate the energy content of foods. Dr. Wilbur Atwater (1844–1907) established the fundamental concepts of energy metabolism—still largely held today—and a better understanding of macronutrients in foods. He also institutionalized agricultural and food research within the U.S. Department of Agriculture (USDA). Dr. Atwater's indelible impacts were many, including the belief that new ideas from science and public institutions should dictate food choice.

Atwater was a reformer, prominent in the temperance movement, and he believed that Americans' food choices were extravagant and wasteful. His ability to measure calories in food quickly led to concern over, and public education about, how to furnish enough calories and protein as economically as possible. On behalf of low-income workers, Atwater favored lower-cost beans, refined grains, cheese, and cheaper cuts of meat over the roast beef, steaks, and other prime meats that people generally preferred to include in every meal.

To teach the public how to eat more cheaply, Atwater teamed up with another remarkable analytical chemist, Ellen Swallow Richards, who founded the American Home Economics Association in 1908. She helped Atwater turn his cheap ingredients into stalwart Yankee dishes such as corn mush, pea soup, and Boston baked beans. Through this partnership, the new field of scientific nutrition became a "kitchen" science housed under the rubric of "home economics," a profession (quite remote from medical science) that created significant changes in American attitudes and eating habits as it spread the gospel of New Nutrition — elevating grains, beans, and other starchy plant foods to essential dietary staples.

Consideration of diet as a medical intervention was further diverted in the early 1900s by the excitement over the newly discovered "vitamines" (as they were first called) and related deficiency diseases, which were understood to be not so much a medical problem but, rather, a public health problem. For example, pellagra (a niacin-deficiency disease) affected mostly poor Southerners in the United States and led to recommendations for food fortification.

Likewise, the dietetics profession, which works directly with patients and designs therapeutic diets, has curious origins. It was founded by a vegetarian and strong adherent to Adventist beliefs, Lenna Frances Cooper. Miss Cooper was the author of the founding 1928 dietetic textbook, *Nutrition in Health and Disease*, which was in use for many decades. The 17th edition was the very textbook I studied while at Cornell University in the mid-1980s. People who believe in plant-centric eating continue to be attracted to the nutrition arena. Even the professor teaching my nutritional biochemistry course was a prominent vegetarian activist, promoting his ideas through his research and advocacy.

Nutrition science as it is practiced today is ill-equipped to identify oxalate toxicity. Researchers investigating the health effects of foods depend heavily on high-volume, low-quality self-reported survey data via food-intake questionnaires that do not sufficiently distinguish high- and low-oxalate foods, and do not associate different oxalate-related symptoms with each other. Meaningful connections between a high-oxalate diet and health problems are completely invisible in that context. Gathering weak data from lots of people and guessing about the connection between foods and health (based on statistical correlation) somehow feels "certain," but it is quite the opposite.

Toxicology has never been an influential voice within nutrition research and education. Regardless of the toxins they may contain, all foods that are "generally recognized as safe" (or GRAS) are considered "edible" in any quantity and frequency. It is rare for any nutritional recommendation to consider the potential toxicity of a familiar food that contains desirable nutrients, especially when the toxin in question occurs naturally. Yet we know that naturally occurring oxalate in many popular foods can exceed our tolerance level. It's important to recognize that our impressions of proper nutrition don't come from careful consideration of what is both safe and nourishing.

Case reports of illness related to oxalate consumption continue to trickle into the medical literature, accompanied by stern cautions not to eat too much oxalate. Yet beyond a subset of kidney specialists, the medical and nutritional professions have remained deaf to these warnings, and they are quite happy to send their patients back to the produce department for another bag of "healthy" spinach without a second thought. At a time when high-oxalate foods are particularly popular and trusted, that blind spot is making oxalates even more dangerous.

The prevailing dismissive view of the risks of eating high-oxalate foods is well represented in this passage from a 1973 review of natural food toxins, by Dr. David Fassett: "It would seem to require a rather improbable combination of circumstances—very high intake of oxalate-containing food plus a simultaneously low calcium and vitamin D intake over a prolonged period—for chronic toxic effects to be noted."

Sadly, Dr. Fassett's "improbable combination of circumstances" is well on its way to becoming the norm. Oxalate overload can seem foreign, confusing, and unlikely because: (1) we're so unaware of it—even the word "oxalate" is unfamiliar; (2) the implications run counter to the nutritional dogma of our times; and (3) our collective ignorance and disbelief promote inattention and dismissive attitudes, even among researchers and otherwise well-informed health-care professionals. Every day, we may be ingesting the very cause of a multitude of symptoms, yet not have any idea. Neither does your doctor.

7

A Confusing Multitude of Symptoms and No Good Tests

*It appears that many persons think it an easy task to
investigate experimentally the physiology of poisoning.
But they are assuredly mistaken. A long apprenticeship
must be passed before any one can observe with accuracy
the phenomena of the action of poisons.*

—R. Christison, MD, and C. Coindet, MD,
Monthly Journal of Medicine, 1823

The oxalic acid syndrome may be absent from contemporary diagnostic schemes, but it has *not* gone away. As the medical field lost its awareness of the oxalic acid syndrome, dietary oxalate poisoning has been subsumed under the diagnostic family of illnesses called *hyperoxaluria*, meaning excessive oxalate in urine. Kidneys keep the blood and body in good condition by helping to manage electrolyte balance and by removing unwanted elements, including oxalate, through urine.

Few of us today are aware of oxalate in our urine, but in the days of bedpans, urinary "gravel" was a well-known phenomenon. Oxalate crust from human urine was beautifully captured in the first microscope studies of the 1600s by two preeminent, self-taught science pioneers: the English early science maverick Robert Hooke (1635–1703) and the Dutch microscopist Antonie Philips van Leeuwenhoek (1632–1723). Every time we pee, we're removing oxalate, principally as oxalate ions and magnesium oxalate, but also as nano- and micro-sized crystals of calcium oxalate.

Kidney Oxalate Output Tolerance

Human and animal bodies are built to excrete a certain amount of oxalate. We make oxalate as a normal low-level waste product of hundreds of biochemical reactions; typical adult humans unavoidably generate roughly 12 mg of oxalate every day. That is a manageable volume, as healthy kidneys' capacity for oxalate excretion is at least twice that amount.

On average, total urinary oxalate traffic leaving the body is 15 to 40 mg per day—the combination of the amount we generate plus any additional oxalate from diet and other sources. The urine oxalate threshold at which hyperoxaluria is identified is 40 mg per day, or sometimes 45 mg per day (see **Box 7.1**).

Current research tells us that we can safely tolerate about 25 mg of oxalate per day in our urine if our kidneys are healthy. That means that optimum levels are 25 mg or less per day. Even small increases in total urine oxalate (for example, from 25 to 30 mg per day) put us at greater risk for kidney damage, kidney stones, chronic kidney disease, and other health problems, even if test results do not indicate hyperoxaluria.

BOX 7.1: URINE OXALATE THRESHOLDS

Oxalate per mg/24 Hours

✦ Well tolerated	< 25
✦ High normal/excessive	26–40
✦ Hyperoxaluria men	> 40–45
✦ Hyperoxaluria women	> 35–40

When oxalate loads surge beyond excretion capacity, the oxalate can crystallize in the minute canals of the kidneys, which collect and handle urine (*tubules*). Healthy kidneys have multiple strategies for preventing oxalates from getting hung up as they pass through. For one, the surfaces of the tubules are built to repel crystals. The kidneys release citrate (which binds to free calcium) and magnesium (which binds oxalate ions), reducing the number of calcium oxalate crystals that form. Kidneys also produce proteins that reduce crystal clumping and help escort calcium and oxalate crystals safely out the urinary tract. When a lot of oxalate crystals do form, stone-resistant kidneys can dilate their tiny passageways to clear out the crystals. This system works beautifully in the majority of healthy people, giving our kidneys a surprisingly high tolerance for excessive oxalate and crystal-filled urine—although there is a limit.

Some folks cannot adequately defend against the higher oxalate loads following meals, which may be due to the combined effects of other toxic exposures, genetic differences, and metabolic stress (chiefly induced by diet). Their kidneys don't fully recover after a large load of oxalate, making them prone to stones or chronic kidney problems. Differences in our individual biology explain why oxalate intake and excretion don't, by themselves, reliably predict the occurrence of kidney stones.

Expecting to see a direct correlation between dietary oxalate and kidney stones in all persons, but not finding that, has led doctors to dismiss the connection—and the value of avoiding high-oxalate foods. Dietary oxalates are a key driver of calcium oxalate kidney stones and kidney disease, but kidney damage is just one type of disorder that may arise from high oxalate loads. A high degree of oxalate tolerance in our kidneys does not protect us from developing oxalate problems else-where.

Difficulties Diagnosing Oxalate Overload

Clinically recognized oxalate diseases include a set of very rare genetic disorders called *primary hyperoxaluria*, in which the liver overproduces oxalate due to enzyme defects.* Ironically, many primary hyperoxaluria patients *do not* have high urine oxalate at the time of diagnosis because by then the excessive oxalate load has damaged their kidneys' ability to excrete it. Because urine testing for oxalate is not performed routinely, the early stages of this disease (when the kidneys can still excrete high loads of oxalate) are almost always missed.

Similar missteps prevent us from diagnosing dietary hyperoxaluria, formally called *secondary hyperoxaluria*. The current diagnostic scheme lumps the dietary cause with all nonhereditary causes of hyperoxaluria, such as renal failure (lost ability to excrete oxalate), hyperabsorption (a high percentage of dietary oxalate entering the bloodstream), and the ingestion of drugs and chemicals that become oxalate inside the body.

Missing from this diagnostic schema, and therefore quite baffling in practice to researchers and clinicians, is the ability of diet alone, even in the absence of diagnosable medical conditions, to create oxalate toxicity. The role of oxalates in the diet is not obvious to doctors, even in cases involving hospitalization and renal failure. Here's a story that demon-strates how this problem plays out in real life.

---

* Primary hyperoxaluria is believed to affect fewer than three people per million. *Primary* is a term used in medicine to refer to "genetic" or "epigenetic" causes.

Hanna's Story

Although Hanna's medical tests seemed normal, her urinary system had shut down — again. Only in her mid-twenties, she had a 16-year history of kidney stones. She was back in the hospital again, having lost count of how many times. Her doctors had no explanation.

Determined never to repeat this misery, Hanna left the hospital and soon after visited a psychic, who told her that she was eating too many vegetables. Huh? Having been a vegetarian since age 5, she did not think that it was possible to "eat too many vegetables." But it got her wondering if all these years of kidney drama and body pain had something to do with her diet. At least she could do something about that.

In her initial note to me, Hanna wrote: "I am 27 now and have been hospitalized with renal colic 3 times — each time, however, the doctors have said my stones are too small [for them] to do anything for me. My ongoing stone issues caused me several kidney infections, sepsis, and urinary retention. I had to have a urethral dilation and have had lower back pain and UTI [urinary tract infection] symptoms intermittently since then. I also bizarrely had golfer's elbow [tendon pain] and a shoulder injury that won't heal, and sensitive teeth. I have difficulty sleeping and I'm tired all the time . . . and then I listened to a podcast you did, and my mind was blown. I have been feeling like I've been going mad with doctors telling me there is nothing wrong with me for YEARS and it's starting to all make sense!"

Hanna had been eating a vegetarian diet for two decades. As astonishing as it may seem, her doctors were not concerned with her dietary choices when designing her treatment plan.

Hanna undertook a low-oxalate diet (including learning to eat meat), and her health has improved considerably. For the first time in years, she now sleeps through the entire night. Not only is her bedtime "brain twitching" gone, her tinnitus — which she used to have every night when going to sleep — is also completely gone. Her bladder stopped feeling irritated, she no longer needs to urinate overnight, and she has not had a kidney stone in over two years.

Hanna's story illustrates our predicament with identifying oxalate illness. We love testing and expect that there are established, objective ways to determine if someone needs a low-oxalate diet. But testing diagnostics provide limited and sometimes misleading information. Hanna's story is just one of a great number of cases where medical testing showed nothing.

Why Is Testing of So Little Help?

In clinical settings today, the early signs of oxalate overload illness are recognized only in retrospect, if at all. Doctors (and health-care workers) don't suspect oxalate overload, don't know what tests might be called for, and don't understand the many limitations of available tests. Until about 30 years ago, accurate measurement of blood and urine oxalate was a major technical problem. Because the tests weren't reliable, they were dropped from medical practice. Now, even though we can measure urine oxalate more accurately, urine (and blood) tests still tell us little about how much oxalate may reside in our bodies.*

The lack of immediate correlation between oxalate intake and excretion has been a constant point of confusion in research and in understanding the effectiveness of low-oxalate eating. Levels of oxalate in the urine rise and fall as the body works to control the strain that high oxalate levels pose on kidneys, blood vessels, organs, and other tissues. Urinary excretion can lag behind food intake by hours, days, weeks, or months. Data from several studies suggest that oxalate excretion is partly delayed during a period of high intake and that excretion will *increase* after intake goes *down* or even stops. Elevated excretion can continue for a long time.

---

* Correctly executing and interpretating oxalate-oriented testing remains a rare skill.

Urine testing is akin to taking a still photo of a moving target. There are daily rhythms, and perhaps monthly and yearly cycles, that influence oxalate movement within the body and its eventual release. One unusually large study associated with the VP Foundation measured oxalate in the urine of nearly 4,000 women with vulvar pain. While most studies combine consecutive episodes of emptying the bladder (voids) into one pooled 24-hour urine sample, that study looked at all the individual urine voids, separately, for 3 nonconsecutive days.* The study revealed that oxalate handling occurs in cycles, appearing as two or three brief but very steep peaks of elevated excretion occurring at the same time on each day in each subject, but at different times for each subject. For many subjects, their symptoms also occurred in cycles. Interestingly, despite the toxic elevations in urine oxalate, 24-hour urine-level totals were normal in all the subjects. Experimental studies of absorption do not generally take such cycles of excretion into account.

In addition to daily cycles, seasonal cycles have been observed. One study followed 13 volunteers in the UK over a full year (circa 1975), periodically collecting 24-hour urine samples.† They found that although oxalate consumption was highest in the spring, the oxalate release from the body is highest in the summer and fall. This study would be less revealing today because our oxalate intake no longer varies with the seasons, as it did when this observational study was conducted. Studies using short-term or one-time oxalate loads and short observation periods cannot detect delayed excretion, or other delayed effects.

Oxalate levels are so variable in the general population that researchers estimate that to really gauge the "average" amount of oxalate

---

* The subjects suffered with chronic pain of the vulva.
† The investigators were looking for factors that might explain why seasonal variations occurred in rates of kidney stones and placenta calcification. Both are higher in the summer and early autumn but decrease in the winter and early spring.

released by any one person, you'd need *nine* 24-hour urinalyses. Even then, averages are not a useful indicator of oxalate-related problems.

The net effect is that results showing urine oxalate values in the "normal range" don't really indicate that the kidneys are healthy. Normal test results are no assurance that the subject is not overloaded with oxalate. In fact, when the kidneys are overwhelmed and damaged by oxalate, less oxalate appears in the urine. The more compromised the kidney function, the worse it gets. In advanced kidney disease, the kidneys can even become oxalate magnets, collecting instead of passing the oxalate, like "a selective sponge that [retains] most of the oxalates." Under these conditions, damage and oxalate accumulation in non-kidney tissues are also accelerated.

In a case report from the Saint Louis University Medical School, a kidney biopsy from a 51-year-old man who had been on a weight-loss diet of spinach, berries, and nuts found an abundance of oxalate crystals and extensive kidney damage. Yet the patient's "serum [blood] oxalate level was undetectable" and his 24-hour urine oxalate was only mildly elevated. The tests of the patient's blood and urine had no correlation with his kidney function and gave no clue as to the chief reason for his severe health crisis: dietary oxalate poisoning.

Functional medicine doctors and naturopaths use a urine test called the organic acids test (OAT) to look at oxalate and many other markers of metabolism. Owing to natural variability of oxalate levels in urine, the OAT, like all urine tests, is prone to false-negative results. The OAT has helped people discover that oxalate may be an issue for them, but it cannot definitively tell you that you *don't* have an oxalate problem, nor can it help you evaluate your progress in undoing it.

Blood testing is even less informative than urine testing. Even in situations of extreme oxalate overload, blood levels tend to spike for about 6 or more hours following high-oxalate meals, but then stay low even as urinary excretion rises and falls.

Standardized clinical testing is done at "fasting"—12 hours after a meal. Yet that is exactly the worst time to find elevated blood oxalate. Researchers have concluded that "[i]n patients with good renal function, plasma oxalate measurement is of little diagnostic benefit."

More invasive tests, like tissue biopsy, also have trouble revealing whether oxalate is accumulating in non-kidney tissues, irritating the nerves, inciting an overactive immune system, thinning the bones, or any of the other things we would love to know about. Luckily, we don't need specialty testing to recognize this disease.

Clinical Recognition: What Your Doctor Should Be Looking For

In an oxalate-aware world, a variety of basic signs would be flags for suspicion of oxalate overload. The most common signs are listed in **Box 7.2**. Any combination of these indicators, perhaps just a few, should raise suspicions and motivate an inquiry into the patient's history (either acute or chronic) of heavy oxalate consumption. If oxalate overload is suspected, the patient should begin a low-oxalate diet and carefully monitor their symptoms. Because the test indicators may not be dramatic, and also because of issues with de-accumulation that I'll talk about later, some indicators listed in **Box 7.2** are not always helpful for monitoring progress.

BOX 7.2: CLINICAL INDICATORS OF OXALATE OVERLOAD

Clinical Signs

- Cloudy urine, indicating excessive crystals in urine
- Recurrent yeast infections or urinary tract infections, complaints of heavy groin
- Episodic irritable bladder, frequent nocturnal urination, painful urination, or high urinary frequency (dysuria)
- Recurrent kidney stones
- Periodic joint swelling, pain, or weakness, including bursitis, tendinitis, arthritis
- Unexplained digestive distress or abdominal pain
- Unexplained brain fog, mood problems, other neurological complaints
- Signs of vasospasm (low blood flow): coldness, numbness, pain, Raynaud's syndrome of hands or feet, angina
- Unexplained pain, such as burning mouth and tooth pain, or burning in the genitals, anus, or urinary tract
- Bone fractures without obvious cause
- Slow or incomplete recovery from injury or surgery
- Low bone density or mixed bone density with one region high and another low
- Unexplained skin or vision problems

Test Results

- Invisible blood in urine (found on urine testing), usually episodic (hematuria)
- Mildly elevated serum creatinine

✦ Glomerular filtration rate (eGFR) on low end of normal or below normal

✦ White or red blood cell counts on the low end of normal or below normal

✦ Anemia, otherwise unexplained

✦ Elevated urine glycolate and l-glycerate (may indicate elevated internal production)

✦ High plasma glyoxal (though test is not widely available)

Source: Kumar, Kinra, and Kashit, "Autopsy Finding in an Infant," 2020; Kuiper, "Initial Manifestation," 1996.

Learning from Studies of Oxalate Toxicity

Published case studies about oxalates' effects on patients with primary hyperoxaluria (PH, the genetic disorder) or acute poisoning from substances that create extreme oxalate levels in the body (such as the anesthetic methoxyflurane, intravenous xylitol, or ethylene glycol) provide invaluable information about the effects of high oxalate loads throughout the body. (Note that while the toxicity of xylitol infusions has led to discontinuation of their use, the limited available research suggests that *dietary* xylitol does not create much oxalate in the body.)

People with PH suffer greatly from various combinations of musculoskeletal pain, a tendency toward bone fractures, joint diseases, skin problems, growth retardation, heart arrhythmias, vascular inflammation, atherosclerosis, eye damage, nerve damage, brain damage, stroke, anemia, low blood cell counts, and low levels of thyroid and sex hormones—all caused by the high levels of oxalate in their bodies. This list is almost identical—not by accident—to the list of conditions that improve with low-oxalate eating in persons who do not have PH.

Another feature of PH that is common to other sources of oxalate toxicity is that each case is unique in its specific symptoms. A team of experts put it like this: "As systemic oxalosis [oxalate accumulation] produces a *confusing multitude of symptoms* partially resembling rheumatoid or autoimmune disorders/vasculitis, correct diagnosis is not uncommonly overlooked for years" (emphasis mine). Oxalate, an established kidney toxin, is also toxic to most other cells, which is why people with all kinds of chronic hyperoxaluria eventually suffer from that "confusing multitude of symptoms."

Poisoning by ethylene glycol (EG) has also taught us a great deal about how oxalate causes damage in living humans. EG is found in many consumer products—notably automotive antifreeze—and leads to poisoning through accidental ingestion or in suicide attempts. The principal toxic effect of ethylene glycol is to produce very high levels of oxalate in the body. That effect is useful to oxalate researchers who use EG to create oxalate toxicity and kidney stones in lab animals.

Cases of ethylene glycol poisoning demonstrate the well-documented biological effects of oxalate toxicity. Because EG continues to convert into oxalate while the body gradually clears it out, and because oxalate damage takes time to unfold, the full effect of EG poisoning can be delayed, taking days or weeks to fully develop. The onset of neurological problems that typically occur 5 to 20 days later include tinnitus, vertigo, facial palsy, difficulty swallowing, hearing loss, lethargy, and lasting neuropsychological problems. The calcium oxalate crystal deposition in blood vessels leads to circulatory problems (especially in the brain), and edema and inflammatory responses—despite relatively normal-looking CT scans or MRI brain imaging.

The slow development of symptoms during many weeks of oxalate being cleared from the body provides some evidence of how symptoms develop, and especially how symptoms of oxalate toxicity appear first in one part of the body and then move to another. Victims of EG poisoning who survive may experience stroke-like symptoms. I have had a few clients report stroke-like symptoms when they are releasing oxalate from tissues, but that's probably rare. It is more common to suffer bouts of joint pain, headaches, tinnitus, cognitive problems, mood shifts, mental and emotional fatigue, reflux, swallowing problems, restless legs, and poor physical coordination.

Case reports of PH and acute poisoning from oxalate precursors provide useful confirmation about the development of symptoms of oxalate overload that can occur from chronic dietary exposure.

Despite the clinical blind spots, we know a lot about what happens to the oxalate we eat before it finally makes its exit from our body. Taking a closer look at the "ins and outs" will help us better understand the important and confusing features of the disease and of the healing process.

How Your Diet
Aggravates Oxalate Overload

*The truth of the ancient adage, that "the knowledge of a disease
is half its cure," is more than confirmed in the diagnosis of the
oxalic diathesis; for, as certainly as we discover the persistent
presence of the characteristic crystal in the urine, so certainly do
we possess the means of a cure in appropriate diet.*

—James Begbie, MD, *Monthly Journal of Medical Science*, 1849

Clearly, oxalate overload is best addressed by shifting to foods
that are lower in oxalate, but to minimize oxalate in the body
we need to understand where it is coming from. There are
three principal sources of oxalate. Based on the expected amount of oxalate that shows up in "normal" urine tests (20–40 mg), at least 50 percent of total body oxalate arrives directly from foods. The remainder
(~12 mg) forms inside the body (*metabolic oxalate*) from two sources.
Vitamin C breakdown accounts for approximately 10 mg. The remaining sliver—approximately 2.5 mg—comes from metabolism of amino

acids and other substances. See **Box 8.1** for a list of ingested compounds that are known to convert into oxalate inside the body.

Metabolic, or *endogenous*, oxalate production occurs primarily in the liver. Red blood cells also produce low levels of oxalate, and researchers are looking at the possibility that the kidneys may themselves produce traces of oxalate.

It is important to understand that the liver *increases* the total oxalate load in the blood, rather than reducing it. A popular misconception comes from recognizing that the liver is an organ of "detox," leading people to wrongly imagine that the liver can "metabolize" oxalate or help with oxalate removal. The liver does neither of those, regardless of whether the oxalate is of metabolic or dietary origin. The excretion job goes mostly to the kidneys, and secondarily to the colon, skin, and saliva glands, and possibly via other secretions such as the fluids of the eye.

As with everything in biology, various interacting factors influence the amount of oxalate our bodies produce internally. Cellular stress (owing to the nutrient deficiencies, toxicities, and chronic inflammation promoted by modern foods and lifestyle) is the prime reason for increased oxalate production. The key features of chronic metabolic stress are chronic inflammation and oxidative stress (excessive free radicals) in cells and tissues, but they are not themselves the cause. Toxicity and nutrient deficiencies are the underlying instigators of chronic metabolic stress.

Today's common foods and dietary patterns are the biggest culprit in metabolic stress, a destructive set of health problems called *metabolic syndrome*, and diabetes. Three key dietary features lead to such stress: (1) use of oxidized polyunsaturated seed oils such as soy, canola, corn, cottonseed, safflower, or sunflower; these so-called vegetable oils are the standard fats used in restaurants and in commercial marinades, salad dressings, mayonnaise, gravy, and baked goods; (2) excessive sugar and starch in the diet, leading to chronically elevated blood sugar and insulin; and (3) excessive calories overall. (Note that because olive oil is predominantly a monounsaturated oil and not heavily processed like seed oils are, it is safe when used in moderation. Obtaining a truly pure olive oil is a tricky prospect, however, and claims that olive oil promotes longevity are not supported by quality research.)

Metabolic problems increase inflammation and our susceptibility to harm from the oxalates in plant foods. A vegetarian diet's inherent health risks include nutrient deficiencies and increased risk of sarcopenia (low muscle mass), weak bones, and mental illness (due to wrong mix of fats and low levels of fat-soluble nutrients and vitamin B_{12}). Because vegetarian diets inherently rely on high-carbohydrate grains, beans, starchy vegetables, and fruits, they tend to cause chronic hunger, high blood sugar, and high insulin levels; these are the elements leading to low muscle mass, a high percentage of body fat, and metabolic syndrome.

The environmental and nutritional factors that heavily influence genetic expression (what is called *epigenetics*) no doubt affect the varying manifestations of oxalate overload illness. Our personal histories and genetics influence our tolerance and susceptibility, which tissues are most affected, the specific symptoms, and their severity. For example, men are more prone to kidney stones than women; women, having more robust immune systems, are more prone to inflammatory conditions like arthritis and fibromyalgia. Timing matters too: growing children are more susceptible to long-term effects of nutritional deficiencies and toxic exposures.

Diet and lifestyle govern our nutritional status and metabolic health: high-sugar, low-nutrient diets and sedentary living create metabolic frailty. Our age, our medication use, our traumatic experiences, and our physical activities all influence what problems appear. With so many influencing variables, we should expect that a toxicity condition harming basic cell functions will take unique forms.

Then there are additional sources of toxic stressors that come from consumer products, building materials, environmental molds, and pollution from vehicles and industry. Dietary and drinking water contaminants include pesticides, plastics, drug residues, and heavy metals, as well as naturally occurring toxins such as oxalate.

Excessive oxalate (coming from any source) may spawn a dangerous and self-perpetuating cycle of increasing toxicity. Excess oxalate lowers nutrient levels and increases oxidative stress and inflammation. The resulting deficiencies, increased inflammation, and metabolic stress hamper liver function, which causes oxalate production to go up. Increased oxalate production encourages greater deficiency, which can amplify the toxic effects of dietary oxalate overload.

Being oblivious to oxalate, we imagine that eating a "clean" organic, plant-heavy diet will protect us from toxic threats by reducing our exposure to pesticides. But when we are eating liver-taxing high-oxalate foods, our ability to process other toxins may be hampered, and we can still find ourselves with a surprising toxic burden, even on an organic diet. Consider the example of a Virginia woman whose breast milk was contaminated despite her "clean" diet:

> It is frightening to see any glyphosate in my body, especially in my breast milk that will then contaminate my son's growing body. It's particularly upsetting to test positive for glyphosate because I go to great lengths to eat organic and GMO free. I do not consume any meats or seafood and only very rarely eat dairy. This really shows me, and should show others, just how pervasive this toxin is in our food system.

Though her contaminated breast milk is indicative of the widespread problem of airborne and waterborne pesticides, as she suggests, that is not the whole story. Her plant-centric diet may have been inherently nutrient deficient, and it was also likely high in oxalate. Both these problems can cause liver stress, which may lead to the bioaccumulation of other toxins. On the low-oxalate diet, we are better able to handle toxic exposure and become less chemically sensitive and more tolerant of fragrances and other airborne toxins, which suggests better liver function.

BOX 8.1: INGESTIBLE OXALATE PRECURSORS

✥ Vitamin C

✥ Collagen amino acids, possibly glycine, hydroxyproline, phenylalanine

✥ Glyoxal

✥ Ethylene glycol (automotive antifreeze)

✥ Drugs: Lexapro and oxaliplatin

Because it is an oxalate precursor, IV xylitol is no longer used in health care. Oral xylitol is probably not a major source of oxalate.

In addition to oxalate coming directly from foods and normal metabolism, substances that become oxalate in the body (called *oxalate precursors*) can elevate oxalate loads (see **Box 8.1**). Vitamin C and amino acids in collagen (from food or supplements) are potentially significant oxalate precursors.

Though our bodies need vitamin C (ascorbic acid), if we take more than we require, the excess increases oxalate in the body. High-dose supplementation with vitamin C (1 gram or more per day) has been shown to increase internal oxalate significantly, and it has been associated with oxalate toxicity and renal failure.

Oxidative stress (an excess of free radical compounds that can damage cellular structures and promote inflammation) can increase internal oxalate production. However, addressing oxidative stress by supplementing with antioxidants (and specifically vitamin C) is likely to be counterproductive. Lowering the oxalate intake, getting adequate B vitamins, and limiting vitamin C to more appropriate amounts will lower the amount of oxalates that cause cell and tissue damage and that diminish the cells' ability to manage free radical compounds and their harmful effects.

The amount of vitamin C we need varies with carbohydrate consumption. If we eat fewer carbs, we need less vitamin C. The U.S. Recommended Daily Allowance (RDA, 75 mg) covers basic needs for a healthy person eating today's typically high-carb diets. Taking 60 to 90 mg every day via low-oxalate foods like lettuce or fresh lemon juice is probably the best strategy for getting adequate vitamin C. Infections or acute inflammation may slightly and temporarily increase our need for vitamin C, perhaps to as much as 250 mg per day.

The use of vitamin C, even for therapeutic purposes, can result in serious damage. For example, the authors of an article in the *American Journal of Kidney Diseases* report a case of "massive oxalate deposits" in a man's kidney and related kidney failure: "Our patient likely had long-term intermittent hyperoxaluria contributed to by misguided use of [IV] vitamin C and [oral] EDTA, ironically in attempts to promote wellness."

The amino acids glycine and hydroxyproline, abundant in animal connective tissues, are also oxalate precursors, but they contribute just a sliver of daily metabolic oxalate production. One source of these amino acids is an elevated breakdown of our own connective tissues—for example, from injury or excessive exercise—and during recovery from oxalate overload.

Normally, the amount of oxalate produced from these amino acids is small, even on a high-protein diet. Protein intake alone does not increase internal oxalate production; and eating meat may decrease it. One study found that on a low-oxalate diet, high animal-protein intake in humans lowered oxalate in the urine. Other studies showed that feeding meat to rats lowered their oxalate production, suggesting that nutrients in meat are good for liver health. Meat and dairy foods convey many critical nutrients and have been shown to improve the gut microbiome and lower inflammation. Researchers, using a rat model, compared soy protein to meat and explain that "the intake of meat proteins may maintain a more balanced composition of gut bacteria, thereby reducing the antigen load and inflammatory response in the host."

Heavy use of gelatin or collagen supplements (1 tablespoon of powder per day or more) may lead to small increases in endogenous oxalate production. A popular source of collagen is bone broth. The effects of culinary amounts of bone broth on oxalate production have not been studied. Bone broth is nutritious and highly digestible; I encourage using it. But in view of its being a potential, though minor, contributor to metabolic oxalate, a general precaution would be to limit the broth consumption to one meal per day in moderate portions (1 cup or so per day).

For several decades, there was suspicion that a high-carb diet contributed directly to internal oxalate production; however, researchers no longer believe that to be the case. Nevertheless, a long-term high-carb diet is certainly associated with metabolic stress (nutrient deficiencies, inflammation, fatty liver disease, insulin resistance or prediabetes, and diabetes itself), and this may increase the amount of internally generated oxalate. Sugar consumption itself is probably not directly responsible—however, routine use of it contributes to the metabolic problems that intensify oxalates' toxic effects.

Metabolic impairments including diabetes and insulin resistance may be partly powered by oxalate damage. People with diabetes or prediabetes have higher levels of inflammation and produce more oxalates, which creates more inflammation and cell distress. That vicious cycle may explain the oxalate connection between diabetes and kidney disease.

A related finding is that an ultra-low-carbohydrate diet increases production of an enzyme (lactate dehydrogenase) that increases internal oxalate production. Other studies suggest that human liver cells produce more oxalate when deprived of sugar. That research is consistent with my own observation that people recovering from severe oxalate overload do better when they keep some carbs in their diet (compared to pursuing a near-zero-carb approach, such as a strict ketogenic diet) and when they limit their use of fasting to occasional periods of 24 hours or less. Depending on activity level, including 75 to 150 grams of carbohydrates may be beneficial most days, but not necessarily every day.

These secondary influences on internal oxalate production tell us that a junk-food diet containing vegetable oils along with excessive sugar and oxalate is a toxic, disease-creating mix. **A healthy low-oxalate diet should be moderately low in sugar and starch, avoid vegetable and seed oils (which cause greater oxidative stress than other fats), avoid routine use of collagen and vitamin C supplements, and include animal-sourced foods.** This holds true even for patients with kidney trouble.

Absorption: Food Oxalate Getting In

The number one source of oxalate in our body is the oxalate in the food we eat. While a lot of that oxalate stays in our digestive tract (causing irritation and inflammation), some amount of oxalic acid passes into our bloodstream.

The amount of oxalate entering the bloodstream after meals influences how fast—and how badly—people get sick on a high-oxalate diet, but the absorption rate is difficult to observe and measure. The estimates of what we absorb have been going up over the last few decades and are now held to be 10 to 15 percent of the amount consumed. Given the level of oxalate intake common today, even a 10 percent rate of absorption is plenty to have important health consequences. When a person absorbs more than 15 percent, it is called *hyperabsorption*.

For some people, the proportion of oxalate getting into the blood can be dramatically higher—as high as 72 percent. Unfortunately, the lifestyle and environmental factors that create hyperabsorption are common and often shared by family members, creating our problems with leaky gut, increasing our absorption, and thus our vulnerability to the oxalates we're eating. Hyperabsorption is a fact of life for those with gastrointestinal inflammation from any cause, be it obesity, insulin resistance, metabolic syndrome, or another inflammatory condition.

Because poor nutritional status and chronic gut malfunction accompany bariatric surgery, anyone electing this procedure should be informed of their extra vulnerability to oxalate in foods—but typically they are not. There are many examples, including the New York City woman mentioned in Chapter 1. Even though she had good kidney function previously, a 10-day "green smoothie cleanse" caused her to lose her renal function permanently. Ten years earlier, she had had Roux-en-Y gastric bypass surgery for obesity.

There are many sources of kidney- and gut-damaging toxins, but one class of popular pain medications is worth pointing out in some detail because these deliver a double hit in terms of vulnerability to oxalates. Nonsteroidal anti-inflammatory drugs (NSAIDs, such as Motrin, Advil, and similar pain medications) can cause serious gut and kidney problems; see **Box 8.2**. Tissue distress from these drugs makes us more vulnerable to oxalate damage and accumulation.

BOX 8.2: SIDE EFFECTS OF NSAIDS

Heart attacks, bowel perforation, heartburn, stomach ulcers, small intestinal inflammation and permeability or "leaky gut," kidney damage

According to a research report in the journal *Arthritis Research & Therapy*, 60 to 70 percent of NSAID users have gut inflammation and 44 to 70 percent have leaky gut. Even a single dose of most NSAIDs can cause leaky gut in as little as 12 hours after ingestion. Over a third of NSAID users have intestinal ulcerations, risking hyperabsorption of oxalate, as well as promoting food allergies and intolerances, generalized inflammation, and other chronic diseases.

How well the gut is functioning has a direct effect on how much oxalate is absorbed. Oxalate ions and molecules enter the bloodstream by "floating" between the gut cells. Healthy gut cells are equipped with membrane *oxalate ion transporters* that limit *net absorption*, the amount of oxalate that passes further into the body. People with gut inflammation absorb more oxalate because (1) the spaces between inflamed cells are wider and oxalate more easily slips between them, and (2) the reduced energy production in the cells leads to fewer active oxalate transporters.

Our food choices influence absorption, as well. The amount of oxalate getting into the blood is greater when our meals contain gut irritants, lack calcium, or have high water content. Examples of such foods include almond milk, vegetable juices, spinach salads, and most smoothies.

Once in the blood, the oxalates mingle with the immune cells, red blood cells, and cells lining the capillaries, veins, and arteries. Absorbed oxalates move with the blood from the gut straight to the liver, then to the heart, lungs, and other tissues, eventually reaching the kidneys. The greater the amount of oxalate moving in or out of the body, the more toxic it is.

Box 8.3 summarizes the prevailing notions about the sources of oxalate measured in urine tests.

Someone on a spinach-smoothie kick or who is heavily into nuts or nut flours might take in 2,000 mg of oxalate daily, which is 13 times that 150 mg tolerance level assumed in **Box 8.3**.

BOX 8.3: HYPOTHETICAL SOURCES OF URINE OXALATE PER DAY

Food Oxalate

⬦ 15 mg absorbed from 150 mg food oxalate intake (at 10% absorption rate)

Internally Generated Oxalate

⬦ 10 mg from vitamin C
⬦ 2.5 mg from amino acid breakdown

Oxalate Excreted in Urine

⬦ 27 mg

And 2,000 mg in food translates into *at least* 200 mg of absorbed oxalate (and could be 5 to 7 times more) entering the bloodstream (but not always proportionally appearing in the urine as expected).

Excessive oxalate in your meals creates spikes in bodily oxalate. The incoming oxalate can't be cleared from the body either immediately or completely. Even though the kidneys are doing their best, high dietary influxes set up a situation (classically) called *transient renal failure,* which is similar to what occurs in chronic kidney illness, except the kidneys can bounce back when exposure drops.

Because we eat fairly frequently, and because absorption takes hours, post-meal spikes can overlap. Our kidneys may not have cleared the previous meal's oxalate load when the next meal delivers an additional oxalate spike. The toxic impact may be higher when adjacent high-oxalate meals compound the exposure. The first meal—say, a cup of hot cocoa (80 mg oxalate) with breakfast—initiates increased urine oxalate levels that peak about four hours after that meal and continue (at lesser levels) for a total of over six hours. Blood and urine oxalate levels will already be elevated when the next oxalate-bearing meal or snack arrives. Be it nearly constant or in discontinuous spikes, elevations of blood oxalate create immediate and delayed problems, especially for our blood vessels and immune system, and every tissue they serve.

People are unaware that such eating induces oxalate overload. Without that information, we have no incentive to change our diet until the overload breaks through as a medical crisis. Such was the case for an active 81-year-old Pennsylvania man who assiduously followed an antioxidant-rich diet for years, with disastrous results.

This patient previously had healthy kidneys, no urinary symptoms of any kind, and no history of kidney stones. An episode of acute kidney injury brought a sudden end to his characteristic enthusiasm and "youthful" vitality. Seeing no other explanation for this abrupt and traumatic health crisis, his doctors blamed his oxalate-heavy diet, which featured daily lycopene (via tomato paste), antioxidants (via vegetables, cocoa powder, and wheat germ), and heavy use of almond milk and whole nuts. His daughter wrote about what happened to her dad, stating, "He became an old man overnight. . . . [H]e is slower moving and less nimble and he seems to have had some type of post-traumatic stress disorder (PTSD). . . . Also, the deficits to his kidneys have come with other problems he has never had to face, including anemia and high blood pressure." The doctors told her dad "to follow a low-oxalate diet, drink plenty of fluids, stop vitamin C, and take calcium acetate to bind oxalate in the intestines."

Assembly-Line Overload

To visualize the limited capacity of our bodies to excrete oxalate, and how that contributes to oxalate overload, let's consider a famous scene from the 1950s television sitcom starring Lucille Ball, *I Love Lucy*. In this scene, the central character, Lucy Ricardo, is working on the assembly line in a chocolate factory. Lucy, working alongside her friend Ethel, is new to the job. They are wrapping the individual candies in paper as the candies travel toward the packaging room. Although it is their first day, the speed of the assembly line quickly picks up, and an incessant stream of chocolates overwhelms them in no time. More and more chocolates glide by them, unwrapped. The ensuing frenzy resembles your body after a high-oxalate meal.

To delay detection by their supervisor, Lucy and Ethel frantically set some of the unwrapped candies aside. At an escalating pace, they stash the yet-to-be-wrapped surplus in their uniform blouses, under their hats, and into their mouths. Those chocolates never make it to the packing room. Lucy and Ethel's management strategies become ridiculously funny—their uniforms and mouths are puffed and smeared with chocolate.

Chronic oxalate deposition diseases, including kidney stones and *nephrocalcinosis* (diffuse calcium deposits in the kidneys), as well as deposits in other tissues, are a lot like Lucy's blouse and puffed-up cheeks stuffed with oxalate—ah, I mean chocolate. Lucy's overwhelm with the incoming chocolates leads to an accumulation problem, with disastrous consequences—getting fired. Who is at fault for the failure here? Is it the able(-ish) workers, so much like our cells and kidneys, working as hard as they can? Is it the speed of the conveyer belt, acting so much like our diets, constantly bringing us an unrelenting stream of oxalate, day after day, with pathological consequences?

There is another set of workers that are said to rescue Lucy and Ethel from their excessive workload. These are the oxalate-degrading bacteria that can break down the oxalate in the colon. The bacterium most adept at this is called *Oxalobacter formigenes*. Although *O. formigenes* can break down oxalates in our foods, its main role appears to be to encourage the colon to excrete more oxalate. When successfully demanding its dinner, this bacterium lessens the constant strain on the kidneys and improves the body's ability to get rid of oxalate that has moved into the bloodstream (coming from cells or meals).

But here's the catch: *Oxalobacter* has gone missing. Fewer than one-third of healthy American adults have detectable colonies of O. *formigenes*. The reason it's missing is either that it did not colonize in childhood or that the population got wiped out by antibiotics or excessive oxalate intake. Even when present, intestinal bacteria don't have much power to stop oxalate absorption. *Oxalobacter* appears to thrive on the oxalate the body supplies, yet not to thrive on a diet overloaded with oxalate. The oxalate in foods enters the blood from the stomach and largely from the upper small intestine, which are places with limited bacterial populations.

Having colonic oxalate-eating bacteria will not spare your stomach and other tissues from the oxalate in foods. Their efforts don't protect the digestive tract from abrasive crystals, nor do they guard other vulnerable tissues from chronic exposure to excessive oxalic acid. Consider, for example, circulating immune cells. Within 40 minutes after a healthy person eats spinach, the absorbed oxalic acid begins harming them—and that's just the beginning of their troubles with oxalate.

The notion that *Oxalobacter* liberates us to eat spinach with impunity is fantasy. Don't fall for the epic myth that gut bacteria protect us from the excessive oxalate we eat.

When we're ingesting too much oxalate, "somebody" must deal with the stuff that does not get excreted because it is coming in too fast. That "somebody" is the rest of the body, which we'll discuss next.

9

How Oxalate Accumulates

It is fair to assume that any accumulation
of foreign material in the body carries risk for health.

—Rostyslav Bilyy, DSc, et al., *Nanomaterials*, 2020

The idea that the kidneys are promptly removing *all* the oxalate we eat (with none remaining in the body) is perhaps the biggest obstacle to medical recognition of dietary oxalate toxicity. The evidence that oxalate stays behind is solid. When we make a careful effort to look, even when kidney function is excellent, we find oxalate deposits in the body (a condition formally called *oxalosis*).

Oxalate accumulation gradually builds over time and sets up chronic, hard-to-reverse problems with three major effects: (1) structural compromise in bones, marrow, tendons, and other connective tissues; (2) ongoing exposure to oxalate even after dietary oxalate is stopped; and (3) immune system activation, encouraging chronic inflammatory disease.

Diet fosters the development—and removal—of oxalate deposits. Not noticing the deposits or the role of diet in their formation has lulled researchers into underestimating oxalates' potential to affect our health. Yet, the relatively simple (but uncommon) choice to abandon high-oxalate foods can unveil a hidden accumulation problem. This is a potential quandary in research studies, as one research reviewer noted: "pre-existent calcium-oxalate crystals adherent to tissue(s) can undergo dissolution under chosen conditions . . . [and be mistaken for] oxalate biosynthesis."

Crystal formation and cellular damage are probably minimal in healthy persons with very little oxalate in their daily diets. But with a history of high-oxalate eating or intestinal hyperabsorption, lowering intake can lead to visible expulsion of oxalate crystals as the body begins a long process of shedding the toxic residue. The surprising symptoms vary widely, but typically involve tissues with excretory functions and are evidenced by changes in urine, stools, skin, nasal mucus, eyes, and dental tartar. Each person's experience is unique, and many have only very mild reactions that do not involve expelling visible crystals.

For some people, reactions in the wake of lowered oxalate intake include gritty snot, fine grit or white crystals coming out of the skin around the nail beds, clouds of white dust emerging from the skin, red bumps, white bumps, "chill bumps," and skin peeling off the toes, feet, and fingers. One client had to wear cotton gloves for six months because the tips of her fingers were so raw with extensive skin peeling. Another woman sent me photos of her body's reaction to her abrupt adoption of a plant-free diet: her legs developed a blistering rash, with each red bump expelling white chunks reminiscent of rock candy or quartz. Some people experience irritated eyes, fluid with fine white grit seeping out of eyes when napping or resting, or eyes becoming glued shut in the morning with thick, gritty debris.

After shifting to low-oxalate foods, people sometimes describe dramatic changes in the consistency of their stools. Days, weeks, months, or even years after their dietary shift, they independently report stools that are gritty or sandy or that contain numerous odd flecks. Several have shared this same report: "I'm pooping out mostly sand!" Boys and men may have white grit at the tip of the penis. Men and women both report urinary urgency and frequent cloudy urine (*crystalluria*) that comes and goes.

The fact that so many people experience grit coming out of their bodies deserves notice. But often doctors have no idea what these crystals are or why they are occurring. Few have the time or skills to find out. And since the condition does not appear life-threatening, and they have no idea what to do about it anyway, they just ignore it. When one of my clients asked her doctor to look at the crystals emerging from her skin, the doctor dismissed her, saying, "That's just some old calcium."

Trigger and Maintenance Doses

So, how did all that oxalate collect without someone knowing it was there? Accumulation is an inevitable response to excessive oxalate. After high-oxalate meals, oxalic acid travels in the blood and may damage cell membranes, bond with calcium and magnesium, and can form crystals—especially at sites of cellular damage. The surfaces of the oxalate crystals are intrinsically toxic, and their positively charged faces link up to cell membrane lipids and proteins. The crystals stick to the cells and cell fragments, leaving ultrafine invisible toxic dust scattered diffusely and indiscriminately in the glands, bones, and other tissues.

A small fraction of that absorbed oxalate may remain in the body, potentially for years, and this accumulation is especially likely when occasional meals "trigger" periods of elevated blood oxalate within a diet that typically delivers moderate, "maintenance" amounts of oxalate. An important study published in 1967 demonstrated the conditions needed for oxalate deposits to develop and persist in the kidneys. Dr. C. W.

Vermeulen, at the University of Chicago, added a derivative of oxalic acid (*diamide*) to rats' diets, and his team determined that a moderate-oxalate diet becomes an oxalate-depositing diet when "spikes" or trigger levels of oxalate are consumed *occasionally.**

BOX 9.1: VERMEULEN'S MEAL PATTERNS

Three Oxalate Exposure Level Scenarios

1. Trigger + Maintenance = Disease
2. No Trigger + Maintenance = Clearing
3. Trigger + No Maintenance = Clearing

Four and a half decades later, an experiment conducted at Case Western Reserve University tested Dr. Vermeulen's trigger-maintenance theory (see **Box 9.1** describing Vermeulen's findings). Researcher Susan Marengo and her team simulated the chronically elevated oxalate levels in the body that result from intestinal hyperabsorption or from a high-oxalate diet. The team carefully implanted tiny pumps under the skin of 12 rats to "feed" them precise amounts of radioactive soluble oxalate at doses low enough to not overwhelm the kidneys. During the study, Dr. Marengo's team measured the levels of radioactivity in the urine and feces, and they determined how much of the oxalate was excreted. After

---

* They created a spike in oxalate levels by feeding a dose of 1.2 grams per 100 grams of food for 4 days. This was the trigger that generates oxalate stones in rats' kidneys. Following the trigger dose, a moderate oxalate intake (0.3 grams oxamide/100 grams food) prevented the rats' bodies from clearing the crystals. Thus, the combination of a high dose for 4 days and a moderate dose for 24 days created kidney stone disease in every rat. Without the moderate dose following the 4 days of trigger, the initial deposits were cleared. Without the trigger dose, the maintenance diet created stones in only 1 of 20 rats.

13 days,* painstaking dissection of the rats and careful detection of radio-active oxalate in the separated body parts revealed a surprise: *4 percent of the injected oxalate was retained in the rats' bodies, scattered throughout many organs and tissues.* Every animal had oxalate in its bones, kidneys, muscles, liver, heart, lungs, spleen, and testes. Some of the rats also had oxalate deposits in their aorta, brain, and eyes. Owing to the short study duration, smaller amounts of oxalate also showed up in the skin and fat.

Dr. Marengo's work suggests that Dr. Vermeulen's trigger-maintenance theory points to accumulation not just in the kidneys but also all over the rest of the body. She demonstrated that a trigger-level dose of oxalate initiates the crystal formation and then the crystals continue to grow even on lower maintenance doses.

The concentrations of oxalate that were left behind in the rats' bodies were well above the ambient levels in their blood. This surprising result tells us two important things. First, oxalate accumulation is *not* evenly distributed throughout the body; and second, accumulation is the result of active mechanisms and does not necessarily result from poor kidney function. In Dr. Marengo's studies, the rats' kidneys maintained excellent function while the oxalate accumulated in their bodies.

To the extent that these rat studies reflect a physiology we share, the results suggest that with a daily moderate intake of oxalate (especially when accompanied by occasional spikes in intake), crystal deposition in the body may be a common or perhaps universal problem, even when kidney function is normal. In a similar rat study in 1986, a German research team also injected their rats with small amounts of radioactive sodium oxalate and used autoradiography to identify the oxalate in the rats' tissues; just 1 hour later, they found oxalate deposits scattered throughout the rats' hearts, livers, and lungs.

For humans, potential trigger doses of oxalate are commonly consumed in real life. Remarkably modest doses of high-oxalate foods cause

---

* The radioactivity required a short-duration study for the safety of the lab personnel.

spikes in urinary oxalate that can trigger accumulation. Once that accumulation is triggered, levels of oxalate intake that might otherwise not have caused problems may further promote accumulation, potentially leading to chronic problems.

In Dr. Marengo's study, all it took for the rats' bodies to become contaminated was a single 5-second injection followed by a moderate, steady stream of incoming oxalate for 13 days. To translate that into human terms, consider a German study of 25 volunteers. When they ate just 60 mg of oxalate per day (plus a 1,000 mg calcium supplement), the subjects absorbed about 5 mg of oxalate daily from their food. When they increased their intake to 600 mg of oxalate per day for just 2 days (adding 150 grams of cooked spinach at lunchtime), the estimated oxalate absorption from the food increased to 84 mg. In other words, eating ¾ cup of spinach was like getting 17 days of "normal" oxalate exposure in 1 day. But triggers do not need to be that high.

Another study showed that eating just 1.6 ounces (50 grams) of milk chocolate (with ~35–40 mg oxalate) can increase urinary oxalate excretion by a remarkable 235 percent. That surge of oxalate can trigger new deposits. Anyone influenced by the dietary trends we looked at earlier is likely to be eating moderate, maintenance-level doses of oxalate daily (150–250 mg). And it's incredibly easy to be eating trigger-level doses at most meals. Remember, even occasional trigger-level consumption can lead to chronic problems if your everyday diet still has moderately high oxalate content.

Hard to See

Oxalate deposits are practically undetectable on high-tech scans or tissue evaluation. Biopsy and tissue studies looking for oxalate deposits have been reserved for the critically ill and the dead. Even then, the technical challenges of direct tissue analysis make it easy to overlook oxalate deposits.

Oxalates assume many physical sizes. The smallest—oxalate molecules and ions—are invisible even with our most advanced technology. The radioactive oxalate studies have measured them, but we can't use that technique for diagnosis. Nanocrystals are also invisible in clinical pathology, and even much larger microcrystals and aggregates are diffuse and hard to see; their detection requires careful preparation and polarized light microscopy, and they can still easily be mistaken for other non-oxalate crystals.

The small size and scattered distribution of these deposits, the lack of attention to specimen age in clinical medicine, and the pathologists' sample preparation process all conspire to make it incredibly easy to miss or destroy oxalate crystals in tissue samples.

Although crystals are the most common form, calcium oxalate deposits can also occur as noncrystalline composites of calcium oxalate and fat, called *oxalate lipids*. Oxalate lipids have been found in liver and intestine specimens, as well as in the joint fluids of patients with gout, rheumatoid arthritis, and traumatic bursitis. Oxalate lipids are resistant to the techniques used to detect oxalate in tissue samples, and perhaps for that reason they are rarely discussed in the literature.

The one accepted way to tell if oxalate is building up in someone's body is to take out a small bit of bone and look for crystals. In practice, this invasive procedure is performed only when doctors suspect advanced disease from primary hyperoxaluria. Because oxalate accumulation occurs unevenly, this test can still miss oxalate deposits if the bone sample is not from a location where the crystals happen to be forming. Even if clinicians were aware of oxalate retention and had access to timely tissue examination (they don't), the technical hurdles effectively prevent reliable diagnosis of oxalosis.

Sometimes magnetic resonance imaging (MRI) scans can show oxalate-induced brain inflammation, but the oxalate crystals usually escape detection. MRIs and computed tomography (CT) scans used in clinical diagnosis cannot reliably see oxalate crystals even when the deposits are large. In a case of oxalate poisoning from ingestion of ethylene glycol, the oxalate crystals that formed caused lasting cognitive impairment. Yet a series of CT scans of the head on the day it happened, and the following day, were essentially normal and an MRI five days later revealed only nonspecific brain abnormalities.

Crystals Everywhere

Oxalate crystals have been found in tissues throughout the body, including the lymph nodes, heart, and other organs—not only as incidental findings during postmortem exams but also in the tissues of the chronically ill, in people who have suffered bodily injury, *and* in healthy people without kidney problems. Crystals are especially likely to gather in the blood vessels, eyes, glands, and bones. Unfortunately, even when oxalate crystals are identified, we don't have any way to quantify how much oxalate might be accumulating in the body.

The blood vessels are prone to damage from oxalic acid and crystal accumulation, which can lead to tissue degeneration, including cataracts, vision problems, and fatal brain aneurysm. Oxalate deposits are found in the arteries and in calcified arterial plaques. Oxalate crystals are associated with blood vessel weakness, vasculitis (inflamed blood vessels), stroke, and cardiac conduction abnormalities and arrhythmia.

Loss of eye health can result from damage to the retinal blood vessels stemming from elevated oxalate. In addition to the eye itself, pathologists have found unexplained oxalate deposits in the eyelids. The specialized photoreceptor neurons at the back of the eyes (the retina) easily attract calcium oxalate. One report documented an unusually massive buildup of oxalate in the damaged eye of a 21-year-old man who, at age 13, had been hit in the eye by some hard plastic that injured his cornea. Recurrent attacks of inflammation and pain in the blind and shrunken eye prompted eye removal surgery. The resulting report described white crystals projecting from the retina inside the excised eyeball as "stalactites." The pathologist describing the case wrote: "Deposition of calcium oxalate crystals in the eye, though not common, is possibly not so rare as the small number of published reports would indicate."

Additionally, crystals commonly occur in the testes, breasts, and thyroid glands. Over 70 percent of normal thyroids show oxalate accumulation. Cells surrounding the crystals lose their ability to produce thyroid hormones, and this can result in ever larger oxalate deposits as we age. People over age 50 seemingly have an 85 percent likelihood of oxalate crystals in the thyroid.

Free oxalic acid or oxalate crystal deposits in breasts can launch a breast cell transformation process that leads to non-oxalate breast calcification and aggressive cancer.

Likewise, teeth, bones, bone marrow, ligaments, and joint spaces are prone to oxalate deposits. Our mineral-rich bones can store massive amounts of oxalate. After finding feathery-looking oxalate crystals within a mass of giant immune cells in their patient's thigh bone, a Korean medical team wrote: "The incidence of [bone oxalosis] may be underestimated because of its benign . . . appearance, which normally does not indicate the need for a bone biopsy." Likewise, the discs, tendons, and other connective tissues that maintain the spine's structure can become oxalate depositories.

Arthritis, bursitis, tendinitis, and gout are all associated with the varied oxalate crystals found in and around the joint spaces, cells, and fluids. For example, rheumatologists noted oxalate in the painful knee of a patient with rheumatoid arthritis and arterial calcifications in the hips and legs. Oxalate accumulation is associated with Parkinson's disease and with the loss of the protective fatty tissue coating on nerve cells (demyelination) associated with multiple sclerosis (MS).

Oxalate deposits, although mostly invisible, are durable and metabolically challenging. Accumulated oxalate has important consequences for our long-term health and our ability to recover. It's likely that prior oxalate accumulation contributed to the death of the Barcelona patient from sorrel soup, mentioned in Chapter 5. Had he lived, the accumulations observed in his heart, lungs, liver, and elsewhere would likely have created persistent problems, such as neurological symptoms and chronic inflammation, as well as severe, irreversible kidney damage.

Though investigations have revealed oxalate crystals in every tissue, researchers still consider the presence of oxalates to be mysterious. Yet we have plenty of clues as to how accumulation occurs.

Why Do Accumulations Start?

Susceptibility to oxalate accumulation varies from person to person and from tissue to tissue. Influential factors include: (1) whether the tissues have enough health and resources to repel, expel, or contain oxalate and avoid death; and (2) whether the tissues have oxalate ion transporters or other oxalate-attracting features.

Healthy, intact tissues that are not undergoing growth, recovery, or regeneration are far more likely to rebuff crystal attachment and successfully repel the oxalate ions. On the other hand, cells and tissues that are undernourished, weak, stressed, inflamed, infected, injured, already holding oxalate, or regenerating can develop more crystals. Cell debris encourages the precipitation of oxalate ions into crystals and creates sites of retention. Researchers have found that inflammation, low oxygen levels, and low pH (acidity) interfere with the cells' management of oxalate ions, increasing the risk of oxalate retention.

When cells cannot repel them, oxalate ions can linger long enough to form calcium oxalate and develop crystals. If the cells cannot generate adequate antioxidants (e.g., *glutathione*), crystal attachment and subsequent crystal growth become more likely. Oxalate then creates additional oxidative stress and causes further cell damage and cell death. Ions or crystals also cling to the membrane fragments of struggling cells and dead cell remnants. If neighboring cells or patrolling immune cells cannot fully contain the damage, initial deposits may amass into larger and larger crystals.

Injuries don't need to be severe to encourage oxalate accumulation—just the daily wear-and-tear of life is enough. When the body is high in oxalate, the routine repair process (much of which occurs while we sleep) may be undermined, leading to tissue weakness and the eventual appearance of symptoms or non-resolving injury.

Crystal accumulation from oxalate in the diet is especially worrisome if the body is stressed, hard at work in some way, wounded, undergoing surgery, or pregnant, or the person has a physically demanding job. Accumulation due to tissue stress is also likely if someone has increased risk of any health problem owing to genetics, obesity, high blood sugar, metabolic stress, or age.

There are also innate tissue characteristics that may attract oxalate. For example, various tissues have membrane transporters that deliberately move oxalate in or out of cells. These tissues include the gut, kidney, liver, and brain. Other tissues with transporters include the cochlear hair cells in the ears, the epididymis of the testis, and the cells of the pancreas, thyroid, and salivary glands. In their daily work of managing ions, tissues may develop oxalate-related stress and oxalate accumulation problems.

When the salivary glands move bicarbonate into the saliva, they also excrete oxalate. Salivary glands concentrate the oxalate under normal conditions at levels 10 to 30 times higher than in the blood plasma. Thus, oxalate may contribute to salivary stone formation, tartar problems, and other dental issues, such as gum inflammation and tooth sensitivity.

The body appears to accumulate crystals actively to divert the oxalate from vital tissues and organs, sparing them from excessive or lasting damage. For example, elevated oxalate in the blood culminates in vascular and nerve damage, arrhythmia, and heart failure. Next to those dire events, retaining blood oxalate elsewhere seems a relatively benign alternative. How the non-kidney tissues of the body help manage oxalate levels in the blood and the role of crystal formation in that process are topics that have yet to be explored.

Accumulation and Inflammation

When oxalate crystals are big enough to see under a microscope, researchers often describe them as beautiful gems, ground glass, sharp splinters, or crystal dust. These "gems" are a problem for the cells and especially for the immune system. When oxalate is lodged in tissues, it acts as an irritant, provoking additional inflammation that can cause pain and fatigue, and may prolong or prevent tissue healing, thereby increasing susceptibility to infection.

Because the immune system has the difficult job of removing them, oxalate crystal deposits can provoke chronic inflammatory disease similar to silica and asbestos nanofibers. The size of the crystals is an important factor influencing their toxic effects. The stealthier nanocrystals are especially destructive to cells and tissues. But the bigger the crystals, the harder they are to degrade. Oxalate deposits above a certain size are most easily seen by researchers. These are harder for the body to remove, but not necessarily the ones causing the most damage.

Oxalate-induced inflammation can occur anywhere in the body. As one paper put it, "oxalate is strongly involved in inflammatory pathways, which makes it a prime candidate to contribute to the progression of CKD [chronic kidney disease] and systemic inflammation."

The presence of oxalate nanocrystals and materials from oxalate-damaged cells incites the immune system to clean them up. When immune cells are not able to neutralize or break up the crystals, they send alarms that may rally more immune cells to gather and clump around the unwanted particles. These compact tumors are called *granulomas*. If the effort fails to dismantle the crystal, the granuloma can turn off, stop growing, and die. The remains of the clustered immune cells become a crystal-containment device, "hiding" the deposits to avoid continuous activation of the immune system. Because infections may attach to granulomas, and because oxalate collects where infections are active, the "buried" crystals may be accompanied by dormant viruses and bacteria.

Oxalate-containing granulomas are often asymptomatic, but they can lead to Crohn's disease, blood vessel inflammation and damage, skin problems, reproductive disorders, postmenopausal bleeding, organ fibrosis, fungal infection, and other troubles. Experts believe that "granuloma-inciting agents" are transported to the lymph nodes and lead to a condition called *sarcoidosis*.

The immune system has another method for shielding surrounding tissues from oxalate crystals: entrapping them with extruded DNA, called a *neutrophil extracellular trap (NET)*. These NETs forming around oxalates may contribute to gallstones, gallbladder "sludge," and other plug-like masses that can occlude pancreatic ducts and small blood vessels. The health problems sometimes become evident after adopting a low-oxalate diet and usually resolve with time. I'll tell you about that in Chapter 11.

The last things you need are invisible toxic crystals in your bones, joints, glands, and organs. Containment efforts by the immune system may turn off inflammation and immune reactions in the short term, even if crystals are not broken down and excreted. If the body also successfully restores oxidative balance, the oxalate toxicity may remain silent or mild until all the reserves are spent. That doesn't mean the problem is resolved, however. Instead, you are building up a toxic debt that no superfood, herbal concoction, or drug has the power to correct. Let's turn next to what happens when the bill comes due.

10

Symptoms and Syndromes

With stockpiled toxicants persistently disrupting normal human processes and physiology, it is understandable that the resulting pathophysiology may induce chronic disease.

—Stephen J. Genuis, PhD, and Kasie L. Kelln, PhD,
Behavioural Neurology, 2015

Two Engines of Illness

Good health requires your cells to control their biochemical environment and activity. Oxalates, however, are *antimetabolites* that interfere with the biochemical basics. They upset cells' control of mineral ions (especially calcium) that are required to coordinate cell activities. They deplete minerals and other nutrients. They block enzyme function. They destroy mitochondria (the power plants of cells). Oxalates can also make it impossible for cells to keep free radicals (reactive by-products) under control, a condition called *oxidative stress*. Oxidative stress damages cell structures, alters genetic expression, consumes antioxidants and nutrients, and triggers inflammation. In addition, oxalate ions and crystals directly damage critical cell structures—the membranes, mitochondria, and genetic material. Cellular membranes are essential structures for life. Without them there is no biochemistry—and no life.

Cell injury, oxidative stress, mineral shortages, and cell dysfunction—this invisible mess becomes disease through what I call the "two engines of illness": (1) *broken energy and repair systems*, and (2) *chronic immune activation* and related damage control. These pernicious problems can lead to insulin resistance, neurological troubles, dementia, fibromyalgia, cardiovascular disease, cancer, and more. In the "engines of illness" sections in this chapter, I briefly survey some of the basic mechanisms behind the metabolic mayhem that erupts into oxalate-induced symptoms. Oxalate toxicity's puzzling and varied array of health challenges fit into a coherent picture. Here, in this chapter—especially for those who want to understand some of the biology—we can make sense of the puzzle.

The First Engine of Illness: Broken Energy and Repair Systems

The body can manage daily wear and tear, recover from injury, and live a long and productive life, but only if cells are able to repair and reproduce themselves. When cells don't have enough raw materials, energy, or structural integrity to support the effort, the normal repair process is undermined. Tissue sturdiness, even in bones and teeth, becomes harder to preserve. Inadequate maintenance makes us prone not only to injury but also to a problem called *fibrosis*—the overproduction of collagen and scar tissue buildup. Alas, excessive oxalate creates basic maintenance problems and an increased need for tissue maintenance and repair.

When oxalate upsets the electrolyte balance, inactivates enzymes and mitochondria, and increases oxidative stress, cells suffer from lowered energy and glucose production. The resulting low energy supply makes it harder for the cells to do their jobs. Cells become lethargic, feeble, confused, and short-lived. They are deficient in needed lipids and glucose. Their protein production slows down. They have difficulty replacing themselves. These energy and repair problems lead to a sluggish metabolism; difficulties with tissue healing, nerve function, and hormone production; and excessive acidity.*

The acidity, called *lactic acidosis*, results in part from reliance on inefficient anaerobic energy production and is especially harmful to bones and kidneys. It also contributes to feelings of malaise. Acidosis promotes microflora imbalance and overgrowth, and it enables infections. Mineral deficiency can make it harder to correct the excessive acidity. When the lungs and kidneys can't clear the excessive acid, calcium and potassium are released from the bones to maintain a correct blood pH. Chronic acidity frustrates bone maintenance and leads to thinning bones (osteopenia and osteoporosis).

Injured mitochondria are a likely factor in most illnesses, including mood issues and gut function problems. Sporadic symptoms of mitochondrial disorders include migraine, muscle pain, gastrointestinal symptoms, tinnitus, depression, and chronic fatigue. Episodes are triggered by mental and physical stressors (such as illness, injury, surgery, toxic exposures, fasting, and overexercise) that create an increased energy demand that can't be met because the mitochondria are unable to generate sufficient energy.

Circulatory problems, vascular diseases, and the development of atherosclerosis are also related to low cell energy.

Critical tissues with high energy needs, such as the brain and other

---

* Oxalate inhibits pyruvate carboxylase, pyruvate kinase, and lactate dehydrogenase.

nerve cells, are especially vulnerable to cell death from low energy supplies. The nerve cells need a lot of energy. For example, the adult human brain requires energy at a rate 10 times more than other tissues. Nerve cell distress contributes to muscle weakness, fatigue, poor physical coordination, abdominal pain, twitches and muscle spasms, headaches, memory problems, irritability, and dementia.

Oxalate also interferes with the enzymes that replenish the *glycogen* (stored carbohydrate) in the muscles and in the liver. When glycogen is low, the muscles lower their energy demands to maintain normal blood sugar levels. This sacrifice typically prevents low blood sugar, but the low glycogen makes the muscles prone to cramping and compromises their physical performance and recovery. Chronic low glycogen and low cell energy levels can make fasting and long-term zero-carb diets stressful and unhealthy, and can lower exercise tolerance.

Damage to glands can lead to hormone problems that affect sleep, reproduction, mood, energy, and performance. A rat study found that diets high in oxalic acid caused hypothyroidism, elevated thyroid stimulating hormone (TSH), lower body weight, and low body fat. The rats' livers, spleen, kidney, and endocrine glands were all undersized.

Cell damage and low energy also impair our self-defense systems, including the immune system. Oxalate in the bone marrow injures the immature blood cells and immune cells as they form. Circulating immune cells also sustain injury in the blood stream after high-oxalate meals. One research team looked at blood cells after giving spinach smoothies to volunteers, and they wrote: "it is likely that oxalate-rich meals could cause inflammation and monocyte [immune cell] mitochondrial dysfunction . . . [which] could compromise the immune system over time," as well as increase the propagation of free radicals that contribute to disease and aging. A compromised immune system may explain the occurrence of chronic infections among the oxalate-injured. Infections (such as repeated sinus infections, UTIs, yeast overgrowth, and even infection with the *C. difficile* bacterium that causes life-threatening inflammation of the colon) often "miraculously" disappear after changing to a low-oxalate diet.

The Second Engine of Illness: Chronic Immune Engagement

Illness emerges when our protection and defense forces get overworked. Recall from Chapter 9 that the immune system works hard to contain oxalate crystals and their damage, as well as to remove oxalate crystals from the tissues. Problems occur when the perpetual presence of toxic crystals incites chronic (pro-inflammatory) immune engagement— meaning the immune system is always turned on in ways that perpetuate metabolic stress generally.

Immune responses to oxalates generate additional biochemical mayhem, including a process called the *inflammasome,* which coordinates immune-cell responses and prompts the release of hormone-like *prostaglandins.* Prostaglandins dilate the blood vessels and allow large immune cells to reach their oxalate target—the crystal deposits. To improve their mobility, the immune cells forge a path by generating enzymes that break down the connective tissues. But that path can also enable oxalate to reach more tissues. If the immune response is not promptly effective and oxalate exposure remains high, the inflammatory process increases the likelihood of continued tissue injury.

Prostaglandins can also elicit muscle contractions (pain and cramping) in the intestines, uterus, bladder, and elsewhere, as well as stimulate estrogen production. If high oxalate levels prompt chronic high prostaglandin levels, this may promote "estrogen-sensitive" conditions, including endometriosis and some cancers.

When the crystal containment I described earlier is working, we don't see a lot of symptoms. In the challenging effort to remove the crystals, a healthy immune system turns off the inflammatory processes that prove to be unproductive. For example, gout attacks stop when the body's own enzymes digest molecules that otherwise would keep the inflammation going. In chronic inflammation, the immune system loses the ability to turn itself off.

Building granulomas around crystals may create long-term changes to the immune function by teaching the adaptive immune cells (cells with memory) to attack a given immune activator (which can be anything the immune cells react to). This training lowers the tolerance for other provocative *antigens* and sets the body up for *autoimmune disease*—an extensive family of illnesses where an overactive immune system interferes with normal tissues, often generating pain, fatigue, and weakened body functions.

A simplistic interpretation of autoimmune disease is that the body is "attacking itself," but autoimmune-like symptoms also occur because of constant immune provocation from foreign threats like oxalate nanocrystals. The primary driving force of the immune system "is the need to detect and protect against danger," and the "chronic autoaggression seen in autoimmune disease is most likely due to the inappropriate presence of a low-lying stimulus" (not the loss of the ability to discern self from non-self, as is commonly conceptualized). Oxalates are persistent low-lying disrupters that distress and overwork the immune system.

Such "autoimmunity" is a factor in dozens of illnesses, including Hashimoto's thyroid disease and painful skin conditions such as lichen sclerosus, which tends to afflict the genitals. Happily, these and various other "autoimmune" conditions tend to abate in individuals who follow a low-oxalate diet.

More Ways Oxalates Stir Up Trouble

In an effort to cope, the body enlists some techniques and helpers that can put the body on a path to pain and disease. These include a protein called *osteopontin*, fibrosis (mentioned earlier), and overly busy immune cells, especially the *mast cells*.

Osteopontin

When protecting the kidneys from stones during oxalate overload (following high-oxalate meals), the body makes a protein called *osteopontin* (OPN).* Ironically, despite OPN's inhibiting mineralization and preventing tissue calcification under (short-term) conditions of injury and disease, the chronic production of OPN fosters crystal retention, inflammation, calcium deposits in tendons, and disease elsewhere in the body. Even periodic spikes in serum osteopontin may be a sign of inflammation and cancer and can help transform normal cells into malignant, metastasizing tissue invaders. Osteopontin is also suspected of causing metabolic damage that fosters diabetes and obesity. Serum osteopontin is elevated in people with muscle-pain syndromes like fibromyalgia and other inflammatory diseases such as Crohn's disease, atherosclerosis, and aortic aneurysms, as well as autoimmune diseases including lupus, multiple sclerosis, and rheumatoid arthritis. Elevated OPN promotes scar tissue formation (*fibrosis*) in the heart, lungs, skin, and muscles.

Fibrosis

Remember the lame horses, mentioned in Chapter 3, that developed distorted and swollen faces from their high-oxalate forages? "Big head" is an oxalate-induced fibrotic disease whereby the loss of tissue integrity sets off uncontrolled scar tissue growth. Fibrosis is normally a temporary stage essential to the tissue repair process, being necessary for holding the damaged tissue together. But fibrosis becomes a problem when the replacement of normal cells is impaired by oxalate damage. Over time, the normal cells diminish, but the scar tissue continues to be produced because the fibroblast cells continue to flourish despite the high oxalate levels. The resulting fibrosis can occur in organs, joints, skin, bone

---

* Osteopontin is needed for bone metabolism and immune functions, and is also produced in non-kidney tissues (glands, lungs, GI tract).

marrow, and in malignant tumors, and can lead to organ failure and death. While normal fibrosis is a healthy response to cell death, *non-resolving fibrosis* is a feature of many chronic and painful diseases, and is blamed for at least one-third of natural deaths occurring worldwide. Understanding how fibrosis gets out of hand could save lives.

While high inflammation leads to fibrosis, inflammation is not the true source. Taking anti-inflammatory agents doesn't stop fibrosis. As researchers put it, "The [e]limination of the inciting stimulus is the first and most efficacious approach." Research has demonstrated that oxalate crystals cause fibrosis. My client Dori wrote me: "I had my first blood test since going low-ox, and guess what? My fibrinogen is normal, which has never happened; even my doctor is shocked! That's a miracle. I struggled with really, really high fibrinogen for so long!" She was sick and in pain for years with joint problems, gastritis, bleeding gums, burning tissues, eye and skin issues, and a huge amount of abdominal scar tissue. She ate "a ton of almond flour, almond milk, spinach, sweet potato, beets, chia, cocoa, and turmeric." Organ fibrosis recedes and patients feel better when normal cells regain their ability to reproduce.

Other cellular repair functions can be overstimulated by oxalate crystal damage, as well. For example, oxalate may cause other cells to multiply excessively (as in patients with Crohn's disease) and may trigger the shedding of living epithelial cells (seen in kidneys).

Mast Cells

Oxalate is a powerful *mast cell* activator. Mast cells are large immune cells with many roles. They sense environmental cues, allergens, and psychological stress, and engulf materials destined for removal. They exist everywhere, including the brain, glands (such as the pineal, pituitary, and thyroid), and tissues facing the external environment, such as the throat and bladder. They cluster near nerve fibers, where they help nerves and the immune system communicate.

Mast cells are provoked into action by injured tissues, inflammatory molecules, or other triggers such as fungi, bacteria, foods, toxins, antibiotics, and pain medications. Active mast cells secrete over 200 response chemicals, including *histamine*, which can cause many unpleasant symptoms, such as itchy rashes and asthma attacks. Histamine, of course, is well known thanks to the antihistamine medications used to curb allergy symptoms. Mast-cell activation can lead to muscle spasm, cold sensitivity, and unpleasant numbness, tingling, prickling, and burning pain. An enormous array of conditions are associated with mast-cell activation, including: osteoporosis, gum disease, leaky gut, food allergies, cancer, restless leg syndrome, migraine, interstitial cystitis, menstrual disorders, and autoimmune hypersensitivity diseases such as multiple sclerosis, Guillain-Barré syndrome, and Sjögren's syndrome.

Mast-cell symptom patterns (see **Box 10.1**) are common among my oxalate-overloaded clients. There is no cure for excessively busy mast cells. Our best option is to recognize and avoid triggers such as oxalate.

> **BOX 10.1: SYMPTOMS OF MAST-CELL ACTIVATION**
>
> Chronic fatigue; strong reactions to cold, foods, and chemicals; flushing, hot flashes; itchy skin, psoriasis; sinusitis, rhinitis, allergies, asthma; palpitations, light-headedness, dizziness; depression, bipolar affective disorder, anxiety, panic, anger

Sick Without Symptoms

Symptoms are not the most reliable indicators of oxalate illness. Ten percent of primary hyperoxaluria patients show no symptoms. When underlying problems have not yet broken through as pain, fatigue, or functional loss, that does not mean you are not sick or that it will never catch up with you.

Take, for example, the problem of calcium deficiency caused by excessive oxalate intake. Calcium deficiency, even when minimal, is bad for general health and is associated with irritable bowel syndrome (IBS), learning and memory problems, and brain arteriosclerosis. The physiologic stress caused by nutrient deficiency may stay invisible because the body prioritizes ion levels needed to keep vital organs working well. The body maintains normal calcium and magnesium levels in the blood, the brain, and the spinal cord, even while the bones lose minerals because of an insufficient and unbalanced diet. This prioritization, while important for daily function, uses up nutrients and silently erodes the body's resilience.

The overall effect sweeps oxalate-related problems under the rug—for a while. At some point, some additional stress overwhelms the shrinking reserves and defenses, and symptoms suddenly break through. That (long-abused) ability to cope finally falters—often in the wake of an incident that raises energy demands or oxidative stress in the body. Inciting events may be a traumatic accident, tragic loss, a course of a strong medication, giving birth, or major surgery. Alternatively, the onset of illness may come and go in vague complaints that gradually intensify to disabling proportions.

There is a sound reason the original syndrome was tagged as a "diathesis" or a "constitutional tendency." When and where specific symptoms break through depends on a person's individual constitutions, health history, and environmental factors. From tiny invisible beginnings, the struggles of cells in coping with toxic, hard-to-remove particles finally blow up into unique cases of multisystem, multi-symptom illness. To add to the confusion, the same person can experience different symptoms at different times.

When sudden symptoms do emerge, we assume an acute problem, without considering the possibility of a hidden and progressive chronic condition behind it. Recall the example in Chapter 8, of a hearty 81-year-old who seemed fine for years during a long period eating high-oxalate foods, until suddenly he wasn't fine. That case made it into the medical literature because the collapse centered on his kidney problems. Other such cases don't get written up because most doctors don't know that serious symptoms or organ failure in other parts of the body can originate in oxalate overload. We do not notice the body-wide cumulative effects that led up to the crisis.

Symptoms and Syndromes

By undermining the basic functions of cells, oxalate buildup is an "everywhere" problem. Wherever there are cells or connective tissues, oxalate can cause damage, leading to a diverse array of symptoms and syndromes.

The gut, liver, and kidneys take a big hit from high-oxalate meals because they are the points of oxalate's entry and exit. Clinically, the most common first symptoms of primary hyperoxaluria are blood in the urine, abdominal pain, kidney stones, or repeated urinary tract infections. The relationships between oxalate buildup and chronic diseases in other parts of the body are less well known. **Table 10.1** summarizes the symptoms and diseases that oxalate can set in motion and that can recede on a low-oxalate diet.

The toxic effects of too much oxalate are interdependent and mutually enabling. Oxalate damage may start in one area of the body, but it can exacerbate other conditions, become self-perpetuating, spread elsewhere, and cascade into diverse diseases. Shared stressors connect seemingly different diseases that arrive in overlapping clusters. For example, people with IBS or depression also tend to suffer from rheumatoid arthritis, muscle pain, fatigue, migraines, anxiety, or other brain-function issues. Persons with celiac disease or IBS are more likely to also develop osteoporosis and bone fractures.

A disorder in one area of the body can turn on generalized reactions. For example, a study at Case Western Reserve University demonstrated that oxalate crystals injected into only *one* back foot of rats produced swelling in *both* back feet. Likewise, tissue damage and inflammation in one place (such as endocrine glands) can engender symptoms elsewhere. That is not to say that oxalate is responsible for all ills, but we should not be shocked that *many* diverse problems arise from, or are aggravated by, too much dietary oxalate.

Table 10.1: Body Systems and Oxalate-Associated Symptoms

System Type	Issue / Mystery Syndrome	Signs
Digestive	Irritable bowel syndrome (IBS) Inflammatory bowel Gastric reflux Rectal/bowel function problems	Trouble swallowing, reflux Bloating, belching, indigestion Cramping, pain, constipation Frequent bowel movements Diarrhea, alternating constipation and diarrhea
Metabolic/Glandular	Gland function suppressed Hypothyroid (or other glands low) Liver function issues Diabetes Metabolic syndrome Poor resistance to infection Systemic acidosis Mitochondrial dysfunction Cystic breasts	Low energy Tiredness, chronic fatigue Weight issues Brain function sluggishness Weakness, muscle cramps Cold hands and feet Slow healing
Immune	"-itis" issues Autoimmune disorders Allergies, asthma, sarcoidosis Fibrosis Hypersensitivities Mast-cell activation	Rashes, itching, pain, migraine headaches Food intolerance, cold intolerance Allergies Fatigue Hot flashes, flushing

System Type	Issue / Mystery Syndrome	Signs
Cardiovascular	Atherosclerosis Vasculitis Arteritis Raynaud's syndrome	Difficulty with venipuncture/rolling veins Cold intolerance Stroke/heart attack Breathing problems or COPD Blood pressure irregularity Heart arrhythmias
Neuro/brain	Pain/burning Oral sensitivity Poor sleep (insomnia, night waking) Headaches/migraine Autism	Light and noise sensitivity, vision issues Burning pains (anywhere) Hiccups Mood issues, indifference/loss of motivation, depression, anxiety Cognitive issues, mental fatigue, brain fog/lack of focus Poor physical coordination/clumsiness
Joints/muscles/bones/teeth	Arthritis Gout Osteopenia Fibromyalgia Excessive tooth tartar Jaw pain, jaw popping, TMJ Carpal tunnel/tenosynovitis Gum disease	Muscle spasms Stiffness, weakness, twitching joint (knee, hip, shoulder, elbow), foot pain Unstable joints, frozen shoulder Injury, slow healing Tightness or looseness of fascia, joints, etc. Weak bones, loose teeth Swelling, heat Bleeding, infected, or inflamed gums

(table continues)

Type	Issue / Mystery Syndrome	Signs
Skin	Lichen sclerosus Scleroderma Dermatomyositis Ehlers-Danlos syndrome	Frail skin, weakness, cuts, or splits White spots, red or purple sores Sun sensitive, difficulty tanning, flushing Bruising from within Rashes, eczema, peeling
Eyes	Sties Deposits	Eyelid redness and tenderness, vision problems Crusty secretions, hazy corneas Watery, itchy, or dry eyes Cataracts
Ears	Tinnitus, vertigo, Ménière's syndrome	Ringing or buzzing, dizziness, hearing loss
Pelvic	Genital pain, vulvodynia Sexual dysfunction	Heaviness, pressure, soreness, itching, sharp pain, stinging or burning in the pelvis, vulva, or scrotal areas Genital redness, rashes, blisters Painful intercourse
Urinary	Kidney stones/kidney calcification Excessive frequency, urgency Burning, cystitis, burning bladder, urethra pain	Incontinence, bedwetting Cloudy urine, sediment-filled or powdery urine

Digestive Troubles from Oxalate

Cell stress and inflammation occurring in the gut owing to chronic oxalate exposure can reduce nutrient uptake and break the intestines' *barrier function*, which opens a path for toxins to incite chronic diseases of all sorts, including cancer. The gut is a major sensory organ regulating bodily health by "reading" and conveying information about the environment so the body (and mind) can respond appropriately. If the immune cells, nerve cells, and hormonal cells in the gut are damaged, there are ripple effects elsewhere.

Oxalate can damage the digestive tract and the healthy bacteria that live there, causing both increased permeability, or "leaky gut," and dysbiosis. Oxalate has been associated with gut inflammation and digestive dysfunction since before the 1850s. For instance, in 1849, a review of 11 cases of accidental ingestion of oxalic acid reported that a "large proportion" of those who suffered "from stomach and nervous complaints . . . have been the subjects of the oxalic diathesis." The *Lancet* medical journal in 1925 described two cases in which intestinal symptoms—pain, vomiting, abdominal distension, and complete constipation—were resolved by "careful dieting by excluding all those foodstuffs known to be rich in oxalates." In both these cases, the intestinal paralysis (digestive muscle contractions unable to relax) was initially misdiagnosed as intestinal obstruction.

According to the Mayo Clinic, abdominal pain is common in primary hyperoxaluria patients. An oxalate connection with Crohn's disease and ulcerative colitis is also evidenced by the similar urinary patterns: acidic urine low in magnesium and citrate.

For 13 years, my client Debra was tortured by fecal incontinence. Her frequent "accidents"—8 to 10 episodes per day—were accompanied by flatulence, cramping, nausea, fatigue, and back and hip pain. Over the years, she tried every diet idea she could find, including strict avoidance of gluten and dairy and heavy use of almonds and sweet potatoes—all in vain.

The pain in her groin and hip area intensified over the years. Numerous medical visits and tests found nothing wrong, except blood in her urine. Eventually, scans found a large gallstone. Later, an ultrasound revealed crystals in her kidneys, vascular calcifications, and two distinct calcium deposits in her pelvis. Within weeks, she found herself in the emergency room with excruciating groin pain, and the doctor said she "probably passed a kidney stone." A few months later, surgeons removed her gallbladder.

The blood in her urine and the abdominal pain continued for years after the surgery. A third colonoscopy found a polyp and diverticulosis— uninflamed pouches (diverticula) in the colon. An exam of her esophagus and stomach found patchy red irritation, granularity, and a fragile, inflamed, injured stomach lining, yet no bacterial infection. Her doctor recommended a higher-fiber diet and prescribed Librax (for possible irritable bowel), but that increased her bowel problems.

After meeting me, she adopted a low-oxalate diet. Astoundingly, normal bowel function returned in just three days. Debra's speedy recovery from spastic bowel suggests that her problem was due to acute toxic effects on the nerves and muscles controlling contractions of the bowel, rectum, and anus.* Thirteen years of misery were finally resolved with a diet that was more diverse and easier to follow than the ones she'd tried before.

In addition to digestive issues and calcifications, Debra was battling anxiety and body pain. Science doesn't offer good explanations for the known associations between gut problems and pain, depression, anxiety, and insomnia. All these nerve problems can arise directly out of toxicity from oxalate overload.

---

* The complete reversal of these symptoms over a few days implies a functional, rather than structural, impairment.

Nerve Damage

Oxalate is a neurotoxin depleting the ability of brain and nerve cells to generate energy and function properly. Direct damage to cells and the hard-to-observe crystals that oxalates leave behind in tissues produce periodic, repeated, or chronic immune activation, which readily leads to malaise, anxiety, depression, migraines, brain fog, and other cognitive issues. Nerve problems can also resemble digestive problems because they have the same source. Excitable (overactive) nerves and muscle spasms are signs of ion disruption in cells.

Muscle and nerve spasticity can occur anywhere. In the digestive tract and the diaphragm, spasticity can mean reflux, difficulty swallowing, excessive belching, and hiccups. Hiccups are common with oxalate poisoning from starfruit, appearing just before death in both rat studies and human case reports. I had painful uncontrolled nightly hiccup attacks prior to adopting a low-oxalate diet! Like Debra's spastic colon, my problem quickly resolved with a shift to low-oxalate eating and it never returned.

Brain Damage

The damage to nerves and the instigation of inflammation by oxalates can lead to facial paralysis, lost speech, anxiety, depression, migraines, cognitive issues, and more. The neurological and psychiatric symptoms of oxalate poisoning are repeatedly noted in the medical literature but are ignored in clinical practice. Sometimes noticeable changes can be apparent soon after changing the diet, as in the case of a 79-year-old man with persistent anxiety. His wife wrote: "so we decided that he too would try low oxalates. From the very first day, no more nightmares each night. No more rushing to the bathroom with bowel or bladder urgency. He has a large senile keratosis on his cheek which is disappearing before our eyes. And he is much less anxious . . . it's been amazing. We were eating a ton of swiss chard, black beans, beets, carrots, and potatoes. We were just doing what we were told." More often, it takes time for these symptoms to resolve, but even adult autism seems to abate.

As noted in a 1994 review of oxalate's toxicity in the *Journal of Applied Toxicology*, "Symptoms of neurological effects [of oxalate poisoning] can be . . . drowsiness, stupor, cramps, exaggerated tendon reflexes, muscle fasciculation, fall in blood pressure, depressed cardiac contractility, tetany, convulsions and coma." Low energy and calcium imbalance are factors in age-related memory loss and other forms of nervous system degeneration, including stroke, dementia, schizophrenia, amyotrophic lateral sclerosis (ALS), Huntington's disease, Parkinson's disease, Alzheimer's disease, and multiple sclerosis (MS). MS is a disease in which the energy-hungry insulating myelin sheath (nerve fiber covering) degenerates and nerve transmission is slowed. Energy metabolism problems in brain cells promote depression.

One source of problems with mood and brain function is that elevated levels of oxalate may "starve" cells of sulfur ions. Through disrupting and depleting ions such as sulfur, oxalates can have wide-ranging effects throughout the body, including the brain. Sulfur-bound steroids—called *neurosteroids*—are hormones made in the brain and are necessary for cognitive functioning, mental health, overall brain health, and even our longevity. A sulfur shortage may compromise brain development and performance. Sulfur deficits can also harm liver function and hamper the hydration and structural integrity of connective tissues, the gut wall, and the function of red blood cells.

Pain

Pain involves tissue instability, inflammation, and unhappy nerves. In the peripheral nerves, oxalate depletes their calcium or magnesium, which causes pain by interfering with the creation or control of nerve impulses. Another way oxalate produces pain is by triggering inflammatory "storms" anywhere in the body—even in the glands. These mobile assaults produce transient bouts of heat and swelling. Mast-cell activation also causes pain and burning sensations.

Being mast-cell activators, nerve toxins, and connective tissue destabilizers, oxalates play a role in various pain syndromes, including burning mouth, migraines, arthritis, fibromyalgia, interstitial cystitis/bladder pain, genital pain, and hemorrhoids—even tooth and bone pain. Effects on intestinal neurons help explain the anxiety, fatigue, and other symptoms associated with painful digestive diseases such as IBS.

Oxalate-related brain inflammation could cause distress for the pituitary gland or hypothalamus, leading to metabolic distress and symptoms far from the brain. Migraines tend to cluster with other oxalate-related symptoms, including those not associated with brain inflammation.

Vascular System

Oxalate-related damage, metabolic stress, and inflammation also contribute to narrow, stiff blood vessels and diseased arteries. The vascular endothelium, the continuous cellular lining of the cardiovascular system, is a critical regulator of health. This distributed organ supports the normal functioning of all the tissues and organs of the body. Elevated levels of oxalate inhibit normal endothelial cell function and repair. That is, the cells can't replace themselves at a fast enough rate, so the vessels degenerate. Injured endothelial and other cells, the development of hypertension, atherosclerosis, vascular degeneration, and related problems are products of oxidative stress and mild chronic vascular inflammation. Endothelial dysfunction in turn promotes a proinflammatory environment that is sticky to oxalate crystals, forming a positive feedback loop.

Vascular inflammation, or *vasculitis*, is an immune response to problems in the arteries and veins, and it frequently occurs in primary hyperoxaluria. Chronic oxalate-induced vascular inflammation is associated with arterial muscle spasms, including Raynaud's syndrome, whereby spasms set off by cold temperatures block the blood flow to the fingers and toes. Problems with the fine capillaries in the heart starve the heart cells of oxygen and nutrients. This is an aspect of a condition called *vasospastic angina*, which can cause pain, shortness of breath, and weakness, and leads to a heart attack.

Oxalate-instigated calcium dysregulation is linked to abnormal blood pressure. A diet chronically low in calcium or high in calcium binders like oxalate disturbs the mineral metabolism systemically and depletes the cell membranes of calcium. Ironically, these changes brought on by calcium deficiency can cause vascular calcification and hypertension.

Because oxalic acid ions upset the mineral management in the cells and the oxalic nanocrystal damage increases the calcification-promoting proteins (including osteopontin), the gene expression is changed in susceptible vascular smooth muscle cells, thereby altering how the cells read the genetic code. As a result, vascular smooth muscle cells with disturbed calcium metabolism start following the wrong "recipe" and behave like bone cells—mineralizing the blood vessels (and making them weak).

To make matters worse, inflamed and damaged vessels directly collect calcium oxalate deposits in the cells and the atherosclerotic plaque, but the most common type of vascular calcium is calcium apatite (the structural mineral of bone and teeth) owing to epigenetic reprogramming. Vascular damage and related inflammation increase the crystal deposition not just in the vessels themselves but also in the tissues they serve. As noted, "high plasma oxalate levels . . . launch a vicious cycle of inflammasome-mediated systemic inflammation. . . . In particular, the cardiovascular implications of high oxalate levels in the circulation are of great concern. In our model of dietary oxalate-induced Chronic Kidney Disease, mice develop a clear presentation of cardiovascular disease including cardiac fibrosis and profound arterial hypertension."

In patients with primary hyperoxaluria who are dependent on dialysis, the oxalate causes "vascular obliteration" and poor blood flow visible on the skin surface, giving the skin on the arms and legs a purplish mottled and netlike discoloration called livedo reticularis.

Heart Attack (Heart Block)

When oxalate levels are too high in the blood or heart tissues, that can lead to an irregular heartbeat, or arrhythmia (even without obvious crystal deposits in the heart muscle). The heartbeat is synchronized by a network of specialized muscle fibers and nerves that conduct electrical signals. This cardiac conduction system includes a tissue bundle called the "pacemaker," which is especially sensitive to electrolyte disturbances. Problems with the heart's electrical system, or heart block, can occur when there is either heart tissue damage or electrolyte problems, such as low blood levels of potassium, calcium, and magnesium. Oxalate overload can damage heart tissue (causing fibrosis) and also disrupt electrolytes either through acute magnesium or potassium deficiency or by electrical failure in the heart conduction system, leading to sudden death. Related symptoms (seen in PH patients) are shortness of breath, chest pain, palpitations, and fainting.

Chronic overconsumption of oxalate can lead to electrolyte disarray and cardiac conduction mayhem. Heart conduction problems are associated not only with renal failure and dialysis but also with other oxalate-related autoimmune conditions, including lupus, rheumatoid arthritis, and scleroderma.

Elevated serum oxalate is a risk factor for cardiovascular events and sudden cardiac death in patients on dialysis. Indeed, the association between elevated blood oxalate levels and heart attacks is so strong that it could be a useful marker for predicting heart attacks in dialysis-dependent patients (whose pre-dialysis blood oxalate levels can be 10 to 100 times higher than in people with healthy kidneys when fasting).

Keep in mind that the body doesn't like oxalate in the serum, yet direct tests of blood (which are never done owing to impracticality)* rarely find oxalate there. There are at least two reasons for this. First, tests of the blood are not reflective of the load of oxalate in the body. Also, although red blood cells contain oxalate, blood cell oxalate is not included in blood oxalate tests, which measure only oxalate in the liquid portion of the blood (the serum and plasma) after the cells are removed. More important, researchers and doctors almost never try to capture the transient effects of the person's meals.

Musculoskeletal System

Oxalate overload is associated with unstable or degenerating connective tissues involving skin, joints, fascia, lungs, and the liver, as well as the bones, joints, and muscles. In a tragic case report, doctors found extensive degeneration of the skeletal muscles of a 16-year-old German girl who died quickly (of cardiac arrest, brain damage, and renal failure), after being accidentally injected with sodium oxalate in the hospital.† Muscle damage is often seen in fibromyalgia patients with muscle fatigue, weakness, and pain. Fibromyalgia sufferers have a lower density of mitochondria, lower levels of ATP, abnormal capillary blood flow (microcirculation), thickened capillaries, and low tissue oxygen. They also tend to be magnesium deficient. All these factors

---

* Blood oxalate is not easy (practical) to measure accurately. Blood samples must be either immediately analyzed or immediately frozen to -80°C.

† The pathologist also found dead cells in her brain and spinal cord, small bleeds in her pelvis, and immune-cell reactions in her heart.

interfere with energy production and can be induced or aggravated by excessive oxalate.

Joint Damage

Arthritis, gout, and joint damage are inflammatory responses to oxalate crystals. Patients on dialysis (which can increase oxalate retention in the body) develop oxalate-calcified cartilage and joint pain. Oxalate arthritis typically occurs in previously damaged joints, but it can be asymptomatic until the oxalate crystals grow large enough to incite local inflammation.

Interestingly, brief gout attacks may commence in the wake of the adoption of a very-low-oxalate diet—probably a sign of tissue clearing efforts by the immune system. Immune reactions to the oxalate crystals in the blood vessels are known to cause the pain of gout and lead to more joint damage and fibrosis. In the 1930s, when someone's arthritis pains flared after eating high-oxalate foods, it was called "oxalate gout." In 1988, Dr. Peter Simkin, the editor of *the Journal of the American Medical Association (JAMA)*, explained that the phenomenon of "microcrystal-induced arthritis" is obscured by the contemporary tendency to confine the term "gout" to a single type of crystal (urate). Simkin reminded readers that gouty arthritis results from any of five types of crystals, including oxalate crystals. But the narrower definition of gout has persisted, which prompted Simkin, in a 1993 article, to again explain that arthritis, bursitis, and tendinitis can be due to oxalate crystals.

Hard Yet Fragile Bones

Bones and teeth can become mineral deficient owing to oxalate overload and are common sites of crystal accumulation. The physical consequences of these crystal deposits include microscopic structural imperfections that disrupt the normal bone architecture. The bones become harder and denser, yet more porous, brittle, and prone to fracture. An oxalate-disturbed metabolism may lead to spinal stenosis and other bone deformities.

In addition to oxalate's direct interference with bone nutrients and bone structure, the crystal deposits promote bone loss owing to immune-cell reactions. The impact of immune reactions to crystals is even more destructive than low blood calcium. When the blood calcium is low, parathyroid glands instruct the bones to release calcium to maintain the blood calcium levels. In response, specialized bone cells (*osteoclasts*, a type of immune cell) issue acid and enzymes to dissolve minerals and eat holes in the bone matrix. Too much mineral mining leads to thin, fragile bones. High parathyroid hormone is associated not only with thin bones but also with bone pain, with calcium deposits in the blood vessels and kidneys, with gastrointestinal problems (ulcers, constipation, nausea, pancreatitis, and gallstones), and with neurological effects including depression, lethargy, and seizures.

Ideally, bone-building cells restore the lost bone later. For complete regrowth of healthy bone, there needs to be a supportive nutritional, hormonal, and electrochemical environment. A high-oxalate diet interferes with all of those, preventing bone recovery.

Sensitive and Mobile Teeth

Teeth and gums are especially vulnerable to oxalate damage. Inflammation targeting the oxalate deposits may become shockingly severe. A 1988 case report observed the "progressive and unrelenting" nature of oxalate problems occurring in the wake of ileojejunal bypass surgery, which induces hyperabsorption of oxalate, resulting in oral pain, mobile teeth, tooth destruction, and jawbone loss.

Hearing

Mineral disturbances can impact the inner ear, resulting in tinnitus, dizziness, and hearing loss. While there isn't much research directly blaming oxalate, these conditions often resolve on a low-oxalate diet. A health coach specializing in tinnitus sent me this note:

> *I've been silencing people's tinnitus for years, and vegans and vegetarians have been my most common clients. I show them your interviews. I've had so many of my clients get incredible results with their ears when they reduce or completely cut out plants that contain oxalic acid. Regardless of whether my clients' hearing problems occurred after noise trauma, medication, or stress, some form of oxalate toxicity always sits at the root cause of hearing loss.*

Anemia

Anemia can result from oxalate crystals displacing bone marrow and interfering with the production of healthy red blood cells, or from oxalic acid traveling in the bloodstream, thus interfering with enzymes needed for red blood cell energy production and causing the red blood cells to explode (called *hemolytic anemia*). Together, oxalate's one-two punch on blood cells can cause untreatable anemia.

Urinary System

The urinary tract sees a lot of oxalate traffic, as it removes oxalate from the body. Kidney problems involving oxalate include: (1) stones that tend to block urine flow, (2) crystal deposits elsewhere in the kidney, (3) chronic subpar kidney function, and (4) chronic kidney failure. Other oxalate-related problems occur throughout the urinary system. When the kidneys are stressed or failing, blood pressure, immune activity, electrolyte balance, and pH become harder to regulate.

Bladder Pain, Chronic Pelvic Pain, and Urinary Urgency

Bladder pain syndrome (interstitial cystitis) and urinary control problems can arise from mast-cell and other immune responses, as well as from nerve function problems initiated by oxalate crystals and oxalate-induced mineral deficiencies. The immune activation leading to chronic or episodic bladder pain is also a key factor in genital pain (vestibulodynia), fibromyalgia, endometriosis, irritable bowel syndrome, chronic fatigue syndrome, headaches, disturbed sleep, anxiety, asthma, and rheumatoid arthritis.

Chronic Kidney Disease

Oxalate crystals cause acute kidney injury and can lead to chronic kidney failure. In chronic kidney disease, diffuse oxalate crystal deposits in the kidney cause tissue damage and fibrosis without stone formation.

Kidney Stones

By now you are aware that kidney and urinary tract stones are predominately oxalate crystal aggregates that form in the urinary tract, leading to tissue damage and infection and obstructing urine flow. With or without painful kidney stones, the waves of oxalate passing through the kidneys after meals cause cellular distress, oxalate crystal accumulation in the kidney tissues, degraded kidney function, and long-term kidney damage. In the presence of kidney stress (damaged cells) and diminished crystal inhibitors, high urine oxalate leads to crystal clumping and slows down (or prevents) crystal removal, resulting in kidney stones.

Kidney stones are a symptom that something is not right in the body.

They are associated with many diseases—perhaps because, as one nephrologist put it, "a common biology underlies calcium stone formation, osteoporosis, and vascular calcification." Stone disease is but one expression of oxalate overload. Like myself, most of the oxalate-injured people I work with naturally avoid kidney stones.

Disturbed cell biochemistry is a root cause of *all* disease. Chronic exposure to cell-disrupting toxins—even in low doses, and especially when deficiency is present—is the central cause of all chronic illness and aging. When oxalate is continually present, attaching to and getting into the cells, even in minuscule amounts, the workings of the entire body are at risk.

The baffling and disparate symptoms of oxalate overload become perfectly comprehensible once you look into the mechanisms of illness; then, the possibility of a common perpetrator becomes more evident. But the point is not to tell you that "everything comes from oxalate." Instead, the message I hope you'll take away is this: if you are having symptoms and have been eating a diet high in oxalate, a simple and inexpensive dietary change can put you back on a path to health. The good news is that by removing the root cause, the repair can begin. However, the recovery process is not always straightforward.

11

Clearing Oxalates from Your Body

*Many assume that in the absence of ongoing exposure, toxicants
are eliminated efficiently. It has recently been recognized,
however, that many toxicants . . . are persistent pollutants with
half-lives that can last for many years or even decades.*

—Stephen J. Genuis, PhD, and Kasie L. Kelln, PhD,
Behavioural Neurology, 2015

We would like to think that if we remove oxalate from our
diet, our bodies will just snap back to good health. And indeed, most people who try low-oxalate eating are rewarded
rapidly with symptom improvement. But we can't just dust our hands
and say, "There, I'm better." The switch to a low-oxalate diet is merely
the beginning of long-term healing that may have its ups and downs. It
took years to build up a toxic load. Now it's time for long-overdue
housekeeping.

How Oxalate Clearing Works

Practical experience suggests that *de-accumulation*—the breaking down of crystals and expelling of their remains—will, and *must*, take time. Clearing out oxalate deposits temporarily increases the oxalates in the bloodstream, kidneys, and elsewhere, and it may have toxic complications, especially if the rate of release is high. The process involves immune cells and inflammation, nutrient and energy consumption, and some amount of collateral damage.

Unfortunately for some of us, additional symptoms—and perhaps even worse ones—appear months or years *after* we stop eating too much oxalate. The symptoms can range in intensity from barely noticeable to severe or even dangerous.

Gwen's Story

Gwen suffered from extreme fatigue, an unstable neck, and connective tissue problems. Her doctors said she had *Ehlers-Danlos syndrome* (a connective tissue condition involving hyperflexible joints, joint degeneration, and pain), but could not tell her the cause.

In hopes of finding relief, she consulted with a naturopath and adopted a nut-heavy gut and psychology syndrome (GAPS) diet, removed all dairy food, and added more green vegetables. For the next six years, Gwen juiced carrots, celery, and spinach and ate high-oxalate stir-fried greens and baby-greens salads. Her health took a dramatic downturn.

After reading about oxalates online, she rapidly eliminated the oxalates from her diet. She felt better at first. But about a month later, new symptoms exploded—insomnia, electrolyte issues, and bladder irritation. Several months after that, heart palpitations sent her to the hospital. Struggling with these problems, she came to me, seeking answers.

Gwen was experiencing severe oxalate-clearing illness. The abrupt diet change incited a valiant but havoc-wreaking effort to unload oxalate.

The messy process of clearing oxalates is akin to digging up micro-sized toxic waste dumps and loading the waste into poorly covered dump trucks. Immune cells perceive the damaging oxalates as a sign of danger, and they respond by whipping up inflammation storms. "Friendly fire" from these storms can damage the vascular system and nerves and cause additional electrolyte loss.

As the oxalate departs, cells along the exit route are exposed to oxalate in its most reactive forms. Symptoms of acute exposure, such as cardiac problems, issues with energy metabolism, and increased *acidosis* (low pH in the cells and body fluids) are especially common. Such effects are typically short-term and pass once the immune system declares the problem resolved, but clearing efforts will resume, often cyclically, and can pop up in any location, at any time. Toxic stress and inflammation, and consequent symptoms such as persistent pain, mood problems, and fatigue, can continue for as long as excess oxalate remains in the body.

Using tools presented in Part 2 of this book, Gwen did successfully stabilize her situation. As I taught her how the clearing works and what to do about it, she was able to stay on a healing path of reduced oxalate intake and she continued to improve her overall health.

The Experience of Oxalate Clearing

For the vast majority of people who start low-oxalate eating and enjoy benefits from it, the clearing will be intermittent and minor, or even imperceptible, if the amount of oxalate moving around the body is small. Even if you do have symptoms, you may not think of them as anything other than an occasional bad day or a cranky hip joint. How would anyone know to connect today's fatigue, headache, bad moods, tooth sensitivity, or joint pain with the chocolate, spinach salads, black beans, and french fries you used to love (and don't eat anymore)? But now you know: they just might be connected. The Vulvar Pain Foundation calls such problems "flare-ups." Susan Owens, the leader of the Trying Low Oxalates community, calls them "dumping."

Some people notice reactions immediately. For others, months pass before signs and symptoms appear, perhaps not happening until the body's clearing capacity is working well again.

Symptoms of clearing can hang on for months at a time or come and go in an hour. And sometimes the effects are anything but mild. Clearing episodes usually occur in waves, often on their own recurring schedule. For people with a lot of clearing to do, the process can be unrelenting, with difficult symptoms. The symptoms can continue off and on for 7 to 10 years, or more.

When clearing is very active, life can become a roller-coaster, as symptoms flare up without warning and change every day. It can be like living inside an amusement park fun house, with dark uneven floors below and warped mirrors all around—you feel disoriented, lost, and without steady, reliable points of orientation. Though it may feel like it, this stage doesn't last forever!

Even when severe, clearing symptoms are usually accompanied by improvements in other areas, and there's a greater sense of overall sturdiness and well-being. However, improvements may be hard to fully appreciate when other things are going wrong. For example, a swollen ankle that makes it hard to walk will get your attention and make you forget that you are sleeping better and having fewer headaches. The situation seems upside down: as your body heals, the side effects of the repair operations can erupt into strange and unpleasant symptoms; you can feel worse even as you get better!

One young woman put it this way:

Dear Sally,

For my 2 years on a vegan diet I ate almond butter, flour, raspberries, chia, celery juice, I mean the whole thing. For the first time in my life, I started getting eye floaters, low grade tinnitus, and fatigue.

Since then, I've returned to an ancestral diet. I felt so good at first, but now not so good. When I rub my eyes now it feels crunchy and grainy like there are little crystals inside. Also having headaches, jaw tension, and fatigue. This oxalate dumping is no joke!! It's affecting bowel movement and blood circulation. I'm feeling awful but also super clean and more energy overall! I'm loving it.

—Yvonne

The Mechanisms of Clearing

A lot of internal factors influence when and how much oxalate our bodies remove. These factors include kidney health, hormonal cycles, nourishment, inflammation, metabolic health, the extent and location of the oxalate damage, genetics, and other factors. Most of these are the same things that influence the formation of the original accumulations. Other factors also apply, including the rate at which different tissues normally regenerate and their overall ability to do so.

The healing process can be paradoxical: while injury and trauma can increase the clearing, so can improved health. Boosting your nutrients, doing healthy activities like exercise and massage, or even getting a good night's rest can be followed by clearing symptoms. When the low-oxalate diet improves kidney function, the improved kidney capacity may encourage clearing, which may temporarily increase urine oxalate and the risk of kidney stones.

The key thing to remember is that the process is unavoidable, and your body is in charge. Attempting to push it may only aggravate the clearing illness. The slower the release, the safer it is.

The Biggest Problem with Clearing

Oftentimes, *we draw the wrong conclusions about what is happening to us, which can be the biggest problem with clearing.*

When I first attempted low-oxalate eating in 2009, which was to address acute vulvodynia, I did not have any awareness that oxalate could deposit itself in tissues and hang around for years. And I had absolutely no idea that the change in diet might instigate oxalate clearing and that I should expect a response from my body.

After several weeks of feeling somewhat better, and having resolved my vulvar pain, I got new flare-ups of old symptoms (joint pain and fatigue), and I mistakenly concluded that I was still on a downward path. If I had known better, I would have recognized that my body was healing. Instead, I slid back into my old habits of high-oxalate foods, and it took several more years before my progressive deterioration led to the crisis and insight that clarified what was really going on.

When oxalate is clearing, it puts additional stress on the body and can lead to complications, especially when a low-oxalate diet increases the oxalate in the bloodstream.

To illustrate that problem, let's look at the medical case report of a 46-year-old British woman. A kidney biopsy revealed that she had fibrotic kidneys loaded with calcium oxalate crystals and immune-cell involvement. "No specific treatment was initiated at this point," wrote the doctors. They did not inquire about what she was eating or inform her that her diet might be a factor in her disease. Six months later, she returned to the hospital very sick. Her symptoms were consistent with high oxalate levels—hyperoxaluria, itching, fatigue, vomiting, postural hypotension, and an abscess on her forehead. A fresh round of testing revealed that her blood oxalate level was 10 times normal and that she was overabsorbing dietary oxalate owing to dilated lymph glands in her digestive tract.

At that point, her doctors prescribed a low-fat, high-calcium, low-oxalate diet. In response, her already-elevated blood oxalate level *tripled*. This jump certainly overwhelmed her flagging kidneys. She eventually ended up on permanent dialysis.

Here are the key lessons from this story:

1. The dietary shift from high-oxalate to low-oxalate eating may trigger the release of accumulated oxalate.
2. The resulting mobilization of oxalate deposits can paradoxically increase oxalate levels in the blood and kidneys, which can be especially toxic when the body is already suffering from chronic oxalate stress or renal disease.
3. It makes sense to start a low-oxalate diet at the first sign of kidney stress, well before any crisis occurs and when there is still time for the kidneys to recover.

Sadly, awareness of oxalate accumulation and the challenges of de-accumulation have not improved in the 25 years since this case was published. Whether the low-oxalate diet is suggested as a practical precaution or prescribed as therapy, it is a critical element in most cases of renal distress—and many other conditions, too. Until doctors (and dietitians) know that significant accumulation is common and that reversing it can *raise* oxalate levels in the blood and kidneys, they will not be able to assist patients through the diet transition and subsequent recovery.

The Symptoms of Clearing

Symptoms of clearing emerge from the difficult and toxic hard work of the immune system, the vascular system, and organs of elimination.

While we may sometimes experience remnants of our earlier problems, the symptoms of clearing are frequently not the same as those that led us to start the diet. They may be entirely new to us, and sometimes truly weird (see **Box 11.1**).

BOX 11.1: POSSIBLE SIGNS OF CLEARING ILLNESS

✥ Rashes, boils, blisters, itchiness, red welts, peeling skin, cold sores

✥ Pain in the bowels, back, bladder, joints, teeth, etc.

✥ Joint inflammation, gout

✥ Chronic diarrhea; gritty stools; hemorrhoids

✥ Indigestion, difficulty swallowing, reflux, gallbladder symptoms, poor fat digestion

✥ Sore throat, phlegm, hoarse voice

✥ Eye grit, eye sties, eye redness and irritation

✥ Poor sleep, poor physical coordination, memory problems, migraines, depression, panic, anxiety, low motivation, irritation, moodiness

✥ Hunger surges/appetite changes

✥ Fatigue

✥ Urine: cloudy, gritty, irritating, stinky, or dark

✥ Kidney stones

Clearing leads to higher internal exposure to oxalate ions and higher levels of inflammation. The symptoms arise from electrolyte or mineral deficiencies, tissue acidity, and nerve or brain inflammation, as if we were being acutely poisoned all over again. These effects can cause pain, anxiety, low mood, irritability, insomnia, and brain fog, or heart palpitations, dizziness, and fatigue. Cell energy metabolism issues can persist, and joint pain and inflammation can periodically return, even in joints not previously afflicted.

Clearing symptoms can be spectacularly variable, appearing out of nowhere and disappearing just as suddenly. Certain types of symptoms show up more often during clearing, corresponding to the three major pathways of release: skin, colon, and urine. Skin symptoms are common; rashes and peeling skin occur very frequently. Bowel function problems such as diarrhea may occur. In the urinary tract, transient urinary tract infections (UTIs), urinary urgency, or darker urine than normal may occur. Cloudy urine (crystalluria) is especially common, and often accompanies clearing in other parts of the body.

Some people report strong-smelling urine for several days, despite drinking copious amounts of water, and strong ammonia release in armpits or elsewhere on the skin. We don't know why that happens, but there are possible explanations in the medical literature. Urea (the principal source of ammonia smells) has antioxidant effects and may dissolve calcium oxalate in tissues such as at the joints. Uric acid may also assist in the removal of oxalate from joint spaces, which leads to a greater production of uric acid and increased amounts of ammonia coming out of the body.

Other tissues that expel crystals include the salivary glands, glands around the eyes that produce tears (copious grit is common), and the gallbladder. Mucous membranes lining the mouth, throat, and GI tract may release oxalates, as well as in the lungs. One client reported coughing up daily mucus plugs followed by a hard white object that was about one-third the size of a grain of rice and shaped like a fingernail clipping. That continued for two weeks, with periodic bouts over the next several months.

Clearing may also activate transient infections. Cold sores and flares of Epstein-Barr virus or other infections may surface (but may also clear more rapidly than usual). Eye sties—to which I have recently been prone yet never had before I began following a low-oxalate diet—may occur when the ducts of these small glands get clogged in the clearing process, or because immune actions just under the surface are intensely engaged.

Flare-ups may also occur anywhere that oxalate has accumulated: areas of wear and tear, including sites of old infections or injuries, and inherited "trouble spots" (like my back). Your own body will probably have a preferred place where symptoms most commonly occur.

A healing body can be fragile and hard to live with, even as health returns. As much as clearing may make you miserable, the symptoms are an indication that your body is reaching for better health. Once you understand what is happening, and that clearing is part of the path out of a toxic situation, you can notice many other improvements and stay motivated to continue low-oxalate eating long enough to truly heal.

Even though severe clearing illness may sound terrible, it is not common. The alternative is to keep harming your health by continuing to overeat oxalate. We know a lot about how to make clearing safe and manageable. The benefits of low-oxalate eating are enormous and the practice is simple, so let's roll up our sleeves and see what it takes.

PART 2

THE LOW-OXALATE PROGRAM

12

Assessing Your Oxalate Health

The best treatment of oxalosis is prevention.
If patients present with advanced disease, treatment of
oxalate arthritis consists of symptom management and
control of the underlying disease process.

—Elizabeth Lorenz, MD, et al., *Current Rheumatology Reports*, 2013

I s your health issue oxalate related—or is it something else? This question can become a real conundrum.

There is no one symptom or set of symptoms that says "oxalate." Oxalate overload affects each person differently. The damage from oxalates often takes years to emerge, and in many cases longer still for it to be recognized as what it is (if it ever is recognized). Symptoms are often delayed, variable, and changeable. The effects can go unnoticed even in very sick people.

If you are ill, that illness might be caused by other chemical exposures, medication, malnutrition, unresolved trauma, an infectious pathogen, or (most likely) some combination of factors. The body has only so many ways to complain, regardless of the root cause. When things do expand into serious illness, we can't easily track the symptoms back to their origin. But you don't need to, because even if your physical distress didn't start with oxalates, eating too much of them can make it worse. *Oxalates may not be the original reason you got sick, but they may still play a role in why you're not getting better.*

Even if oxalates are a big instigator of your health issues, changing to a low-oxalate diet will not necessarily yield *complete* symptom relief that is also immediate or constant. But the frequency, duration, and intensity of your symptom episodes typically improve.

Revealing Diet: Helen's Story

The low-oxalate diet can be a path of discovery, revealing some of the consequences of oxalate toxicity.

At age 72, Helen was (*still*) trying to drop stubborn pounds while overcoming a lifelong battle with nagging hunger. Despite her recent success in sticking with a strict no-sugar, no-gluten diet, she was discouraged. The excess pounds hadn't dropped. To make things worse, some of the advice from her nutritionist and weight-loss counselor conflicted with what her body was telling her. The vegetables they insisted she must eat often gave her stomach pains.

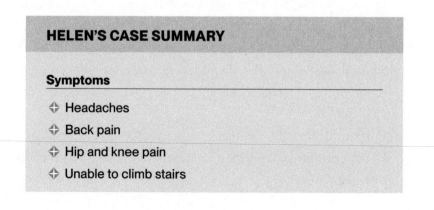

HELEN'S CASE SUMMARY

Symptoms

⬥ Headaches

⬥ Back pain

⬥ Hip and knee pain

⬥ Unable to climb stairs

- Walking difficult
- Disturbed sleep
- Long-standing addiction and emotional issues

Her High-Oxalate Foods

- Almonds (15; 2 times/day)
- Other nuts: pecans (2 times/week)
- Sweet potatoes (2–3 times/week)
- Mashed potatoes (2 times/week)
- Potato chips (2 ounces/day)
- Tomato sauce and salsa (3 times/week)
- Black beans (1 time/week)
- Spices: curry, black pepper (heavy use)
- Amaranth stew or amaranth spaghetti (1 time/week)
- Artichokes or parsnips (1 time/week)

Results of Low-Oxalate Diet

- Improved digestion
- Relief from cravings and addictive urges
- Weight loss
- Restored ability to walk
- Back pain relief
- Improved outlook

Time to Symptom Relief

1 month

At the height of her predicament, Helen shared her frustrations with me and pleaded for my input. I told her that my own physical energy and mental focus were much better on a low-oxalate diet, which involved simply avoiding certain vegetables, fruits, and most nuts. She insisted that I suggest specific dietary changes. Particularly, she wanted to know what *not* to eat. Instead, on a napkin I wrote a list of low-oxalate vegetables she *could* have and told her to eat more real butter.

A few weeks later, a much happier Helen called me. "I feel like I've got my life back," she enthused. "I know this sounds like an exaggeration, but this approach has worked miracles. I feel better, and I'm not getting headaches. I've stopped taking Advil. My stomachaches are better, and my digestion is finally working. For once, I feel as if I'm actually digesting and absorbing my food, and for the first time in years, I don't feel hungry."

Helen was eating less and found it easy not to binge—which was a huge breakthrough for someone who'd endured a lifelong struggle with compulsive eating. "I no longer feel out of control," she said, practically crying in relief.

As we talked, Helen mentioned other benefits. For instance, the daily chronic pain that had followed an auto accident 13 years prior had been relenting, and she was now using the stairs. That excited *me*, because weakness in her knees, legs, hips, and back had made stairs impossible for her for over five years. But Helen insisted that freedom from food cravings was far more valuable. She described how her struggle with obsessions, emotions, and patterns of denial had abruptly come "crashing down." She felt free, hopeful, and victorious.

Helen had spent decades seeking help from medical doctors, nutritionists, chiropractors, energy healers, and herbalists, all without success. She poured incalculable amounts of time and money into these efforts, with only aggravation to show for it. No wonder it seemed like a miracle that selecting a few different vegetables, avoiding spicy foods, eating more fat, and using a few simple supplements enabled her to turn around a self-described food compulsion, reduce her medication, and dramatically reduce her pain levels, all of which increased her independence. She eventually lost a total of 50 pounds, and her confidence soared! Helen had found the critical missing piece that helped explain a lifetime of struggle.

I initially found Helen's results hard to believe, but hers (like others) kept me exploring and reading biomedical papers for an explanation. This process, by the way, is how science is intended to work. First, we observe reality, and then we experiment to reveal the processes and phenomena behind the associations we see. The low-oxalate diet can be your own experiment.

Try It Out

The most affordable, informative, and useful way to determine if a low-oxalate diet will work for you is to just try the diet. If you get your oxalate consumption down and keep it there consistently, your body will eventually speak. And having read this far, you are now well equipped to listen to your body with greater understanding. You know oxalate is "a thing," you know the foods that deliver it, you're equipped to monitor your intake, and you know the hidden effects and signs of trouble. Those basic tools help you listen to your body and learn from it. You may be surprised at what starts to feel better, and it may not be at all what you expected.

The Three-Month Trial Run

As mentioned in Part 1, think of your low-oxalate eating trial as a two-part experiment. First, work your way through Phase One, as I describe in Chapter 13, and stay consistent for three months. Second, if you are still unsure, see what happens when you reintroduce a higher level of oxalate into your diet for 3 to 5 days.

By now, you probably know which of your favorite foods are high in oxalate, but double-check that by reviewing the *worst offender* foods listed in **Table 3.1** (and in **Table 14.1**) as often as you need to. Which of the worst offenders do you eat routinely? Of these, which do you like the least? Simply start there: eliminate or replace one or two of those least-loved, high-oxalate foods with something low-oxalate (cabbage, arugula, onions, turnips, white rice, coconut). (The *safe bet* foods are listed in **Table 14.1**.) If you have a diverse diet already, you don't necessarily need a direct replacement for many high-oxalate foods; you might just skip them and eat more of the (confirmed) low-oxalate foods you already know. See the **Swap Chart** in the Resources section.

You don't want to aim for zero oxalate (that's asking for "trial by fire" through clearing illness; see Chapter 11). You don't even need to get especially low in oxalates when you're starting out. Just arriving at what researchers think is "normal" will do you a world of good, even if you never go further down the discovery path.

Chapter 13 lays out the concepts underlying the two-phased approach and provides tips on how to stay consistent for at least three months, once you have lowered your oxalate intake.

The shift to low-oxalate foods doesn't have to be permanent, but if you're going to try it, commit to following it consistently. Unlike a weight-loss diet, you don't get "cheat" days. If you decide a high-oxalate food needs to go, it needs to stay gone. Remember that because oxalate levels go up in the blood and urine after you lower your intake, adding more oxalate is especially toxic. Also remember that a periodic high intake of oxalate works as a trigger, so even when you return to eating lower levels, you may end up continuing to accumulate oxalate.

Think of the three-month trial period as a chance to learn how to detect your body's response to lowered oxalates. Your symptoms may lessen as you eat less oxalate. But also you may have odd reactions, perhaps a sudden "flu," a rash or other strange skin symptoms, acute pain in one joint, or diarrhea. These can be signs of a healing response to the diet change. If eating less oxalate does nothing for you, and it seems like too much trouble, you can always go back to what you were eating before, with nothing lost (except perhaps your future health!).

Is It Doing Anything? The Oxalate Challenge Test

If, after a few months of consistent low-oxalate eating, you are still not sure about the benefits, you can try a slightly risky experiment: add higher levels of oxalate back into your diet. Ideally, you would do this *oxalate challenge test* intentionally. More commonly, though, owing to a simple lapse of attention, the challenge test happens accidentally — with sometimes dramatic side effects.

Several of my clients have reported lessons they learned the hard way. One woman accepted a single small piece of keto chocolate cake at a birthday party, and she suffered a huge flare-up of diarrhea. Another started a new protein powder for two weeks, without realizing that the rice bran in it was high in oxalate; her increased foot pain alerted her. A third had three distressing days of frequent urination and bladder pain after grazing on ripe fruit from her mom's fig tree. In each case, the price paid was the sudden return of symptoms, sometimes with harsh effects that lasted for days.

If your health is good and you still want to try the challenge test, be intentional about it. Prepare a method for documenting your specific foods, portions, and symptoms. Be careful not to overdo the amount of oxalate you add back in. The challenge is effective adding as little as 300 mg of additional oxalate a day for 2 to 5 days. For example, 1 cup of mashed sweet potato has about 200 mg; ½ cup of cooked red stem chard (or beet greens) has about 400 mg.

As you increase your oxalate intake, carefully watch how you feel. Did any of your issues return? Did you get a sudden bout of joint or muscle pain? Did you have an energy crash, mood swing, or bad night's sleep? Did you get some sudden skin breakout? Spiking your oxalate intake can often lead to new reactions, sometimes stark ones. When obvious symptoms emerge, it's conclusive evidence that oxalates are worth paying attention to.

Isn't Going Low-Oxalate Really Hard?

"This is the easiest diet in the world!" So says Debra (who had a spastic colon and had strictly avoided gluten and dairy), and so say many others. You may not agree, at least not at the start.

You can invest as much or as little effort into refining your approach to oxalate-conscious eating as you like. At worst, it may require you to rethink your "must have" foods and to find new ingredients. It is mostly a matter of developing a new filter for skillful food selection.

Take heart: you don't have to adopt low-oxalate eating perfectly to get results. In the chapters that follow, I'm going to offer guidance to help you get the best possible outcome. I'm going to show you how and why you should be deliberate, consistent, and persistent.

13

A Phased Transition

[T]he significant can only be revealed through practice.

—Nassim Nicholas Taleb, PhD, *Antifragile*, 2012

Low-oxalate eating is simple: find the high-oxalate foods in your diet and gradually replace them with lower-oxalate alternatives. How you get there—what foods you eat—is yours to decide. I offer recipes on my website to help you get started trying out new foods and finding new favorites to add to your routine. Before you begin building your own version of a low-oxalate diet, it's important to understand the big picture.

Guiding Principles

Zero is not the goal. Your first aim is to consistently reduce but not completely eliminate foods with oxalates. Oxalate toxicity is not like celiac disease or a peanut allergy, which require the total elimination of specific ingredients. Don't think of your low-oxalate diet as an "oxalate-free diet." In fact, it should *not* be a "no-oxalate diet," especially at the start.

Go slow. *Any* drastic diet change has the potential to upset your body, your microbiome, and your life. If you have health concerns and you've been routinely using high-oxalate foods, you may be loaded with oxalate. An abrupt jump from a high-oxalate diet to a very low-oxalate one can elicit heavy oxalate mobilization that can provoke difficult and potentially dangerous symptoms. Overworking "Lucy and Ethel" (see Chapter 8), your body's essential excretion workers, will only make it harder on you. Unloading stockpiles of oxalate will demand energy, disturb electrolytes, and increase inflammation. In short, you can't get completely better all at once. An accelerated pace is especially toxic. In fact, that could get so unpleasant that you might be tempted to think that going off oxalates was the problem, not the solution. But there is an easy answer . . .

Use a two-phase approach.

1. *Get out of danger.* In the first phase, you gradually lower your oxalate intake to moderate or "normal" levels. You p*ause there for a while.*

2. *Repair your health.* In the second phase, you carefully move into the low-oxalate diet. This allows the years of oxalate accumulation to begin to clear, which is hard, ongoing work for your body. Once you get to a low-oxalate diet, you avoid haphazard use of high-oxalate foods.

Be deliberate and keep it simple.
Use foods with known oxalate content.

Be consistent.
Don't jump on and off a low-oxalate diet.

Be persistent.
The most important benefits unfold over the years as you stick to the diet. Take the long view.

One Step at a Time: Ron's Story

To illustrate an effective use of the phased transition, consider Ron's story. Retired and in his seventies, Ron, a musician, struggled with thumb pain that made composing at the piano difficult, but he was otherwise in great health. Ron and his wife, Kitty, preferred quality, healthful foods and a satisfying diet, but they were in a tussle.

Kitty, being the head cook in their house, had converted their shared meals in the direction of low oxalate over the previous year. Ron patiently tolerated the shifting menu to keep the peace, but he was not about to abandon the two most revered moments of his day: an afternoon bite of gourmet dark chocolate and his evening peanut butter and celery snack. Together, Ron's two daily snacks delivered 180 mg of oxalate—120 mg from the 2 ounces (56 grams) of 86 percent dark chocolate and at least 60 mg from the 2 tablespoons of peanut butter and a small stalk of celery.

One Saturday afternoon, both Ron and Kitty attended my brief oxalate presentation. Hearing my husband share his story of recovering from carpal tunnel pain convinced Ron that forgoing the chocolate and peanut butter was worth a try. Soon after, Ron's piano playing became pain free. Chocolate lost its charm and he never looked back.

Why was Ron's approach a good one? He and Kitty had been eating a sky-high 700 to 2,500 mg of oxalate, or more, every day. Kitty's initial efforts to convert their shared meals initiated a first phase during which Ron's intake dropped to about 250 mg per day. That "normal" level was a safer height from which to jump into the low-oxalate pool, especially when compared to the Olympic heights he had started from. When Ron later made the decision to lower his intake further, it was a smooth dive into his low-oxalate Phase Two and his pain-free future.

Ron's stepwise progression allowed body, mind, and life's daily rhythms to adjust easily, without mental and physical anguish. So, you don't have to give up all your current favorite foods right away. Continuing some of them in moderation at the beginning is a *good* strategy.

Kitty, being the enthusiastic low-oxalate warrior, took the daredevil high dive and quickly went as low as she could. She felt better, but after about 18 months of oxalate clearing, she developed a kidney stone for the first time. She was one of my very first students, and at that time I did not know enough to warn her that going very low too fast could overwork the kidneys. Some of us who are eating for our health, myself and Kitty included, have little patience for consuming foods we now know are harmful. We instinctively choose the deep dive, risks and all.

Not everyone has a partner to do the heavy lifting of learning and changing the household menu. If you are the kitchen leader or making this change by yourself, take your time and have a relaxed yet attentive mindset. A few pointers from this book, some good data, and your own willingness and determination will take you far. As you're learning, expect to encounter minor frustrations and confusions until low-oxalate eating becomes second nature.

Oxalate Intake Zones

The value of making gradual and deliberate changes becomes clear if we understand how the body's responses to its oxalate levels must be managed. Is oxalate entering at such a pace that it is building up? Or, is its rate of entry so low that oxalate deposits can be broken down and moved out?

The stepping-stones that lead to oxalate overload start with individual meals. A single high-oxalate meal can trigger the start of those deposits, and a more modest intake can maintain or grow those deposits. **Table 13.1** lists the approximate levels of oxalate in one meal that might *trigger* deposits, *maintain (or grow)* existing deposits, or lead to sustained *reduction of deposits* when minimal intake is maintained at every meal over multiple days.

Table 13.1: Oxalate Intake Thresholds

Effect	Oxalate per Meal
Trigger	60 mg or above
Maintenance	30–50 mg
Reduction	Under 30 mg, maintained in all meals for at least 4 days

Additionally, **Figure 13.1** can help you think about how the body handles oxalate over longer time periods. Think of your typical daily intake levels as zones. Each zone describes the level of toxic threat to the body.

FIGURE 13.1: Dietary Intake and Zones of Oxalate Accumulation and Deaccumulation

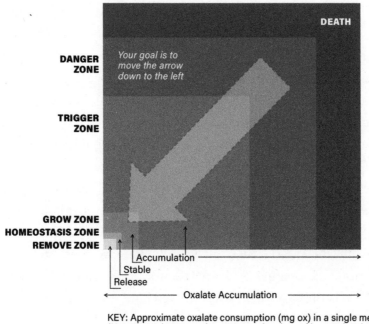

KEY: Approximate oxalate consumption (mg ox) in a single meal. (Note that release requires consecutive days of low oxalate intake.)

- Reduce/Release 0–10
- Homeostasis/Release 10–30
- Grow/Maintenance 30–60
- Trigger 60–800
- Danger 800–3,500

The chart in **Figure 13.1** has two dimensions. The vertical axis represents your level of daily oxalate intake, from zero at the bottom to extremely high at the top. The horizontal axis represents your body's response over time: releasing or accumulating oxalate. The arrow pointing down to the left represents the direction you are heading with a low-oxalate diet: consistently lowering your daily intake (and avoiding trigger meals). The arrow crosses the boxes that represent the zones of intake and toxic response, from Danger down to Remove.

The **Danger** zone (approximate daily intake over 800 mg) causes toxic stress that puts all your critical organs at high risk for damage. Eating in this zone forces your body to sequester oxalate and make other compensations that will eventually lead to serious health problems.

Below the Danger zone is the **Trigger** zone (approximately 250 mg to 800 mg per day), where intake also outstrips excretion capacity. Intake in the Trigger zone initiates new sites of oxalate accumulation after trigger meals, and the deposits become larger and more numerous.

The **Maintenance** zone (100 mg to 250 mg per day) is where the existing deposits remain in place yet may still grow. This zone is at the high end of "normal" intake. A high-oxalate diet often has you bouncing between meals that grow oxalate deposits and those that trigger new deposits, despite a generally moderate daily intake.

Below the Maintenance zone is a thin zone of **Homeostasis** ("staying the same," 60 mg to 100 mg per day). At this level of intake, the deposits do not grow. Tissue and kidney healing can both occur.

Finally, the lowest level of intake is the **Remove** zone. Intake at this level promotes clearing of deposits but asks the kidneys ("Lucy and Ethel") to perform at a high level. To overcome chronic illness, you may want to get to the upper end of the Remove zone. Moving too rapidly or too deeply into the Remove zone sets off clearing illness. *This process typically involves cyclic bouts of increased inflammation that may aggravate individual tendencies toward mast cell activation syndrome, food allergies, and even cancer.* It is important to enter that zone with care.

As your diet changes, your body moves through these zones. The body is an adaptive, dynamic organism that does all it can to defend itself, so when you change your oxalate intake level, the *relative* difference influences how your body responds. Likewise, the specific amounts of oxalate corresponding to your body's zones will vary. The amounts mentioned here and listed in **Table 13.1** are conceptual (with fuzzy edges) but will help you understand and track what is happening in your own situation.

The Two Phases

As mentioned in Ron's story earlier, moving to low-oxalate eating is best done in phases, giving the body time to adjust.

In Phase One of low-oxalate eating, the goal is to stop accumulations from forming and growing. You would stay in Phase One long enough to rebuild your body's ability to cope with clearing. In Phase Two, the goal is to release the accumulations. The first phase moves you out of the Danger zone and Trigger zone, while the second phase eases you from the Maintenance zone toward the Remove zone as your body heals.

Phase One: Moving from Danger to Maintenance

If you've been on a modern "first world" diet, chances are you have been eating at least 250 mg oxalate daily, probably for years (in the Trigger zone). If you eat a lot of extremely high-oxalate foods, like potatoes, nuts, peanuts, spinach, and chocolate, you could be consuming as much as 2,000 mg per day or more (in the Danger zone). Your initial goal is to move toward the Maintenance zone, stepping gradually down to 150 mg per day.

In the first phase of reducing your oxalate intake, you are going to accomplish four major things: (1) getting out of the Danger zone and stopping acute dietary assaults; (2) slowing the accumulation process; (3) learning to select and enjoy low-oxalate foods; and (4) avoiding significant clearing of oxalate too soon and too fast. In Phase One, you'll continue eating some foods with significant oxalate to protect yourself as the oxalates start moving out, which is stressful to the kidneys and vascular system.

To achieve that step-wise transition, you will gradually taper your oxalate intake until you reach 150 to 200 mg oxalate per day, or about 45 mg per meal. If you are starting at a Danger level of, say, 3,000 mg per day, the decrease might be from 3,000 to about 1,000 mg in the first week, then reduce by halves, perhaps on a weekly basis. For example, in week 2, you would drop from 1,000 to 500 mg and then in week 3, you would drop down to 250 mg. Later, you take that last fine adjustment to reach the 150 to 200 mg target.

During this time, if you are taking vitamin C supplements, you also taper off to avoid "reactive scurvy" from a sudden withdrawal. For example, you would cut your daily doses of vitamin C supplements down by half every 5 to 7 days, until you reach 50 mg twice a day, or discontinue entirely. Remember that packaged foods and beverages are fortified with vitamin C. Check their labels for stated amounts.

Table 13.2 shows the theoretical Phase One oxalate-reduction schedule. If you can manage it, rest at the Phase One "median" for at least a month—maybe even six months—before crossing over into Phase Two, shown in **Table 13.3**.

Table 13.2: Phase One: Get Out of Danger

Week No.	Daily Oxalate Intake (mg)	Per Meal Target (mg total oxalate per meal)	Predominant Effect
0	3,000	NA	Extreme danger
1	1,000	< 300	Very high danger
2	500	< 150	Danger
3	250	90	Trigger
4–24 or longer, as needed	150–200	40–50	Maintenance (kidney recovery/ symptom relief)

Phase One allows your body to adjust and begin to recover from routine high-oxalate exposure, with minimal side effects. Metabolic gains at this level of oxalate consumption include better kidney function and less inflammation. These metabolic improvements put your body in a more advantageous position to handle the next phase. Phase One includes enough oxalate to (usually) restrain your body from aggressively clearing out the oxalate from your tissues.

Observe how your body is responding at this level of oxalate intake. If you're just trying to prevent future illness, you can stay in Phase One for the long term. If you're not feeling better and not having many clearing symptoms, consider moving to Phase Two, which will eventually be half the intake level you've gotten comfortable with during Phase One. Remember that every body is different. In some cases obvious clearing symptoms may not occur for as long as two or three years. You will need to judge when (or if) it's time to move lower.

Table 13.3: Phase Two: Nuance Your Low-Oxalate Diet

When	Daily Oxalate Intake (mg)	Per Meal Target (mg)	Predominant Effect
Weeks 9–24+, as needed*	100	25	Homeostasis: symptom flares
Begin when ready. Feel free to intentionally return to a *slightly* higher level, if needed	< 60	< 15	Reduction; overall improvements *and* symptoms of clearing

Adjust Your Oxalate Intake as Needed

Maintenance dose, 3 to 5 days in a row	100	Extra 35–50 in one meal daily for 3 to 5 days	To limit clearing symptoms
Mild trigger dose, one meal, up to twice a week	100+	Extra 60–70 in one meal weekly or occasionally	To limit clearing symptoms

* The week numbers listed here indicate time passed since the start of Phase One. They are intended to convey the principle of gradual reduction. You can spend as much time as needed at any level.

Phase Two: Moving from Maintenance to Remove

In Phase Two (see **Table 13.3**), the mission is to heal by gradually and safely clearing out the oxalate deposits. In this phase, you are heading toward an oxalate intake of 100 mg per day, or under 30 mg per meal. Now is the time to be aware of medium-oxalate foods and eat them only in portions that will keep your total intake near this lower level.

Stopping at 100 mg may be enough, or you can keep lowering your numbers and eventually drop to under 60 mg daily. However, lower levels of oxalate can provoke stronger clearing reactions (see Chapter 11). Look for a level of intake that puts you in your "sweet spot," where your body tissues release the oxalate deposits at a tolerable pace, which minimizes heavy clearing. You can't know for sure where the sweet spot is until you go below it. If you find yourself "too low," where the clearing symptoms are intense and relentless, you can adjust by adding some *modest* amount of oxalate. Nevertheless, as much as you might like to use moderated oxalate levels to curb the clearing, you don't have complete control over the process. Sometimes, just keeping your oxalate low (and managing the symptoms) is the best you can do. Chapter 15 will help you with that.

Phase Two is when you experiment and build a diet you can live with forever. Remember, this is an idealized program based on theory and generalizations from observations, and so is intended to offer some structure for reaching the goal of safely lowering oxalates. Please don't try to be overly precise in conforming to the consumption numbers, as that is not realistic or essential, and it will make things needlessly stressful.

Be Consistent and Persistent

Once you have established your new way of eating, know that consistency is key to regaining health and vitality. Here are a few things to watch for:

Avoid strong trigger doses. Avoid flipping on and off your low-oxalate diet. Adding strong trigger doses (~100 mg or more) at the wrong time might spike oxalate levels and throw the clearing process out of balance. Remember to stay aware—don't absentmindedly accept a piece of chocolate fudge pie at a party. "Cheats," intentional or not, can produce unpleasant and prolonged symptoms!

Use mild trigger doses if needed. Paradoxically, an intentional low-oxalate trigger dose of 60 to 70 mg in *one* occasional meal might be useful to stop the clearing symptoms (see **Table 13.3**). We get into the specifics of this in Chapter 14. See the **Dosing Estimates for Selected High-Oxalate Foods** table in the Resources section to gauge portion sizes needed to achieve mild trigger doses. Here, the idea is to make use of the trigger-and-maintenance theory (discussed in Chapter 9; see also **Box 9.1**) so as to rein in any aggressive clearing of oxalate from the tissues. Try this occasion-ally when lower amounts of oxalate (25 to 50 mg in one meal) don't give symptom relief. Also, see the section below about new reactivity poten-tially prompting responses to high-oxalate foods; this partly explains why the mild trigger dosing strategy can give mixed results, and why it doesn't always provide symptom relief (and sometimes makes things worse).

Eat enough. How do you resist the temptation of high-oxalate foods? If you let yourself get too hungry, it will needlessly test your willpower and self-discipline, and make it especially difficult to resist your old habit-forming high-oxalate foods. It's better to plan ahead and make medium- and low-oxalate foods the default choice in your life. You won't feel deprived if you are getting enough nutrients and calories, so *eat enough at mealtime*. And keep learning and growing. Try new foods and new recipes to expand your palate and your culinary talents. In Chap-ter 14, you will learn about low-oxalate options.

Watch for new sensitivity. Many low-oxalate dieters tell me that after being low-oxalate for a time, they have dramatic negative reactions to high-oxalate foods, as if they now have an extra "sensitivity" to oxalate. That happened to my husband (after about nine months of maintaining a low-oxalate diet), when the fig tree we had at the time called to him like apples in Eden. He ate about 20 figs! That night he could not sleep, and the next morning he was possessed with an uncharacteristic angry mood. It took him a few days to feel like himself again.

There are at least four reasons why people get a new "reactivity" to high-oxalate foods after having adopted a low-oxalate diet.

First, with your newfound awareness you now pay attention and recognize the connection between your foods and your body's reactions.

Second, when your body is accustomed to a low-oxalate diet, your relative absorption of oxalate is a bit higher (perhaps 14 percent instead of 8 percent); that is, when your body isn't expecting it, a high-oxalate food may have a slightly greater impact.

Third, your body may be working at full capacity when removing oxalate. This is a different metabolic state from sequestration (that is, collecting oxalate deposits in the tissues). During this time, oxalate levels in the blood and urine may be elevated. Adding more oxalates would push the body into a toxic "overcapacity" state.

Fourth, your immune system may have been trained to go after oxalate crystals while doing its clearing. Adding more oxalate to the gut or bloodstream might set off an immune storm, increasing inflammation and mast cell reactivity throughout the body (including the brain).

Pay attention to ups and downs. Learn to recognize the ups and downs in your health as your body cleans out the oxalate deposits, possibly for years. Stick with the low-oxalate diet and keep coming back to it if you stray briefly. It can be easy to get lulled into thinking you are over your oxalate problem. If you drift back to routine higher-oxalate eating, you may feel better for a while because it will have slowed the clearing and calmed its symptoms, but it will be restarting a chronic process of oxalate accumulation that in the long run will only make things worse.

How to Use Oxalate Content Data to Meet Targets

We think of numbers as precise things, like how much cash is in your wallet, but with the biology of oxalates, the numbers have fuzzy edges. Precision is an illusion, owing to the variability of food and of testing methods.

All worthy foods come from living things, which means they vary in oxalate content, so the numbers are always ballpark estimates. Trying to get more precise can be a waste of time. It's never possible to know *exactly* how much oxalate you are eating or how much you may be absorbing (because you can't directly measure it).

Nonetheless, ballparking can work wonders. You can check the numbers for oxalate content in the tables available on my website. Also see the abbreviated **Dosing Estimates for Selected High-Oxalate Foods** table in the Resources section of this book. These tables will allow you to learn which foods to eliminate or reduce to suitable portion sizes.

Remember, the portion sizes determine how much oxalate you're getting from a particular food. Many lists identify foods as low, medium, and high in oxalates, but that is misleading because how "high" a food's oxalate content is depends on how much you eat of it. For example, spinach can be considered low if you eat only one leaf (see **Box 13.1**); that is, you could eat one leaf a day and have a very low-oxalate diet (depending on what else you're eating).

BOX 13.1: THE IMPORTANCE OF PORTION SIZE: HOW TO MAKE SPINACH A LOW-OXALATE FOOD

Very High	High	Low	None
40 leaves →	10 leaves →	1 leaf →	Zero
(200 mg)	(50 mg)	(5 mg)	(0)

In contrast, **Box 13.2** lists the formal thresholds that designate food servings, meals, and daily intake as either high or low. When you evaluate the oxalate content of the servings you are eating, these numbers will give you a sense of scale. You'll see the differences between a diet that causes oxalate accumulation, a diet that puts you near a stable level, and a diet that allows for de-accumulation.

BOX 13.2: SUMMARY OF PORTION THRESHOLDS

Food Servings

✛ High-oxalate food: over 10 mg/serving

✛ Very high-oxalate food: over 15 mg/serving

Meal Totals

✛ "Normal" meal: 45–70 mg

✛ Mild trigger meal: 60–70 mg

✛ Maintenance meal: 30–50 mg

✛ Low-oxalate meal: under 25 mg

Daily Totals

✛ "Normal" diet: 130–220 mg

✛ High-oxalate day: over 250 mg

✛ Low-oxalate diet: < 60 mg

The **Dosing Estimates** table in the Resources section will help you determine how to use high-oxalate foods intentionally, if needed. Remember that consistency and awareness are much more important than precision in numbers. The real focus should be on paying attention to how your body is adjusting and responding to the food portions you're eating.

14

Converting Your Diet

There has been, of late years, much said and written respecting the benefits of adhering to a strict vegetable diet, and many excellent people are sadly perplexed about their duty in this matter, and whether they ought to give up animal food entirely.

—Sarah Josepha Hale, *Early American Cookery*, 1839

Imagine meals without spinach and beets. What do you have instead? Watercress and radishes can stand in. If you love vegetables, quitting chard and spinach is not hard, because there are plenty of other leafy options, such as turnip or mustard greens.

Whatever your motives for adopting an oxalate-aware eating pattern, the starting point is right where you are. The endpoint, then, is an updated, informed way of eating that you can sustain with consistency. With a bit of study and practice, you will see your foods through new eyes as you navigate a world so peppered with high-oxalate landmines.

Selecting Foods

If you're already eating healthy home-cooked meals made with whole, fresh ingredients, use my list of Safe Bets (see **Table 4.4**) to fill your pantry and fridge with safer foods. While there's no reason to dive straight into a detailed data table, you do want to build your new diet from foods that have been tested. Start by limiting and removing the Worst Offenders in **Table 3.1** and also view the **Swap Chart** in the Resources section of this book. Scan the lists for the foods you eat. If a particular food you're wondering about is not in these simplified lists, look for it in the Food Oxalate Content Data Resources available on my website. Remember that reliable test data do not exist for all foods. **Table 14.1** shows the worst offenders and safe bets side-by-side.

Table 14.1: Worst Offenders and "Safe Bets"

Worst Offenders *Very High-Oxalate Foods*	Safe Bets *Low- and Very Low-Oxalate*
Animal Products	
	Meats, dairy, butter, eggs, fish, shellfish, fats (seafoods are presumed to be low, but most have not been tested)
Beverages (8 to 12 oz servings)	
Almond beverages, beet juice, carrot juice, chocolate-flavored beverages (chocolate milk, hot cocoa, mocha coffees, chocolate plant drinks), tea (black or green), V-8 vegetable juice, starfruit juice	Apple cider, beer, coffee, coconut milk, fruit juices (apple, cherry, cranberry, lemon, lime, orange), ginger ale, herbal teas, dairy milk, kefir, sparkling water, wine
Desserts, Snacks, and Treats	
Carob products; chips made with banana, plantain, potato, sweet potato, or taro; crackers containing nuts, sesame, poppy, or chia seeds; chocolate or cocoa products (brownies, cake, ice cream, etc.); rhubarb desserts	Flax crackers, pickles, pork rinds, toasted coconut flakes, blueberry jam, candied ginger (4 tsp.), dates (6), ice cream (vanilla or coconut), whipped cream, white chocolate

(table continues)

Worst Offenders *Very High-Oxalate Foods*	**Safe Bets** *Low- and Very Low-Oxalate*
Fruits and Berries (serving size: ½ cup whole fruits, 1 cup juice)	
Apricots, avocados (underripened), blackberries, clementines, elderberries, figs, guava, kiwifruit, lemon (zest), olives, pears (Anjou), plantains, pomegranates, prunes, raspberries, rhubarb, star fruit, tangelos	Apples, blueberries, cherries, coconut, cranberries (fresh), dates, grapes (seedless) Hass avocado (ripe), melon (cantaloupe, honeydew, watermelon), kumquat, peaches, fruit juices (apple, orange, lemon, lime, pineapple) Banana, mango (fresh), papaya, plums (fresh)
Grains and Grain Substitutes, Grain Products (dry ¼ cup; cooked ½ cup)	
Amaranth, arrowroot, barley flour, buckwheat flour, green banana flour, potato flour, rice bran, tapioca flour, teff, wheat germ Corn grits, quinoa, shredded wheat cereal Pumpernickel breads, rye breads, whole-grain breads	Coconut flour, cornstarch, potato starch (not flour), rice starch; cooked white rice (½ cup), Uncle Ben's Minute Rice; cellophane (mung bean) noodles, kelp noodles, shirataki "rice" or "noodles," white rice spaghetti, corn on the cob, coconut wraps Kelp noodles, pearl barley
Greens and Other Vegetables (½ cup servings)	
Artichoke hearts, beets, beet greens, carrots, celery, chard, cactus/nopal, okra, parsnips, sugar snap peas, potatoes (sweet and white, fries, chips, etc.), spinach, tomato sauce, yams	Alfalfa sprouts, arugula, bok choy, chives, red bell pepper, cabbage, capers, cauliflower, celery root (celeriac), cilantro, cucumber, escarole, kale (lacinato or purple, boiled), kim chee, kohlrabi, lettuce (romaine, Bibb, butter, and iceberg), mizuna, mushrooms, mustard greens, onions, radishes, rutabaga, turnips, winter squash, watercress, water chestnuts, zucchini Asparagus, broccoli (boiled), Brussels sprouts (boiled), collards, endive, green peas (boiled), green bell pepper, kale (raw), pumpkin

Worst Offenders *Very High-Oxalate Foods*	Safe Bets *Low- and Very Low-Oxalate*
Seasonings and Herbs	
Black pepper, caraway and poppy seeds, cinnamon, cumin, Indian-style curry powder, parsley, turmeric	Salt, white pepper; Frank's RedHot Sauce, Tabasco; horseradish; garlic (fresh or dried); sweeteners (honey, stevia, sugar); dried herbs (bay leaf, dill, marjoram, onion powder, poultry seasoning, rosemary, sage, savory, tarragon, thyme); spices (cayenne, mace, mustard seeds); extracts (chocolate, lemon, peppermint, vanilla) Ground cardamom Italian seasoning Oregano (dried)
Legumes/Beans	
Black, Great Northern, pinto, and most other legumes Soy flour, soy milk, soy protein Vegetarian burgers and meat analogs	Black-eyed peas, butter beans (Use in modest portions. Always soak legumes prior to cooking them with high heat to disarm lectins.) Green peas (fresh or frozen), mung beans, split peas (yellow or green)
Seeds and Nuts	
Seeds: chia, hemp, poppy, sesame Nuts: almonds, cashews, pecans, pine nuts, walnuts	Seeds: coconut, flax, pumpkin, sunflower, watermelon and their oils (Although they are low in oxalate, avoid oils from soy, corn, cottonseed, sunflower, and safflower as much as possible owing to inflammatory breakdown products and the unstable/rancid nature of these oils.)

If you're committed to eating a plant-heavy diet, achieving your target goal calls for good data, awareness of serving size, and bit of math. The data can be hard to remember, so you'll have to keep going back to your sources. Nevertheless, developing and maintaining an awareness of the oxalate content of foods is a valuable, lifelong skill. Keep coming back to it.

If you're *not* cooking all your own food, it gets just a bit more challenging. That's because most commercial products and restaurant foods have not been tested for oxalate. If there are no numbers available, what do you do? You look at ingredient lists online that have been posted for chain restaurants, or you quiz the waiter (or call ahead to the restaurant), or you read the labels on packaged foods to identify their main ingredients. You don't have to do a detailed analysis, but it is important that you can recognize high-oxalate ingredients. Scrutinize those labels with special attention to the first three or four ingredients, as label ingredients are listed in order of greatest amount.

For a simple example, consider three varieties of the Jimmy Dean Egg'wich, which the VP Foundation had tested in 2020. The Broccoli and Cheese Egg Frittata and the ham variety (with bell pepper, mushroom, onion, and turkey sausage) had under 20 mg of oxalate, which makes them a reasonable choice for Phase One. But the Bacon, Spinach, Caramelized Onion, and Parmesan variety (with turkey sausage and processed American cheese) had over 80 mg! If you were guessing based on the ingredient list and didn't have a food test available, all you would need to know is that spinach is very high in oxalate, while ham, cheese, and broccoli are not. If the product includes spinach, it's not a good choice for a low-oxalate diet—ever.

While there is a lot of bad diet advice out there, one worthy diet rule is to limit your consumption of packaged foods generally and to select only products that have very short ingredient lists. These Egg'wich products contain seed oils and a long list of ingredients, many of which you might want to avoid. Your health will be improved if you eat foods that you prepare yourself from better ingredients.

When you are unsure about a food, you have three options: (1) Skip it, knowing there is always something else to eat. There is no food you must eat; "No, thanks" is the phrase that will pay the greatest dividends. (2) Use "mystery foods" only in very modest portions and not daily. (3) Test how a given food makes you feel, but bear in mind that this is not always a safe and reliable indicator, especially in the first year or so while you're learning to recognize how your body is responding to lower-oxalate intake.

Replacing Foods

Take a glance at the foods that have been categorized by oxalate levels, listed in **Table 14.2**. You'll find many of the extremely high-oxalate foods that you'll discontinue using listed in the left-hand column. Better choices are listed in the middle column, featuring (technically) high-oxalate foods that you *can* safely use in appropriate serving sizes. Items in the middle column are especially useful in Phase One, when your goal is to lower, but not completely eliminate, oxalate. They can also be used later, if you find yourself needing to slow the oxalate clearing process. As mentioned, portion awareness is key to success.

The right-hand column of **Table 14.2** lists medium-low-oxalate foods, which are appropriate in both phases of the diet. Just for now, imagine a fourth column on the far right, featuring near zero-oxalate foods. That fourth column would list meats, eggs, cheese, butter, and other nutrient-rich animal foods. Those foods make the oxalate math much easier and provide the nutrients critical to your recovery. Learn to eat more of them, at your own pace, of course.

You may continue to find the foods in the middle column useful in Phase Two, especially if you experience heavy clearing symptoms. Portions of foods with 20 to 50 mg of oxalate can sometimes help in slowing the rate of oxalate clearing. See the **Dosing Estimates** table in the Resources section.

Table 14.2: Replacement of Extremely High-Oxalate Foods

Note: The following are ideas for using foods with moderate levels of oxalate, which will help you avoid going too low too soon, and for adding maintenance amounts of oxalate to avoid excessive clearing symptoms. You can find additional ideas in the **Swap Chart** in the Resources section.

Note on volume unit abbreviations: C = cup (8 fl. oz., or 240 ml); Tbs. = tablespoon (15 ml).

Foods to Avoid	Phase One Food Servings (with care in Phase Two)	Food Servings to Use Anytime
Extremely High Oxalate (Omit) ≥ 50 mg	High Oxalate (Beginners and "Adders")	Low and Moderate Oxalate
Salads		
Spinach salad (~500 mg): 1½ C raw baby spinach (480 mg) 1 Tbs. sliced almonds (35 mg) one 13 g scallion (3 mg) (50 g spinach = 500–600 mg)	Spring greens salad (~55 mg): 1 C mixed baby greens (48 mg) 6 black olives (6 mg) (50 g mesclun mix = 85 mg)*	Romaine salad (5 mg): 2 C sliced romaine (2 mg) sliced red onion (0) sprinkle of Parmesan cheese (0) 6 croutons, 15 g (3 mg) (100 g romaine = 2 mg)
Fruits (Raw)		
1 C sliced kiwifruit (55 mg) 1 C fresh blackberries (74 mg) 1 C pomegranate arils (60 mg) 1 tangelo, medium (80 mg)	1 clementine (20 mg) 1 Anjou pear (20 mg) 1 C fresh pineapple (22 mg) 1 navel orange, small (20 mg) ½ pink grapefruit (17 mg)	1 Bartlett pear (5 mg) 1 peach (3 mg) 1 C honeydew, cantaloupe, or watermelon (5 mg) ½ C mango (5 mg) ½ C orange juice (<1 mg)

* Mesclun mixes vary tremendously; remember that the oxalate comes from the spinach, chard, and beet greens. The relative concentration in the mix will determine the oxalate content.

Foods to Avoid	Phase One Food Servings (with care in Phase Two)	Food Servings to Use Anytime
Nuts and Seeds		
½ C almonds (290 mg) ¼ C chia seeds (260 mg)	20 macadamia nuts (20 mg) ⅓ C sunflower seeds (20 mg)	½ C pumpkin seeds (3 mg)
Potatoes		
8 oz. russet / Idaho potato (110 mg) 5 oz. orange sweet potato (140 mg)	6 oz. parsnip (30 mg) 5 oz. red new potatoes (30 mg) 3 Tbs. orange sweet potato (30 mg)	6 oz. rutabaga (7 mg) 8 oz. turnips (3 mg) 8 oz. cauliflower florets (5 mg) 6 oz. baked butternut squash (8 mg) 3 oz. canned celery root (6 mg)
Vegetables		
½ C steamed red chard or beet greens (880 mg) ½ C steamed spinach (670 mg)	3 oz. artichoke hearts (30 mg) 1 C cooked asparagus (20 mg) 1.5 oz. (¼ C) steamed red beets (20 mg) 1 C steamed broccolini (20 mg) 1 C steamed Brussels sprouts (20 mg) ½ C chopped raw celery (15 mg) ½ C steamed or boiled carrots (15 mg) 1 C cooked spaghetti squash (9 mg) 1 C boiled dandelion greens (16 mg) 2 plain grape leaves (15 mg)	½ C cooked mustard greens (6 mg) 1 C cooked cabbage (5 mg) 1½ C raw watercress (6 mg) 1 C boiled lacinato kale (3 mg) ½ C boiled Brussels sprouts (5 mg) ⅓ C dandelion greens (5 mg)

(table continues)

Foods to Avoid	Phase One Food Servings (with care in Phase Two)	Food Servings to Use Anytime
Beans (cooked)		
½ C black beans (65 mg) ½ C white beans (65 mg) ½ C Great Northern beans (70 mg) 1 Boca burger (75 mg)	½ C chickpeas (10 mg) 1 C canned green peas (10 mg) ½ C lentils (5–20 mg)	½ C mung beans (3 mg) ½ C black-eyed peas (3 mg) ⅓ C green peas (4 mg) ½ C cauliflower hummus made with pumpkin seeds (2 mg)
Beverages		
1 C hot cocoa (45–80 mg) ⅔ C beet juice (100 mg)	1 C black tea (20 mg) 1 C green tea (15 mg) 1 C yerba maté tea (7 mg) 1 C carrot, celery, or tomato juice (15 mg)	1 C herbal tea (<1 mg) 1 C coffee (<2 mg) 1 C herbal coffee substitute (<5 mg)
Treats		
2 oz. milk chocolate (> 30 mg) 2 oz. dark chocolate (> 100 mg)	2 Tbs. chopped crystallized ginger (5 mg) ½ C fresh or dried pineapple (10 mg) ½ C chocolate ice cream (20 mg)	2 oz. white chocolate (4 mg) ½ C vanilla ice cream (dairy or coconut types) (1 mg)
Pasta and Grains		
1 C cooked elbow macaroni (45 mg) 1½ C cooked whole wheat spaghetti (40 mg) 2 slices pumpernickel or whole wheat bread (35+ mg)	½ C cooked spaghetti (12 mg) 1 C cooked egg noodles (18 mg) ½ C cooked brown rice (12 mg)	1 C cooked white rice spaghetti (5 mg) 1 C cooked shirataki noodles (4 mg) ¾ C cooked jasmine white rice (5 mg)

Reformed Menus

To think in terms not only of individual foods but also of whole meals and daily total consumption, let's look back at the three eating styles featured in Chapter 4: Whole-Foods, Pescatarian, and Paleo. Here, we'll adjust those menus to illustrate the transition from a high-oxalate menu to a Phase One menu and then to a Phase Two menu. We'll look at our three menus in **Tables 14.3, 14.4, and 14.5** respectively. The first column in each table shows a baseline high-oxalate menu. The second column, for Phase One, reduces the portions of some oxalate-containing ingredients and replaces others to achieve a daily intake of about 150 mg. The third column, for Phase Two, further reduces high-oxalate foods and aims for a daily intake of under 60 mg. **Table 14.3** contains a "whole foods" diet with no particular restrictions: it includes meat, wheat, dairy foods, and vegetables in **simply prepared** recipes. **Table 14.4** is for pescatarians who avoid meats except for fish. **Table 14.5** shows a Paleo menu that avoids all grains, legumes, and most dairy foods but allows meat.

Table 14.3: Whole-Foods Diet Transition

Meal	High-Oxalate Diet		Phase One Oxalate Diet
	Food	**Mg Oxalate**	**Food**
Breakfast	1 cup oatmeal (20 mg) 1 Tbs. raisins (1 mg) 1 Tbs. cashews (23 mg) and dash of ground cinnamon (0) 1 cup coffee (2 mg)	45	Breakfast burrito: 1 large flour tortilla (10 mg) ¼ cup pinto beans (20 mg) ¼ cup grated cheese (0) 2 large eggs (0) 1 slice ham (0) chosen spices (3 mg) 1 cup coffee (2 mg)
Lunch	Tuna salad (10 mg) on multigrain bread (32 mg), 1 celery stalk (8 mg) 1 oz. potato chips (20 mg) 1 cup V-8 juice (20 mg) OR Applebee's Paradise Chicken Salad (55 mg) 3-inch brownie (37 mg)	90	6 oz. blackened salmon fillet (5 mg) ½ cup mashed potatoes (20 mg) 1 cup steamed broccoli (20 mg)
Snack	1 clementine (20 mg)	20	1 cup honeydew melon or 1 large apple (5 mg)
Dinner	Small romaine salad (5 mg) with pickled beets (25 mg), 1 Tbs. pine nuts (17 mg) Chicken thighs (0), with 6 oz. roasted potato wedges (80 mg) ½ cup cooked chard (500 mg) or spinach (500 mg)	625	6 oz. fried pork chop or meatballs in ¾ cup red sauce (20 mg) 1½ cups cooked white-rice angel hair pasta (17 mg) Small romaine salad with cucumber slices (3 mg)
Dessert	2 small chocolate chip cookies (20 mg)	20	3-inch brownie (37 mg)
~Total		800	

	Mg Oxalate	Low-Oxalate Diet	Mg Oxalate
		Food	
	35	Breakfast burrito: 1 large flour tortilla (10 mg) ¼ cup grated cheese (0) 3 large eggs (0) 1 slice ham (0) chosen spices (3 mg) 1 cup coffee (2 mg)	15
	45	6 oz. blackened salmon (5 mg) 1 ear corn on the cob (3 mg) 1 cup romaine salad (3 mg) 5 black olives (6 mg)	17
	5	1 cup herbal tea (2 mg)	2
	40	6 oz. fried pork chop or meatballs in ½ cup white sauce (1 mg) 1 cup cooked white-rice angel hair pasta (11 mg) or spaghetti squash (9 mg) or shirataki noodles (4 mg) Small romaine salad with cucumber slices (3 mg)	15
	37	½ cup vanilla ice cream (0)	0
	160		**50**

Table 14.4: Pescatarian Diet Transition

Meal	High-Oxalate Diet		Phase One Oxalate Diet
	Food	Mg Oxalate	Food
Breakfast	Chia pudding: ¼ cup chia (265 mg), 1 cup almond milk (30 mg), and 1 Tbs. strawberry jam (3 mg) Starbucks White Chocolate Latte, made with skim milk (10 mg) OR 4 Boca breakfast patties (120 mg) 2 slices multigrain toast (32 mg) and 2 Tbs. almond butter (120 mg) 1 kiwi (30 mg) Small coffee with ⅛ tsp. turmeric (7 mg)	310	3 oz. smoked salmon or sardines (0 mg) on toasted sourdough English muffin (11 mg) 1 Tbs. cream cheese or butter (0 mg) ½ pink grapefruit (17 mg) 1 oz. sunflower seeds (9 mg)
Lunch	1½ cups black bean soup (45 mg) 1 bagel (15 mg) 1 cup green tea (15 mg) 3 oz. carrot sticks (40 mg) OR Chickpea, mint, and green pea tabbouleh (43 mg) 1 clementine (20 mg) 3 oz. carrot sticks (40 mg) 1 cup green tea (15 mg)	115	1½ cups split pea soup (10 mg) 1 bagel with butter (15 mg) 1¼ oz. cheddar cheese (0 mg) ½ cup fresh pineapple (11 mg)
Snack	1 oz. dark 86% Ghirardelli chocolate (90 mg)	90	1 cup black tea (20 mg)
Dinner	Indian-spiced salmon (10 mg), with cumin-spiced carrots (30 mg) and pear chutney (5 mg) 1 cup quinoa (100 mg) 1½ cups mesclun salad (75 mg) Decaf tea (10 mg)	230	6 oz. pan-fried whitefish (0 mg) ½ cup brown rice with diced carrots and 7 black olives (24 mg) ½ cup cooked dandelion greens (10 mg)
Dessert	10 vanilla wafer cookies (10 mg) 2 Tbs. peanut butter (50 mg)	60	1 clementine (20 mg) OR ½ cup peachy blueberry crisp (15 mg)
Daily Ox		805	

Mg Oxalate	Low-Oxalate Diet	
	Food	**Mg Oxalate**
37	2 scrambled eggs topped with 1 Tbs. minced cilantro (1 mg) ⅓ cup chickpeas (3 mg) 2 corn tortillas (14 mg)	18
36	1½ cups split pea soup (10 mg) 1 Singoda Indian flatbread or 2 soft crackers (3 mg), with 1¼ oz. cheddar cheese or boiled egg (0 mg) 1 Gala apple (3 mg) OR 1 cup black-eyed pea salad (9 mg) ½ cup with cottage cheese (3 mg) over 1 cup romaine salad (3 mg)	15
20	5 large shrimp with cocktail sauce (0)	0
34	6 oz. pan-fried blackened salmon fillet (8 mg) ½ cup mashed celery root and rutabaga (2 mg) 1 cup sautéed bok choy (3 mg) 1 ear corn on the cob (3 mg), or ½ cup green peas (1–5 mg), or 1 cup romaine salad (3 mg)	18
20	½ cup vanilla or coconut ice cream (0 mg)	0
150		**50**

Table 14.5: Paleo Diet Transition

Meal	High-Oxalate Diet		Phase One Oxalate Diet
	Food	Mg Oxalate	Food
Breakfast	Shake (150 mg total): 1½ cups almond milk (46 mg), 1 cup mixed fresh berries (25 mg), 4 Tbs. hemp powder (50 mg), ½ banana (5 mg), ½ tsp. ground turmeric (24 mg) 5 Tbs. Paleo granola (60 mg)	210	⅓ cup sausage hash: sausage with grated carrot (10 mg), diced turnip or celery root (4 mg), seasoned with rosemary and pepper (1 mg) 1 fried egg (0 mg) ⅓ cup rosemary-scented walnuts (17 mg)
Lunch	Kale salad: 1 cup chopped kale (5 mg), ¾ cup mashed roasted sweet potato (140 mg), dressing (3 mg), 1 Tbs. sunflower seeds (5 mg), and 7 black olives (8 mg) OR 1½ cups Paleo clam chowder with cashews (80 mg) 1¼ cups mesclun baby greens salad (60 mg) 2.8 oz. marinated artichoke hearts (20 mg)	160	1 cup modified Paleo clam chowder (40 mg) 3 red radishes (0.3 mg) 1 oz. fried pork rinds (0 mg) 1 cup black tea (20 mg)
Snack	Trail-mix nut bar (65 mg)	65	Trail mix (1 oz. sunflower seeds [12 mg], dried pineapple [3 mg], shredded coconut [0 mg])
Dinner	Zucchini parmigiana made with nut "cheese," sausage, and a hint of spinach (250 mg) 1½ oz. raw fennel sticks (10 mg) 2 small tapioca-flour garlic rolls (20 mg)	280	8 oz. beef chuck roast with carrots and onion (31 mg) 1 cup julienned raw zucchini (7 mg) ½ cup cranberry juice with 1 Tbs. lime juice and sparking mineral water (1 mg)
Dessert	3 homemade chocolate macaroons (85 mg)	85	1 baked apple with ¼ tsp. minced ginger (6 mg)
Daily Ox		**800**	

Mg Oxalate	Low Oxalate	
	Food	**Mg Oxalate**
30	⅓ cup sausage hash, no carrot (5 mg), 3 eggs (0 mg) OR ½ cup sardine mash in coconut yogurt (1 mg)	5
60	1 cup low-oxalate clam chowder (6 mg) 1 small romaine salad (3 mg) 1 apple (4 mg) OR 6 oz. meatballs (3 mg) 1 cup corn salsa (7 mg) ¼–½ cup peeled English cucumber slices (3 mg)	13
15	1 cup bone broth with coconut milk and white pepper (2 mg)	2
39	8 oz. chuck roast (0 mg), *or* 1 rib-eye steak (0 mg), *or* 2 baked chicken thighs (0 mg) ½ cup cooked asparagus (9 mg), *or* 4 oz. zucchini noodles (8 mg) *and* 4 oz. cauliflower rice (4 mg), *or* ½ cup baked winter squash (4 mg)	13
6	3 vanilla macaroons (5 mg)	5
150		**38**

Implementing Your Low-Oxalate Plan

Here is some additional advice for succeeding at adopting a low-oxalate diet.

Learn how to prepare new foods so you enjoy them. Don't eat foods you don't like. But do give unfamiliar foods a chance, because their gastronomic appeal is often a matter of knowing how to prepare them. Enjoying food is an essential part of embracing your low-oxalate food options, so it's important to bring out the best in these foods with skillful preparation. For example, the taste and texture of vegetables improves considerably when seasoned with enough salt and butter or other fat. (Yes, I know bad information has trained us to cut down on fat and salt. Don't listen to those misinformed voices.)*

Customize food selections to suit your individual needs. If you struggle with food intolerances and need to avoid certain foods, you can still build a diet around the foods you can eat. But our bodies and food sensitivities evolve when oxalate is doing less damage. Many people find that after starting a low-oxalate diet, they can add wheat and cheese, or other previously irritating foods, back into their diets. The fact that you have been sensitive to certain foods does not mean you will continue to be.

To test how well you tolerate a food, eliminate that food for at least two weeks, then bring it back in generous servings for a day or two, and see how your body reacts. If things seem fine, you should continue to keep notes and use your instincts. Listen to your body; some foods may subtly increase pain and inflammation, regardless of their oxalate content. Milk and eggs are great examples of nutritious and versatile foods that work well for some but are certainly not for everyone.

Be nourished. Oxalate overload illness commonly occurs because of consumption of fad foods and diets. Some folks imagine—without any

---

* Recommended reading: *The Big Fat Surprise*, by Nina Teicholz; *The Salt Fix*, by James DiNicolantonio; and *The Vegetarian Myth*, by Lierre Keith.

factual basis—that eliminating high-oxalate foods might lead to malnutrition. Nothing could be further from the truth. Malnourishment is what we are rectifying with low-oxalate eating.

Remember that the oxalic acid in foods like spinach causes malnourishment. Such malnourishment caused infertility and premature death in Dr. E. F. Kohman's rats and serious mineral depletion in human infants (see Chapter 4). These fates are sensible to avoid.

If you're nervous about not getting adequate nutrients, make sure you're considering all the food alternatives available to you, and are not imposing needless restrictions. If you're adhering to a strict vegetarian diet, you should keep assessing whether your diet includes enough protein and other essential nutrients.

The best way to improve nutritional adequacy is to include ample portions of beef and other quality animal foods in your typical daily meals. Try my Easy Creamed Canned Oysters recipe (see my website). Oysters provide an impressive array of nutrients, including omega-3 fatty acids, vitamin D, vitamin B_{12}, high-quality protein, and many important trace minerals, like zinc, iron, selenium, and copper.

Tips for Navigating Your Food Selections

Keep track. You can help yourself make better decisions about your diet if you keep track of the foods you're eating, the symptoms you're having, and any related feelings. Keeping notes about what you are eating can help you make decisions about what to eat based on how you feel in the hours and days after eating certain foods. Tracking your symptoms over time will give you a long-term perspective and a view of your progress. Writing about how you feel as you make that progress toward reaching your goals (or how sometimes you feel you are not) can help you cope emotionally.

Begin by stating your goals and intentions. Why did you decide to undertake low-oxalate eating? What are your feelings about change in general and the learning process? How did high-oxalate foods fit into your former way of eating? What are your feelings about them? What social pressures influence your food choices? Who might support you in reaching your goal? Keep your answers to those questions up to date as you move forward.

Keeping a symptom inventory journal is especially important. It will give you the perspective you need to appreciate your progress on days when you're feeling frustrated. Ask yourself: What are your starting symptoms and what is their impact on your life and daily activities? See how that answer changes over time.

Make new food friends and make them real. Searching for low-oxalate foods that imitate the foods you're already familiar with can make your diet seem much more restrictive than it really is. If you're hunting for that perfect low-oxalate pizza, high-fiber breakfast cereal, or a peanut butter and jelly sandwich replacement, you may be setting yourself up for frustration. You also risk reliance on low-nutrient, imitation foods. Oxalate-wise eating works better if you are willing to set aside long-standing habits and personal food rules, and instead find new tastes, textures, and even "comforts."

Remember the oxalate precursors. Being mindful of metabolic oxalate, remember to moderate your use of oxalate precursors (listed in **Box 8.1**). Limit your use of supplements and foods fortified with vitamin C, so as to keep your daily total C intake under 250 mg. Moderate your use of concentrated gelatin and collagen supplements to about 1 tablespoon a day (or less). The gelatin capsules used in supplements are insignificant, unless you are taking many dozens daily. Recall, too, that moderate use of sugar and complex carbs is safe for non-obese persons and does not elevate oxalate levels.

Enjoy animal foods. Because I've cautioned you to limit gelatin and collagen supplements, it is useful to repeat that greater intake of animal protein does *not* increase the oxalate in the body and urine, nor does it stress the kidneys, despite the common misconception that animal protein is bad for the kidneys. Meats, especially beef, venison, elk, goat, and lamb, are traditional human foods, and are uniquely important sources of many essential nutrients. They may even be vital to metabolic health, long-term well-being, and weight control.

Even though animals may eat oxalate-rich foods, the foods derived from these animals are relatively free of oxalate; for our purposes, they are essentially zero, with only a few known exceptions such as toxic giant snails. Processed and seasoned meats may, however, contain high-oxalate spices and other plant-sourced ingredients. Muscle meats from ruminants (cows and sheep) are very low in oxalate, while meat from other animals (pigs and poultry) and dairy products may contain traces of oxalate. Organ meats have slightly more oxalate, but are still not significant sources of dietary oxalate. Dairy products are very low, though fresh cow's milk is unique in having a great deal of bioavailable calcium *and* traces of *soluble* oxalate; goat's milk seems to have no oxalate. Most fish are generally low to zero in oxalate content, but popular fish like canned tuna and sardines have sometimes tested slightly higher.

Use caution with the brassicas. Cabbage family vegetables can cause digestive distress when eaten in excess. The brassicas can promote bloating, discomfort, cramping, belching, and flatulence, owing to their fiber and an indigestible sugar called raffinose (existing in many plant foods, including asparagus and beans). Maybe this is what makes kale the butt of jokes. The brassicas can also trigger or aggravate symptoms of reflux, small intestine bacterial overgrowth, and irritable bowel syndrome. Brassica vegetables, like most vegetables, are best eaten fermented (as in sauerkraut), or cooked and eaten in modest quantities.

Here is an example: try roasting red radishes. They can be a fun finger food to enjoy while you prepare the rest of your low-oxalate meal — but don't load the rest of that meal with endless amounts of cauliflower, mustard greens, turnips, and so on. To round out a vegetable-heavy meal, add buttered hot spaghetti squash and a small salad made with romaine lettuce, peeled cucumber, slices of red onion, a few leftover steamed green peas, and a sprinkling of romano or Parmesan cheese. May I suggest an omelet or a thick and juicy steak or cheeseburger at the center?

Kale, by the way, comes in several varieties that vary in oxalate content, with Red Russian and dinosaur (also called Tuscan or lacinato) being the lowest in oxalate. Green curly kale, however, has three times more oxalate (at a rate of 30 mg/100 grams). Boiling the chopped kale can reduce the oxalate by half—*if* you throw away the cooking liquid. But even at 30 mg /100 grams, kale is not a huge source of oxalate, compared to spinach and chard. Nevertheless, if you eat a lot of kale chips and kale smoothies, the oxalate will add up! See **Figure 14.1**, which compares the oxalate content of various leafy green vegetables.

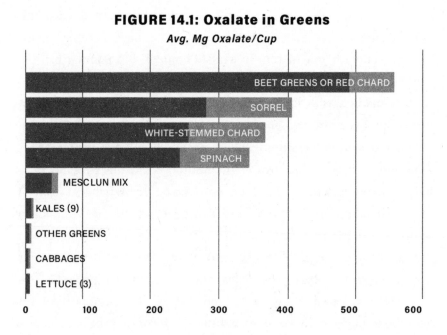

FIGURE 14.1: Oxalate in Greens
Avg. Mg Oxalate/Cup

Be cautious with nuts and seeds. Nuts and seeds (grains and beans are seeds, too) are high-oxalate foods, with a few notable exceptions: pumpkin seeds, watermelon seeds, and flax seeds. Medium-level nuts include macadamia nuts and pistachios. Please don't try to live on seeds or nuts, though. Seeds have other compounds that are hard on the gut and that may not be helpful for some people who need to rebuild their health. For example, in addition to having lectins and phytates, pistachios are prone to mold contamination, which typically means the presence of aflatoxin. That doesn't mean you can't use pistachios in cooking on occasion (chopped pistachios make a great garnish), but don't scale them up to the level of a daily staple.

Remember that oils and fats are oxalate free. The good feature of fats and oils is that they don't have oxalate, even when they come from a high-oxalate food such as peanuts. When oils are prepared, the oxalate sinks and gets filtered out. If you do eat out and a restaurant is cooking with peanut or sesame oil, you do not have to be concerned about the oxalate in the oil. However, vegetable oils are undesirable for other reasons, such as their high concentration of potentially unhealthy oxidized omega-6 fats. In general, animal fats are healthy and nutritious, but seed oils such as soy and canola are not. Finally, understanding that oxalate is not carried in fats should help you feel comfortable that lotions and many skin products are low in oxalate for this same reason.

Use extracts to enhance foods. Know that extracts used in cooking or baking are generally low in oxalates. If you long for the flavor of your favorite high-oxalate spice, extracts can be a good alternative. While the taste that extracts add is often quite different from the raw equivalent, they nevertheless can be a good way to vary food flavors and keep some familiar tastes in your new low-oxalate menus. You can dilute some essential oils and use them very sparingly as seasonings in place of cumin or lemon peel. Also, many herbal preparations are extracts that are very low in oxalate. In cooking, curcumin, an extract derived from turmeric root, can replace ground turmeric (which is quite high in oxalate). There are a few minor exceptions to this rule; olive leaf extract is one such exception, but at typical doses it still doesn't have much oxalate (1 mg/teaspoon).

Choose your cooking starches carefully. A refined starch, like potato starch, is very useful as a thickener and has almost no oxalate. Neither does cornstarch. But it is important to read the fine print on the
packaging and to recognize that not every finely ground white thicken-
ing agent is a refined starch. Potato *flour* (made from powdered dried
potatoes) has a lot of oxalate (11 mg/tablespoon). Arrowroot, another
popular thickener, has 7 mg per tablespoon. Even if the product has the
word "starch" in its name, it may not have been refined. For instance,
tapioca starch is not a refined starch: it is simply dried ground tapioca,
and at 8 mg oxalate per tablespoon, it is rather high.

Watch your spice and herb amounts. Portion size is a significant factor in oxalate exposure, which can work in your favor when it comes to
spices. Allspice is really high in oxalate; 100 grams has over 1,000 mg of
oxalate, which is a lot. However, if you are using ¼ teaspoon of ground
allspice in a recipe that serves two people, you add only 5 mg oxalate, or
2.5 mg per serving. (Allspice has 20 mg per teaspoon.) No problem—
unless you are also adding other high-oxalate spices. If you like spicy or
heavily seasoned foods, the spices can add a significant amount of oxalate. For example, if a recipe intended to serve two calls for 1 teaspoon
of curry powder, the spice can contribute 12 mg of oxalate to each serving! The simplest strategy is to drop or replace the worst offender spices,
which are turmeric, cumin, and black pepper. Certain herbs, notably
parsley and basil, are also high in oxalate, and they should be used only
in small quantities.

Use caution with wheat products. Refined flours are a major (but
nutritionally unfavorable) staple of Western diets. Flours are used to
make breads, buns, macaroni, noodles, pasta, couscous, crackers, pas-
tries, cookies, and cold cereals, as well as to thicken sauces and gravies.
Wheat proteins (and other lectins) can cause gut distress and may be
ill-suited for oxalate-injured people. Even if you seem to tolerate wheat
flour, a healthy diet requires that you not make flour the centerpiece of
your diet.

Every type of wheat product, as well as most gluten-free substitutes, have some amount of oxalate. As a group, refined wheat products have the potential to deliver meaningful amounts of oxalate—especially considering the meager nutritional value they offer. Commercial white sandwich breads made with refined white flour (speedily assembled using industrial processes) are on the low end, containing 6 to 7 mg of oxalate per slice. At 12 mg for two slices, even a white bread sandwich technically becomes a high-oxalate food. The standard white bread bun for a hot dog or hamburger has about 8 mg of oxalate, while a white flour tortilla has 8 to 10 mg. White breads made using artisanal or fermentation techniques such as sourdough are likely to have similar oxalate content.

Whole-grain breads have had the bran included in the milled flour and contain about twice the oxalate compared with white flour breads. One slice of commercially made whole wheat bread has 15 to 20 mg of oxalate; dense whole-grain breads from artisanal bakeries may contain 30 to 40 mg of oxalate per slice. Multigrain breads include variable amounts of high-oxalate ingredients as well, such as chia and poppy seeds; quinoa, teff, or buckwheat; and nuts. When you see any of these items listed on the package, know that the oxalate content will be higher still—50 mg per slice, possibly even more.

Non-wheat breads and gluten-free breads vary widely in their reliance on high-oxalate ingredients, such as tapioca starch, brown rice, potato flour, rice bran, arrowroot, and nut meal. Watch out for these ingredients, as they increase oxalate content. Low-carb almond bread is, of course, off limits. One possible gluten-free, low-carb, and low-oxalate alternative is to make "bread" at home using egg whites and other low-oxalate ingredients such as coconut flour.

Of course, our use of wheat flour goes far beyond bread, buns, and pizzas. Pastas constitute a big group here. In fact, some noodle and macaroni products have tested higher in oxalate than their white-flour base would suggest. For example, cooked Mueller's Elbows (macaroni) has about 40 mg of oxalate per cup, and the tricolor version has 50 mg. A test of cooked Mueller's Thin Spaghetti measured 20 mg per cup. (Spaghetti squash, a gluten-free vegetable substitute for wheat-based noodles, has about 9 mg per cooked cup.) Lower oxalate options for pastas (which are also gluten-free) are Asian white rice noodles, Asian bean thread (cellophane) noodles, and the newly available shirataki noodles (from a plant called konjac). I do not recommend using low-oxalate pastas made with lentils or chickpeas because of their lectin content.

Another popular way to eat highly processed wheat products is ready-to-eat breakfast cereal. And, yes, the "healthier" versions can mean high oxalate content. All-Bran cereal has about 75 mg per ½ cup and shredded wheat has about 40 mg oxalate per 50 gram serving.

The oxalate content of wheat products pales in comparison to that of spinach and nuts, but it's important to be aware of it nonetheless. Even highly refined wheat flour yields a significant amount of oxalate—anywhere from 60 mg to more than 300 mg daily, if you are eating the 9 to 11 servings every day as recommended for 20 years by the 1992 USDA Food Pyramid. That is a lot of empty carbs, too. Importantly, portion size matters; keep your use of breads, pastas, and other wheat flour foods modest. Further, people who have serious health challenges related to oxalate usually do best if they eliminate gluten-containing grains while they are recovering. For bread and carb lovers who have to avoid gluten (and have been using almond flour and other high-oxalate substitutes), see the recipes available on my website for flatbreads or crackers and muffins.

Know the Effects of Preparation Techniques

Oxalates are not destroyed by cooking, but some preparation methods can change the net oxalate content. For example:

Boiling can help. Variable amounts of soluble oxalate are leached out by boiling, provided you discard the cooking liquid. Boiling medium-oxalate foods like asparagus and fresh ginger can be useful, for example. Fresh ginger has 10 mg per tablespoon but crystallized (candied) ginger has very little oxalate because it is boiled for 1 hour in water that is discarded before being cooked and coated in sugar. Tests find that boiling fresh broccoli for 12 minutes will reduce the oxalate content by at least half. People more typically boil broccoli for much less than that (3 minutes is typical), and I have not found a study showing how much oxalate is reduced with shorter boiling times. But boiling extremely high-oxalate foods is fruitless; even after a long boil, the oxalate level is reduced, yet remains extremely high.

Soaking doesn't help. There is no evidence that soaking nuts and seeds will lower their oxalate content. In fact, soaking might even increase the amount of soluble oxalate in nuts, beans, and grains, as the germinating seed accesses calcium. Soaking grains (even relatively low-oxalate ones) is a good idea to remove other plant toxins, such as phytates, but does not remove oxalate.

Lacto-fermentation mostly doesn't help. *Lacto-fermentation* of some foods (the traditional method for creating dill pickles, kimchi, sauerkraut, and yogurt) has been shown to degrade some of the oxalate in the final product versus the raw state. But these fermented foods are typically made using low-oxalate ingredients. Fermentation of high-oxalate leafy vegetables does not result in meaningful reductions in oxalate. Testing has found that after six days of fermentation, oxalate levels went down only 10 percent in amaranth greens and 14 percent in spinach (from 894 to 773 mg per 100 grams). A traditional Hawaiian food called *poi*—a starchy paste made mainly from cooked taro—is often fermented for one to two days, which reduces the oxalate content by ~18 percent, from 86 mg per 100 grams (unfermented) to 70 mg per 100 grams. With typical tunnel vision regarding food effects, some researchers suggest using poi to treat gastrointestinal disorders, on the theory that the starches support "good" bacteria. One example of fermentation making a meaningful difference in oxalate content is kombucha, a fermented tea product that is lower in oxalate (4–9 mg/cup, based on limited testing) compared with the strong tea it is made from (likely to be 25–40 mg/cup).

Now you're on your way because you have much of what you need to get started on converting your diet. It's up to you to make it happen and to keep the changes as simple as you can. But, if you've been an oxalate abuser, you may need to learn yet more about how to support your body's recovery with your lifestyle and a few supplements. That's next.

Summary and Action Steps

1. Assess your status.
   a. Use the Risks, Symptoms, and Exposures Self-Quiz in the book's Resources section and **Table 3.1** Worst Offenders list. Find the foods you eat. Take some notes: How many "offenders" are or have been in your diet? How much and how frequently do you eat them?
   b. Make a ballpark assessment: How far over "normal" (150 mg) is your regular diet?
   c. Understand the oxalate-intake zones, and see **Figure 13.1** and **Table 13.2** to determine where you are starting from.
   d. Understand the phases of transitioning from zone to zone. See **Table 13.2, Phase One: Get Out of Danger,** and **Table 13.3, Phase Two: Nuance Your Low-Oxalate Diet.**

2. Make a plan for your long-term health.
   a. Decide what changes you want to make to your diet. Write them down, along with your reasons for doing so.

b. Document and track what you're doing. Keep records so you can see that you're getting better, so you can identify any clearing-symptom setbacks, and so you can identify other issues you need be aware of.

c. Make notes about your intentions and action steps. Plan for specific actions, and when and how you'll incorporate them into your daily routines. I like using 4x6-inch blank index cards for making reminders for action items.

3. Drop the Worst Offenders foods gradually.

a. Reduce the number of high-oxalate foods you eat, the amounts of them, and the frequency. Aim to cut your oxalate intake by one-half each week until your intake is 100 to 200 mg daily.

b. Use data to meet your targets. For example, pick the one or two Worst Offender foods you will miss the least, and just eliminate them. A week later, look for a few more foods to eliminate. If you're not ready to let go of a particular food, just eat less of it, and eat more of other foods that are *very* low in oxalate.

c. Use low-oxalate foods to replenish your diet and ensure that you're eating enough calories and protein. Learn about the Safe Bet low-oxalate foods (**Table 4.4**) and the medium-oxalate foods that can help with the transition. You can use the **Swap Chart** in the Resources section for ideas. Consult **Table 14.1** for other ideas.

d. Remember that portion sizes matter a lot: practice careful portion control when using medium-oxalate foods. See the **Dosing Estimates** table in the Resources section for help with using high- and moderately high-oxalate foods.

4. Don't rush it. Succeed over time.
   a. Pause once you've gotten to "normal."
   b. Going too low too fast will not get you over the tox-
      icity any faster. In fact, it could very well make your
      symptoms worse.
   c. Take your time and avoid an on-and-off approach.
      Aim for consistency.
   d. Learn to recognize and manage the pop-up toxicity as
      your body unloads its burden.
   e. Expect the healing to take time.

5. Enjoy the new, healthier, more vibrant you with awareness.
   a. Keep self-care at the fore in your choice of foods and
      activities.
   b. Be aware of your relationship with food. Use this diet
      as an opportunity to clarify and simplify.
   c. Food is first and foremost for nourishment. It is,
      however, wrapped in layers of social meanings and
      talisman-like powers. I invite you to step back from
      this psychic jungle and set yourself free of both the
      internal dialogue and the suffocating and manipula-
      tive social pressures, both real and imagined.

15

Supporting Your Recovery

Oxalate in the body is reversible.

—A. Bergstrand et al., *British Journal of Anaesthesia*, 1972

t is quite feasible to get better from oxalate overload just by reducing your oxalate intake, but because so many of us are deficient in essential minerals and even vitamins, it may be worth also considering supplements. Supplements become especially important for people who are ill with oxalate-related symptoms or who may be at risk for kidney stones, and for those who are experiencing disruptive symptoms of clearing illness. Selecting supplements requires a bit of technical detail. I summarize some of the key information for you in this chapter to make it easier.

Adapt as Your Body Heals

The biggest obstacles to reaping health benefits from a diet of good foods with added supplements are the various factors that limit our ability to both absorb and deliver those nutrients to their intended destinations. Gut health, nutrient status, composition of your diet, your general state of inflammation, and genetic tendencies may be blocking you from using nutrients to their best advantage.

Oxalate is a big factor in creating those obstacles. As your health improves on a low-oxalate diet, the relative proportions and specific amounts of supplemental nutrients needed (or tolerated) will most likely change. Remember, your situation is dynamic, and you will need to adapt. The supplements you were taking yesterday may not be quite what you need today, or what you will need tomorrow.

Every recommendation offered here to get you started with supplements should be considered a starting point, not a definitive statement of what you need. I do not promote always using high doses or low doses; I promote using the "right dose," which you will need to determine for yourself. You should listen carefully to what your body tells you, and expect to ease up or down from your starting point. It can be helpful to keep a health journal, in which you track what you're eating, and what you're supplementing, and how you're feeling.

Lifestyle Adjustments

The most important way to support your recovery is to establish some supportive lifestyle changes. Oxalates cause physical and emotional stress, especially when you're removing them. Address the stress with some changes in how you live your life.

Get Rest and Use an Easy-Does-It Approach

Sleep and rest are healing, as is a calm and centered mind. But "calm and centered" can be elusive. Small shifts of thought or action can improve any challenging moment. Think a different thought. Decide on a small action. Engage with music, art, or your own creativity. Close your eyes and take 10 deep breaths. Attend a meditation session. Soothe your soul with compassion. Establish and maintain healthy rituals. Even if no other gain is achieved, when your mind is calmed, your body's repair process is made a little easier. And that is really something.

Bring that gentleness approach to your peripheral supports as well. Dial back the intensity of your workouts, massages, and so on. Trying to rush to the endpoint will not shorten the journey, and it will just make it harder to enjoy the benefits that happen along the way. Remember, too, that if you fall away from the diet or other healthy practices, it is okay to start, restart, and start again.

Lower Your Exposure to Toxins

Oxalate is not the only poison we face. Our modern world is toxic. Our routine daily exposure to noxious environmental toxins is excessive. Avoiding toxins, whenever possible, will help your body gain the strength needed to deal with oxalate clearing. If you haven't already made efforts to limit your exposures to chemicals, pollutants, and allergens, adopt strategies to do so now; this will support your gut health and lower your general metabolic overwhelm. A mineral-hungry and/or inflamed body is prone to absorb toxic minerals such as lead, aluminum, arsenic, bromine, chlorine, tin, copper, and fluoride.

Major sources of toxic metals in water include treated hot tubs, swimming pools, and tap water. It is prudent to avoid treated pools and hot tubs. (Tap water is discussed later in this chapter.) If you use a well for your water source, get the water tested for presence of heavy metals and other contaminants.

Avoid eating large fish that can contain mercury, especially swordfish. Choose wild-caught fish and favor small fish, such as sardines and anchovies.

Be aware that vaccines (and flu shots) may contain aluminum, formaldehyde, and thimerosal (mercury). The immune-stimulating effects of vaccines and the other residual proteins they contain (from eggs, chicken, and human cell cultures) may increase reactivity in persons with chronic inflammation and autoimmune disorders. Vaccine ingredient lists are available at the CDC.gov website.

Inexpensive imported consumer products can contain lead. For example, it has been found in lunch boxes, kids' toys and jewelry, paints and coatings, and even some foods. You can use lead test kits available at hardware stores to check for the presence of lead.

Use Sauna and Cold Therapy

Inconsistent blood flow in the small vessels can slow your healing and get you stuck in chronic pain. Thermal therapies are an effective and inexpensive support for improving your blood flow and lowering any inflammation. The following are recommended therapies.

Heat

Use heating pads wherever you have pain; doing so is great at bedtime, because it is also relaxing. (I like reusable sodium acetate pads.) Preheating your bed with a heated mattress pad can also improve sleep quality—just remember to turn it off (or unplug it) when you get into bed to avoid needless electromagnetic field exposure. If you have a history of having cold hands and feet, or have concern about your blood circulation, always keep your feet warm (for example, by wearing wool socks, even in bed).

Sauna

Heat exposure that activates the sweating process in a relaxed state can gently and safely help eliminate toxic substances of all kinds, including oxalate. A hot sauna opens and stimulates blood flow, improving delivery of nutrients and oxygen to the tissues, with benefits that are similar to exercise but with less energy expenditure. Using a sauna can improve blood pressure, reduce arterial stiffness, improve circulation and cardiac function, aid in weight loss, enhance pulmonary function and immunity, reduce inflammation, and relieve pain.

As one researcher put it, "sauna treatment may be, in effect, a lazy person's exercise with regard to health improvement." That's an important benefit, because energy can be in short supply when oxalates are on the move, and heavy exercise can prompt oxalate release and energy deficits in some people. If you are dealing with oxalate clearing illness, a regular sauna habit can fill in for intense exercise. Sauna use also supports your efforts to improve physical fitness.

Dry sauna options include the classic hot-air sauna (160 to 200°F), which are readily available in most well-equipped gyms or fitness clubs. Infrared (IR) saunas operate at much lower temperatures (100 to 160°F), making them easier to tolerate for those who are not heat-adapted. There are many options for at-home saunas on the market, with differing features and IR light wavelengths. High heat is key for good results from sauna, and near IR is the most desirable for health benefits. Red light in the visible spectrum can be irritating and stimulating to the body, so I don't encourage it as a principal sauna feature. Disadvantages of home saunas are that they do not get hot enough to induce a complete healing response, and they often outgas toxic substances from wood, glues, fabrics, and their electronics.

Note that all types of saunas will come with cautionary language and directions during pregnancy, especially IR sauna. The standard dry sauna is probably fine for use during pregnancy when following the recommendations below.

It is safe and beneficial to have a sauna session every day, but as with most of my recommendations, I urge you to start slowly with sauna therapy. Begin with 5- to 10-minute sauna therapy sessions every other day. If you find you respond by feeling worse (weak, dizzy, faint, nauseous, or headachy), shorten the sessions or try an IR sauna (if you were using a dry sauna). If you tolerate it well, increase the frequency before increasing to longer sessions. Very hot sauna sessions can eventually be up to 20 minutes, or as long as it takes to get a good sweat going, while lower temperature sauna sessions may eventually be 30 to 45 minutes.

After a sauna, it is helpful to rest at room temperature for 5 to 15 minutes to let your body recover. Even more critical, don't skip the cool after-sauna shower, which will remove toxins from the skin surface. It is also important to drink plenty of water (plus sodium and potassium) long before and after a sauna to stay hydrated.

Yoga performed in a heated space (90 to 105°F) has similar benefits to sauna if practiced with a relaxed mind and attitude. It may, however, be more strenuous than a sauna session and thus more of a challenge relative to oxalate clearing.

Cold Therapy

Cold showers, or even cold-water immersion, deliver a superficial but therapeutic cold shock to the body with no apparent side effects and at minimal cost. A 3-minute cold shower has been shown to have mood-boosting and energizing effects, perhaps by activating the sympathetic nervous system, which "primes" the body for action. Cold-stress therapies produce beta-endorphin, a neurotransmitter that's important to one's sense of well-being and pain suppression. Sauna plus a cold shower afterward is very restorative.

Here are some guidelines: Use the coldest water you can. Stay in contact with the cold water for about 3 minutes. Do not direct the cold water at the top of your head, so as to avoid core-temperature hypothermia (which could potentially activate mast cells or trigger Raynaud's syndrome in some people). Daily cold showers are fine, but *avoid* them at night (after 7 p.m.), when relaxation is most needed (nighttime is for hot baths). After a cold shower, put on your socks or slippers to maintain your core body temperature.

Get Some "Vitamin Sunlight"

Getting enough sun exposure is an important part of a healthy lifestyle that supports recovery from oxalate overload. Sunlight exposure is the best source of vitamin D, which has many health benefits, including for the cardiovascular system.

I recommend getting 15 to 20 minutes outdoors as often as you can manage, with at least your arms and face exposed (if not your whole torso) to create a baseline tolerance so that longer periods in the sun are not damaging. The less clothing you wear, the better. Early morning sunrise offers red light, and midday sunshine is especially critical. On rainy days and in the winter, you might want to use a vitamin D lamp with UV-B bulbs. Start with short sessions and work your way up to about 12 minutes every day, either in the morning or at midday, until your skin has acclimated to the UV light. However, understanding your own tolerance and personal sensitivity to sunlight is important, and you should get only as much as you comfortably can tolerate.

Sun exposure is frequently viewed as "all bad" and has been wrongly blamed as a primary cause of skin cancer. Blaming sunlight for cancer development simplistically ignores many other factors that make skin more easily damaged by the sun. People's indoor work and schooling, for example, give them an on-and-off relationship with the sun during the week, then they eagerly take their untrained skin outside on sunny summer weekends and vacations. Additionally, certain supplements, many drugs (including several antibiotics), and some personal care products can increase the risk of sunburn. An often-overlooked factor that may dramatically increase the risk of skin damage is the regular consumption of seed oils such as corn, canola, and soy. Often labeled "vegetable oil," seed oils are rich in oxidized omega-6 fats (specifically linoleic acid) extracted with solvents and heated to extreme temperatures. Seed oils are also used in margarine, salad dressings, mayonnaise, chips, fries, and other common commercial foods. Grain-fed chicken is another source of omega-6 linoleic acid; however, poultry will not have the same detrimental effects as seed oils provided it is cooked with gentle heat.

Heightened *photosensitivity* from drugs, seed oils, and other modern lifestyle factors hampers our ability to tolerate sun without cancer-causing harm. The use of margarine and salad oils has been widespread since the 1970s and may be partly responsible for the huge increase in skin cancers in recent decades. Conversely, the omega-3 fats provided by seafoods are skin protective and may improve our sun tolerance in the context of a low omega-6 polyunsaturated fatty acid diet. The key point here is that avoiding the seed oils and eating salmon and sardines will likely improve your sun tolerance.

In another example of foods influencing the development of skin cancer, know that fruits, berries, beans, peas, and other tannin-rich foods act as co-carcinogens, promoting the effects of other carcinogens that cause skin (and other) cancers. Sunscreens are also problematic. They block an important benefit of sun exposure—vitamin D production—and may be partly responsible for the low vitamin D levels that are so common today. There is also some concern about the direct toxic effects of sunscreen lotions.

Routine exposure to the sun is good for you, provided your lifestyle, diet, and medications are not creating excessive photosensitivity.

Supplements

As we saw earlier, oxalate overload creates a need for extra nutrients. In conjunction with your dietary changes and adoption of a healthy lifestyle, your body probably will continue to need extra nutrients to recover from oxalate overload. Supplemental vitamins and minerals help correct nutrient deficiencies and may lower the amount of oxalate produced in the body. Supplements can ease the symptoms and side effects of oxalate de-accumulation as well.

The need for extra nutrients does not disappear once oxalate intake has gone down. In fact, you may need more nutrients as the oxalate clearing exposes you to oxalate from old deposits. Nutrients, especially minerals, are critically needed to safely escort oxalate out of the body. Oxalate-induced damage to metabolic pathways may also increase the need for nutrients. Diet alone may not be enough to meet those heightened nutritional needs.

For example, when your body is struggling with chronic inflammation, leaky gut, and oxalate overload, you will need adequate calcium. Not many foods are particularly good sources of calcium beyond milk (~280 mg per cup), cheese (~200 mg per ounce), and the bones of animals (3 ounces of sardines have ~300 mg). Cruciferous greens are decent calcium sources (1 cup of boiled cabbage has about 70 mg of calcium; boiled mustard greens have 105 mg per cup; and boiled kale has 170 mg per cup). But greens don't begin to reach the recommended daily intake of 1,000 to 1,300 mg of calcium.

Thoughtful supplementation, when combined with a diet of high-quality, digestible, nutrient-dense food, is the most effective and least toxic route to correct a chronic nutrient shortfall and to rebuild health.

Be Ready to Adjust and Adapt

There is no one-size-fits all protocol for nutrient replacement and supplementation. However, some general information can guide your decisions. Once you understand your options, you will be able to (gradually) find your way to what works for you. Although I mention specific supplements and target amounts, think of these as starting points. What works for many people may not work for you. Pulling it all together takes time, effort, and attention to what your body is trying to tell you.

The safety of the supplements I suggest gives you the freedom to experiment and find what works best for you. Often there is an adjustment process when using supplemental nutrients. Initial effects may involve unpleasant reactions. Remember, too, that the dynamic processes of clearing oxalate toxicity and metabolic recovery are moving targets. What worked or did not work last week may give you a different effect the next time you try it. That means you need to stay open-minded, double back later, and try again in smaller doses if your first efforts did not seem to agree with you. Experiment and see what works.

Also remember that the ability of supplements to nourish you is a double-edged sword. Nutrients can also encourage oxalate release from the tissues! If you get difficult and persistent signs of oxalate release, and you have been taking relatively high levels of supplements, cutting back may slow the oxalate clearing and lead to relief from the acute effects. Likewise, you should be deliberate when adding nutrients to your new health routine, especially if you are experiencing heavy symptoms. Note what you are taking and see how your body responds. Adding more supplements may not always be what you need. Avoid traumatizing your body with abrupt increases or decreases in supplements.

Nutrient "Dependency"

Some individuals may find they need fairly high amounts of certain supplements indefinitely to feel well. Oxalate toxicity can change a person's metabolic pathways (how our cells work), perhaps owing to *epigenetic* influences. Epigenetic means that environmental and lifestyle factors have altered gene expression and have affected cell function. The resulting functional imbalances can even be inherited, and may create *vitamin dependencies*. That altered metabolism may require higher amounts of some B vitamins and minerals to achieve normal functioning and well-being. Increasing your nutrient intake can be like running a lot of fast-moving water onto a rusted waterwheel turning an old-fashioned mill. The waterwheel would turn easily if it were not so rusted, but we can partly overcome its resistance if enough water flows

over it. In adding nutrients to the body, we can help overcome the metabolic blockages—the functional "rust"—that are promoted by oxalate
toxicity.

Essential Minerals

My top, "magical" supplement picks are a handful of basic minerals,
some of which are needlessly controversial. The key minerals are calcium, magnesium, and potassium. Good old salt is also important,
along with sulfur and trace minerals (including boron and silicon).
Minerals may be delivered as capsules, but you can also get them by
dissolving mineral powders in drinking water, and by skin transfer
through foot soaks, mineral baths, even topical lotions or sprays.

Minerals are essential co-factors that activate B vitamins. The value
of calcium has been mentioned throughout this book, but all minerals
are important and are at risk of deficiency. Mineral supplements also
provide an easy way to get citrates (which I discuss on page 256). Minerals generally improve kidney function and lower the risk of kidney
stones, but please note: If you suspect you have compromised kidney
function, have your doctor monitor your kidneys before you begin using
even modest doses of potassium and magnesium, and get your kidney
function checked frequently.

Myths Regarding Minerals

A popular internet myth holds that if you just get enough minerals like
calcium and magnesium in your diet, you can eat any amount of oxalate with impunity. In reality, no exposure management strategy (be it
boiling all your food or taking extra minerals) is any match for the
amount of oxalate we're sending down our throats. No technique or
supplement can work unless you first undertake the most basic step:
lowering your oxalate intake to a level that is aligned with what your

biology can handle. The advice that follows is in addition to low-oxalate eating, not in place of it.

Calcium

In biology, calcium is a mineral superstar. Calcium is involved in a huge range of bodily processes, including bone formation and conduction of nerve signals. Many of oxalate's most dire effects arise directly as a result of interrupting the body's access to and use of calcium. Dietary and supplemental calcium may be the most important nutrient for supporting a safe recovery from oxalate overload. Adequate calcium intake also helps to prevent kidney stones.

Calcium's primary recovery function is to bind oxalate and remove it via the colon, where calcium oxalate is excreted via the feces. Supplementing the diet's calcium can also address deficiencies caused by oxalate's binding the calcium inside the cells. Loss of bone calcium may originate not just in inadequate calcium intake but also because the body borrows calcium from the bones to make up for electrolyte imbalances caused by oxalate.

Claims abound that calcium supplements have some potential for causing calcifications in the body. If you've read this far, you understand that the presence of calcium deposits does not mean that calcium caused the problem. Indeed, supplementing your calcium intake has many documented benefits. For example, according to a recent consensus paper, taking calcium supplements might prevent cardiovascular illness. The authors found that calcium supplement–takers have a lower risk of death in all age groups, have no difference in coronary artery calcification scores, and show no increased risk of atherosclerosis. Another review study found cardiovascular benefits from calcium supplements and slightly lower blood pressure in people with normal blood pressure, while it also found no adverse effects. Calcium is known to be calming and helpful for getting good sleep!

Generally, calcium supplements are an important and safe precaution—even in the context of a diet that normally includes dairy foods like cheese, yogurt, and milk—and have pain-reducing benefits for the process of oxalate clearance.

Dosing Your Calcium Supplements

You can use calcium supplements in any combination of bulk powder, tablets, or capsules. And you can use any combination of types (citrate, pyruvate, or others) as long as there is no vitamin D added (see page 238). Here is information on the types of calcium supplements.

Calcium citrate (with no added vitamin D and no added herbs). Citrate is a good way to provide minerals in supplements, which is why calcium citrate is popular and is considered by some to be the optimum calcium supplement. NOW Foods, Pure Organic Ingredients, and several other brands sell it as bulk powder. There are many options for buying it in tablets, too (including KAL Vitamins, Allergy Research Group, Vitamin Shoppe, and GNC brands—select one with the least amount of fillers possible).

Calcium pyruvate (with no added vitamin D). I find this is a good, well-tolerated supplement if calcium citrate does not agree with you for any reason (such as constipation). Calcium pyruvate is available in capsules; look for NOW Sports brand.

The base dosage. If you are not already taking calcium, start low— about 400 mg a day in divided doses. If that is well tolerated, gradually work up to a maintenance dose of 1,000 to 1,600 mg/day. If you eat a lot of milk and cheese, your maintenance dose may be lower—600 to 800 mg. If you're timid about taking calcium owing to fears of constipation, try the following step approach.

In three or four daily steps: Start with 200 or 250 mg calcium (as citrate or pyruvate) at bedtime for about a week, then double that amount by also taking it before breakfast for three to five days, then increase it again, with an afternoon dose. Maintain that for least a week, and if you tolerate that dose, double the evening dose and continue to increase at other convenient times until you reach about 1,200 mg daily.

Other timing options: Take calcium 15 to 30 minutes before meals or 1 to 2 hours before your "worst time of day"—times of low energy, low mood, increased pain, and so on. Dr. Clive Solomons's research and reports from the members of the VP Foundation suggest that you might "preempt" or proactively take the edge off of pain or relieve other symptoms associated with oxalate clearance by timing the calcium supplement prior to periods when the symptoms periodically intensify. The pain-reducing benefits may come from the alkalizing effects of the citrate and the calcium.

Adjusting your dose and schedule: When oxalate-related symptoms are occurring, it might help to temporarily adjust your calcium dose either up or down by 200 to 400 mg. It's fine to take as much as 1,800 mg daily, if you find that it helps with symptoms. If the calcium citrate seems to create symptoms or unpleasant side effects, take less; if a lower dose doesn't help, try a different type of calcium.

Vitamin D in Calcium Supplements

There are many forms of calcium available, and the most important feature you need is the *absence* of vitamin D. Keeping your vitamin D separate (by 2 hours or more) allows more of the calcium to remain in the colon, where it lowers net oxalate absorption and supports oxalate excretion. Calcium's benefits are optimized when taken without vitamin D.

In cases of low vitamin D status, the ideal approach is to optimize your sunlight exposure while boosting the sulfur levels in your skin. (I explain how to do that on page 231). The vitamin D created in the skin following sunlight exposure occurs in a bioavailable form that is more easily delivered to the tissues.

If you have a vitamin D deficiency and feel you need to take vitamin D, take it as a stand-alone product at least 2 hours away from the times you take your calcium. For those who need it, I usually suggest taking vitamin D on a periodic schedule (weekly or monthly) in moderate-to-high doses (5,000–20,000 IU), depending on need.

Magnesium

The mineral magnesium is important to cellular energy and thiamine metabolism, both of which can be impaired by oxalate. And while calcium helps oxalate not enter the body (and leave via the feces), magnesium helps oxalate get out without crystallizing.

Good food sources of magnesium are fish, crab meat, molasses, and yogurt, but foods can't begin to make up for magnesium deficiency, which is common. If you are prone to headaches, migraine, or depression, low magnesium may be contributing to the problem. Without adequate magnesium, recovery from oxalate toxicity is difficult. In the gut, magnesium can also bind oxalate and reduce absorption.

Dosing Your Magnesium Supplements

Magnesium is available in many forms, including citrate, carbonate, chloride, malate, gluconate, L-threonate, and others. Different forms vary in their magnesium content, bioavailability, and tolerance. One option is to take a combination product, but I suggest you try different forms separately to see which and how much works best for you. Magnesium gluconate (or calcium gluconate) is acceptable, but the glycinate form is less desirable if used in large amounts because high levels of glycine could be partially converted into oxalate in the body.

L-threonate has increased ability to cross into the brain and might be therapeutic for pelvic pain, depression, and memory problems. Magnesium citrate is a convenient way to get both magnesium and citrate. But magnesium can act as a laxative; if you don't want this effect, choose liquid magnesium chloride, magnesium malate, magnesium L-threonate, or magnesium carbonate, and adjust the amount to avoid watery stools or diarrhea.

A starting dose of magnesium may depend on the form you choose and if it prompts loose stools. Begin with ~200 mg and gradually add doses at other times, increasing to ~600 mg per day (in three doses). The amount tolerated without diarrhea is very individual. Unless you have kidney failure, oral magnesium cannot cause excessive magnesium in the body.

As with calcium and potassium, you can use tablets or capsules, or bulk powder. Start at the lower dose and increase over a week or two to bowel tolerance. If your stools become very soft or you have diarrhea, just cut back. Magnesium is good to take at bedtime because it has relaxing effects and may improve sleep. Magnesium is a key ingredient in mineral baths, as I later explain (page 252).

Potassium

Hardly anyone gets enough potassium in their diet, especially women. The Recommended Dietary Allowance (RDA) is 4,700 mg, but women in their 20s and 30s average only about 2,300 mg. And, based on my experience, cellular shortages of potassium seem to accompany oxalate clearing. Cellular potassium deficiency can lead to fatigue, weakness, muscle knots, cramps, and constipation. Potassium is especially important while the body is undergoing metabolic stress such as removing oxalate from the tissues (which goes on for years as long as a low-oxalate diet is maintained).

Medical science is clear on two points: (1) taking supplemental potassium has many potential benefits, although health-care workers are generally unaware of the broad need for potassium; and (2) potassium can be dangerous for people in chronic renal failure, who cannot clear excessive potassium from the blood. If you are in the hospital with kidney problems, be very wary of potassium. For the rest of us, the benefits of higher potassium intake are far-ranging, from improved carbohydrate tolerance to rebuilding demineralized bones and the prevention of bone loss in the first place.

High potassium intake prevents fibrosis and kidney-stone formation and reduces urine calcium levels. It also protects the cells by directly inhibiting free radical formation by immune cells. Potassium can reduce muscle knots and cramps, prevent headaches, lower blood pressure, stabilize blood sugar, rebuild thinning bones, and improve muscle and nerve performance. But be aware that it can take weeks to months of supplementation to restore healthy levels in the heart, muscles, and connective tissues.

BOX 15.1: POTASSIUM (MG) PER 50-CALORIE PORTIONS OF SELECTED FOODS

Item	MG Potassium	50-Calorie Serving Size
Avocado	150	2.2 Tbs.
Banana chips	50	2 Tbs. (0.33 oz.)
Bananas	100–200	½ medium fruit
Bok choy (boiled)	1,550	2½ C
Broccoli rabe	650	1½ C
Brown rice (boiled)	35	3¼ Tbs.
Cantaloupe	395	1½ C
Coconut water	430	1 C
Corn Chex cereal	20	7 Tbs. / 13 g
Egg (large)	40	⅔ large egg
Honeydew	315	¾ C
Milk (whole)	120	⅓ C
Mushrooms, portobello	920	23 oz.
Mushrooms, white button	260	8 oz.

(box continues)

Item	MG Potassium	50-Calorie Serving Size
Onions	190	0.6 C chopped
Papaya	330	0.5 C
Parsnips	250	⅓ C mashed
Pineapple	108	⅔ C
Potato, Red Skin (boiled)	310	2 oz.
Rutabaga	420	¾ C mashed
Steak, flank	90	1 oz.
Turnips (cooked)	405	1½ C pieces

Source: J. A. Pennington and J. Spungen, Bowes and Church's Food Values

Low-oxalate food sources of potassium include bok choy, mushrooms, milk, coconut water, and many fruits such as cantaloupe. **Box 15.1** compares the potassium content of various foods per 50-calorie portion. Incidentally, half the potassium in a banana is in the peel. Claims of banana's high potassium content are based on old testing of *un*peeled bananas. (I still can't be sure that testing reported for bananas is for peeled banana, so it is indicated here as a range.) Still, you'd have to eat about 1,200 calories of bananas (with 200 mg potassium per 50 calories) to meet the recommended daily potassium intake. That would be a formula for developing diabetes, protein malnutrition, and many vitamin deficiencies.

Dosing Your Potassium Supplements

Potassium is typically taken either as potassium citrate, potassium bicarbonate, or potassium chloride (the latter is a frequent ingredient in low-sodium salt substitutes). If you have any doubt about your kidney function, you should get it evaluated by a doctor. And persons with chronic kidney disease should consult with a doctor about any limits on potassium intake. The *estimated Glomerular Filtration Rate* (eGFR) is one standard indicator of how well your kidneys are doing, and this is included in the standard comprehensive blood test. As long as the eGFR is over 60, your kidneys are clearing excess potassium easily.

If your kidneys are working adequately, it is safe to begin taking 800 mg of potassium per day. A recommended and available supplement is 99 mg *potassium citrate* capsules. Begin at a modest dose of one (99 mg) or two capsules (198 mg) three or four times a day. Gradually increase to ~2,500 mg per day in divided doses—which is well under the Recommended Dietary Allowance (RDA; 4,700 mg) and is less than half the dose used in clinical trials for lowering blood pressure and cardiovascular disease risk factors.

Timing and delivery method can make a meaningful difference. One of my clients made his own gelatin caps with pure potassium citrate powder and wrote this: "After taking the potassium caps with lunch, I did not get any type of headache. I also had my first normal bowel movement in a long time. It could have been coincidence, but I plan on using the potassium this way from now on." Potassium citrate is best taken with food to avoid stomach irritation and improve assimilation into the cells. If you notice stomach irritation when taken in higher doses, cut back and take the capsules only with meals.

If you tolerate potassium citrate well and want to make taking sufficient potassium convenient, try adding modest amounts of bulk powder to your drinking water and sip it all day long. I suggest you first try my formula for enhanced alkaline drinking water (**Table 15.3**, page 251). That water supplies about 70 mg potassium per 8 fluid ounces. Add additional bulk powder as needed, or you can use my Salty Sport Drink (**Table 15.2**, page 246). If you are taking capsules and adding bulk powder dissolved in water, be sure to keep track of the total dose. For mixing larger quantities, **Table 15.1** (page 244) shows how to estimate mineral amounts in bulk supplements.

Table 15.1: Volume-to-Mineral Conversion for Bulk Supplements

	Potassium		Calcium Citrate	Magnesium Citrate
	Citrate	Bicarbonate		
Weight per 1 tsp. (5 ml)	3,900 mg	4,200 mg	1,520 mg	3,000 mg
Percent of mineral	38%	39%	24%	16%
Mineral per 1 tsp. (5 ml)	1,480 mg	1,630 mg	365 mg	480 mg
Mineral per ¼ tsp. (1.25 ml)	350 mg	408 mg	90 mg	120 mg
Mineral per ⅛ tsp. (0.63 ml)	175 mg	205 mg	45 mg	60 mg
Recommended Daily Intake	4,700 mg		1,300 mg	400 mg (Male) 310 mg (Female)

Source: Dietary Reference Intakes (DRI) for minerals, Food and Nutrition Board, Institute of Medicine, National Academies.

Salt and/or Sodium

Sodium, in concert with other key electrolytes and minerals (especially potassium), has the power to maintain the battery-like electromagnetic charges that power life's biochemistry. Sodium is very important to the proper function of the adrenal glands. Additionally, too little sodium can contribute to low blood sugar, lethargy, and heart palpitations. In short, you need sodium—and a lot more of it than you might guess.

High oxalate creates conditions that deplete sodium, and too little sodium in the body turns on the sodium-retaining hormones that may increase fibrosis. To have a good electrolyte balance, it may be important to match your potassium intake with your sodium intake and vice versa. Potassium belongs inside healthy cells (especially muscle and bone cells), and sodium is high outside of the cells.

Salt is the principal source of sodium in our diet. When I recommend "salt," I mean mineral salt such as Redmond Real Salt or Himalayan pink salt. Both these salt types naturally contain traces of many important minerals, including iodine. (Avoid table salt because it is overly purified, treated with excessive heat, and has undesirable additives.)

Begin using mineral salt as a nutrient by introducing the healthful practice of salting your food to taste with good-quality mineral salt. In addition to diet, take salt in water or make an electrolyte drink that includes potassium as well. Experiment with using salt as a nutrient and/ or supplement. Go beyond what you use to season your food by at least ½ teaspoon per day for the first five days. (See **Table 15.2**, Salty Sport Drink, for one option for doing this.)

Salt can also lower your cravings for sweet stuff, and maybe hunger in general. You can suck on coarse grains of Himalayan pink salt to "treat" those cravings for sweets, wine, chocolate, and other stuff you wish to avoid. Introduce the healthful practice of salt supplementation gradually. Work up to as much as 2 teaspoons added salt per day.

BOX 15.2: SUPPLEMENTING YOUR SALT INTAKE IMPROVES THE FOLLOWING

- ✦ Hydration (good for kidneys)
- ✦ Blood circulation
- ✦ Exercise tolerance
- ✦ Brain function
- ✦ Stress tolerance
- ✦ Heat tolerance
- ✦ Fatigue
- ✦ Joint pain

How do you judge how well your body likes the salt? Remember, getting the nutrients you need can trigger oxalate release and launch feelings of unwellness. However, in general, you should feel more consistently energetic and more mentally focused thanks to salt supplementation. Back off on the salt if you have signs of water retention, such as swelling ankles. If you are salt-sensitive in terms of blood pressure, it may indicate a need for potassium (and calcium). If you are an endurance athlete or practice regular sauna, increase your salt intake to meet this extra need.

Try the electrolyte/sports drink recipe in **Table 15.2**. Drink it throughout the day (between meals) and especially in the evenings (instead of evening snacking). Drink it during the hour prior to exercise for a better workout. Becoming hydrated with salt may make you less thirsty and more able to tolerate longer periods without water because you are not depleted. (This can be helpful when traveling by plane.)

Salty Sports Drink

My approach to getting therapeutic doses of salt, along with potassium and other trace minerals, is this formula for a Salty Sport Drink (**Table 15.2**). The directions are for preparing one portion.

Table 15.2: Salty Sport Drink

Place the ingredients in a clean large glass jar or bottle. Add water, cover tightly, and shake well. Allow to sit for at least 30 minutes before consuming. Consume within 48 hours.

Ingredient	Amount	Source
Reverse osmosis or ionized water, prepared as in **Table 15.3** with potassium and trace minerals	24 ounces (3 cups or 710 ml)	Local source, plus minerals
Organic vinegar or lemon juice	2–3 tsp. (to taste)	Grocery

Ingredient	Amount	Source
Salt	½–1 tsp. (1.8–3.5 g)	Himalayan pink salt or Real Salt
Potassium bicarbonate (powder)*	¼ tsp. (1.5 ml, 0.7 g)	Bulk online, multiple sources
Potassium citrate (powder)*	¼ tsp. (1.5 ml, 0.7 g)	Bulk online, multiple sources
Magnesium citrate*	⅛ tsp. (1 ml, 0.5 g)	Bulk online, multiple sources
ReMyte Mineral Solution (optional) †	½ tsp. (2.5 ml)	RNAReset.com
High-quality pure maple syrup or other unrefined natural or organic sugar (optional). Avoid stevia and zero-calorie sweeteners.	4 tsp. (20 ml) (adds 18 g carbs)	Multiple sources

* Buy bulk powder online for use in drinking water and also use bicarbonate for bathing.

† If not using ReMyte, consider taking trace minerals in capsules or try other liquid electrolyte formulas, such as LyteShow, or E-Lyte if the taste is acceptable. Note: If you can't get used to the taste, there are options: (1) omit the ReMyte and magnesium citrate for a few weeks, then try smaller amounts after that; (2) add coconut water, maple syrup, or minimal amounts of another sweetener until you get used to it; (3) swallow salt and minerals as you would capsules taken with ample water or food.

Keep in mind that if you add sweetener as one of the options, drinking sweetened fluids is generally not recommended and can be habit-forming. However, it is unlikely to pose any issues if you maintain a low-carb diet (under 150 grams per day) and are physically active. This sports drink is one way to increase your carbohydrates if you are following a very low-carb diet, such as the carnivore (all meat) diet, or are otherwise limiting consumption of plant fiber owing to gastrointestinal issues. Alternatively, adding coconut water to the mix has the benefit of contributing valuable potassium and is very refreshing after a workout or a hot sauna. Coconut water has 2 mg of oxalate per cup, whereas the basic Salty Sport Drink has none.

Sulfur

Sulfur is an essential mineral needed throughout the body. We need a lot of it, yet sulfur's role in human well-being is generally overlooked. Sulfur metabolism and sulfur deficiency are not discussed in most nutrition textbooks, for example. Sulfur requirements are assumed to be met by the sulfur-containing amino acids that are abundant in animal proteins, including eggs, meats, and milk. Although hard drinking water, cabbage-family vegetables, onions, and garlic also contain sulfur (especially if grown in sulfur-rich soil), deficiency of the sulfur amino acids (methionine, cysteine, cystine, homocysteine, homocystine, and taurine) can occur in vegans, children, or persons with HIV. Our need for sulfur is yet another reason that animal foods are important to human health.

Sulfur has great therapeutic potential for many conditions related to oxalate overload. Sulfur-containing compounds can lower oxidative damage and inflammation and promote healing. For example, MSM (methylsulfonylmethane, also known as dimethylsulfone or DMSO2), penetrates cells readily and can be used topically and orally for treating allergies, pain syndromes, arthritis, gastritis, post-exercise soreness, athletic injuries, interstitial cystitis and other bladder disorders, and inflammatory conditions generally. MSM is also good for the skin, vascular system, and stomach lining; it may have anti-cancer benefits; and it supports the repair and regeneration of bones and teeth. Other sulfur compounds, such as SAMe, dimethylsulfoxide (DMSO), taurine, and glutathione, may also help with fibromyalgia, arthritis, interstitial cystitis, injuries, depression, diabetes, and cancer.

My clients vary widely in their initial tolerance for sulfur supplements such as MSM—even though it is nontoxic, many don't tolerate it. In addition to baths (discussed on page 252) using magnesium sulfate (Epsom salts), I generally suggest beginning using MSM in a topical lotion or gel applied to the feet, hands, and areas of pain at bedtime and after bathing.

If good results occur, regular mineral baths may be adequate for boosting sulfur and for pain relief and at times of elevated inflammation, and to support connective tissue repair. Or you can experiment with taking MSM or other sulfur compounds orally. The suggested dose of MSM is to begin with 0.5 gram or 1 gram twice daily, and, if well tolerated, gradually increase to as much as 3 grams twice daily—perhaps on an as-needed basis. If it makes you feel worse, you may need to take a trace mineral supplement containing molybdenum for a month or so before taking MSM; molybdenum facilities sulfur metabolism.

Silicon

Connective tissue symptoms can persist or recur over the course of the oxalate clearing. Some people may experience hair loss, tendinitis, or joint and back pain. Bone repair and connective tissue formation require many trace nutrients, including the nontoxic mineral silicon. Although breathing silica crystals is toxic, taking silicon orally is not toxic.

Supplementing with bioavailable silicon (for example, BioSil) seems to have a number of benefits, helping with joint instability or pain, thinning bones, back problems, hyper-mobile joints, wrinkly skin, and poor circulation. Silicon can be more effective than collagen for connective tissue health, and it may be an especially important supplement for older people. In combination with low-oxalate eating, potassium citrate and silicon may help arrest and reverse bone loss in postmenopausal years.

Trace Minerals

There are several trace minerals that may support your return to better health. Consider use of a trace mineral complex supplement containing boron, iodine, zinc, selenium, copper, manganese, chromium, and molybdenum. Designs for Health, Pure Encapsulations, and Klaire Labs brands offer full-spectrum trace minerals in capsules.

Water

In addition to taking sensible daily precautions regarding environmental toxins, taking some control over the water you use can reduce your exposure to toxins and help increase your intake of minerals.

Tap water may contain not only toxic metals but also many other additives (acrylamide, bromate, fluoride, chloramines, etc.) and contaminants (the pesticides 2,4-D and glyphosate, asbestos, atrazine, benzene, chlordane, cyanide, lindane, styrene, vinyl chloride, etc.). Carbon filters can remove a limited number of contaminants, notably bacteria, particulate impurities, and chlorine.

Drinking bottled water is not a good solution. Most bottled water contains plastic residues picked up from its packaging, and it may contain other chemicals as well. (I call bottled water "plastic tea.") That's because bottled waters are frequently sourced from tap water; the effort the manufacturer spends in fixing it up is usually focused on taste, not removing toxins.

The best alternative for reducing your exposure to toxins in tap water is to drink filtered water with adequate minerals added. There are many effective filters and water products available to consumers. Carbon filtration is better than nothing for showering or bathing, but I recommend more highly purified *and* mineral-enhanced water for drinking. If you use any type of home water-filtration equipment, it is important to replace the filters and perform other maintenance regularly. If you are using well water, it is important to have it tested by a reputable lab for toxins and mineral content.

Reverse osmosis (RO) water filtration removes most contaminants in tap water. You can get home equipment, or you can buy RO water in bulk from dispensers in many health food stores. Good water is fundamental to health, but it's not free nor easy. Naturally sourced water, such as clean well water or true spring water, is great if you can get it, but for most uses, highly filtered water is a good starting point.

Improving Purified Waters

The RO process strips out the toxins, but it also removes the nutritive minerals, including calcium, magnesium, and sulfur. That is not good in the long run, as water is an important source of minerals. Some RO systems and similar de-ionized water filters restore trace amounts of the calcium or magnesium that would normally be present. But manufacturers of these systems often do not report the mineral type or the amounts in the water.

Being exceptionally low in necessary minerals, purified water can be improved by adding trace minerals and a touch of potassium. See **Table 15.3** for ways to improve your water so it is healthy for the whole family. You can use it as a basis for all drinks, including the Salty Sport Drink (**Table 15.2**), or in tea and coffee. Being slightly alkaline, it makes coffee taste smoother.

Table 15.3: Potassium-Enhanced RO Purified Drinking Water (per Gallon)

Instructions: Combine the listed ingredients in a clean glass jar and consume within one week. To sterilize glass jars after washing, bake the jar at 250°F for 20 minutes.

Ingredient	Amount	Source
Reverse osmosis water (or tested well water)	1 gallon (3.8 L)	Local source
Potassium bicarbonate (powder)*	¼ teaspoon (1.5 ml, 0.7 g) ~400 mg potassium For ionized waters, decrease the bicarbonate by one-half	Bulk online, multiple sources

(table continues)

(Table 15.3 continued)

Ingredient	Amount	Source
Potassium citrate (powder)*	¾ teaspoon (4 ml, 2g) ~1,050 mg potassium	Bulk online, multiple sources
Electrolyte liquid—trace minerals such as LyteShow (omit when using well water)	1 teaspoon (5 ml)	Online, multiple sources
ReMyte Mineral Solution or equivalent product (optional)	1 teaspoon (5 ml)	RNAReset.com— other brands may suffice

Note: Measuring these powders by volume is imprecise; weight measures are more accurate. In mixing at home, aim for ballpark figures, even though specific numbers are given here. Or get a digital milligram scale for about $25.

*Buy bulk powder online for use in drinking water and also use bicarbonate for bathing. Can use sodium bicarbonate too. For alkaline (hydroxide-enhanced) ionized waters, decrease bicarbonate by half. (Note: A water ionizer uses electrical current to artificially break the water molecule into positive hydrogen atoms and negative hydroxide ions.) The amounts of added minerals I suggest are based on taste. If you don't like the flavor, add about half the nutrients listed. Once you get used to that level of minerals, increase to about ¾ of amounts suggested. And once you are used to that, try increasing again.

Mineral Bathing

Immersion in mineral-rich water, such as a hot mineral spring, is an ancient form of spa hydrotherapy, used for restoration, pain relief, and to lower stress. By soaking in a mineral solution, your skin absorbs minerals, which helps address acute symptoms of oxalate overload. This practice may also support the longer process of restoring minerals to many tissues of the body without causing gut irritation. Magnesium, potassium, sulfur, bicarbonate, and other electrolytes are readily absorbed through the skin. Sulfur and other minerals also help the skin produce vitamin D.

For therapy bathing, I suggest a broad spectrum of minerals to support absorption of whatever is most needed. See **Table 15.4** for a basic formula. Start with what you can easily find, such as sea salt, Epsom salts, baking soda, and a touch of borax (for the essential nutrient boron). Potassium bicarbonate (easily purchased online) is a useful addition.

How to begin: For a gentle start, the right "dose" is about one 15-minute foot soak every other day. To make a foot bath, use about one-fourth of each of the ingredients listed in **Table 15.4**. This solution will be more concentrated compared to a full-body tub bath, as a crude adjustment for the relatively small body surface area involved in the foot bath. Use very hot water. Increase the soaking time to 20 or 25 minutes if it feels good to do so. If that does not aggravate your symptoms, progress to a full-body hot mineral bath as often as time allows and your symptoms dictate—I suggest at least twice a week. If you are sure the bath is helping, take them daily. Some of my clients find they benefit from mineral baths twice a day when clearing symptoms are heavy.

If you lack a tub or haven't the time, mix a solution of the minerals and use a spray bottle to apply it to your skin after a daily shower, then let it dry.

Table 15.4: Mineral Bath Formula for General Use

Ingredient	Amount	Source
Potassium bicarbonate (powder)	½ cup (120 ml)	Bulk online, multiple sources
Sea salts	½ cup (120 ml)	Bulk source, sold at natural food stores
Baking soda	⅓ cup (80 ml)	Buy in bulk (e.g., Costco)
Epsom salts (no additives)	2 cups (480 ml)	Buy pure in bulk (e.g., Costco)
Borax (for boron) (common laundry additive; optional)	3 tsp. (15 ml)	Grocery store

Note: Consider swapping bulk magnesium chloride for the Epsom salts, if you are sulfur-sensitive.

Citrates for Lowering Acidity

Citric acid is a ubiquitous metabolic molecule, and the namesake of the *citric acid cycle* inside the mitochondria where the energy from food becomes cell energy. Citric acid (or citrate) in the urine and elsewhere binds to calcium oxalate crystals and weakens them, helping to dissolve the deposits in the kidneys and elsewhere. Oral intake of citrate is a well-established, highly effective, and well-tolerated treatment for kidney stones. Whether the source is a supplement, a food additive, or lemon juice, citric acid is helpful for getting the oxalate safely out of the body.

The citrate sticks to and softens oxalate crystals. Citrate also increases the protective effects of other anti-clumping molecules in the urine. Citrate may help you feel better because it also reduces osteopontin levels (see Chapter 10), protects against oxalate-induced oxidative stress, and corrects acidic conditions that can cause malaise. Citrate also promotes strong bones and teeth and, along with potassium, may stop or even reverse the loss of bone in osteopenia, osteoporosis, and other disorders of bone fragility in both stone formers and non-stone-forming people. As a client noted, "I can't thank you enough; 24 hours and the juice of 5 lemons later and I am so much better! Nausea is gone. I made some other adjustments too but this is dramatic and unexpected."

Unchecked acidic conditions from any cause can lower urinary citrate, which can then increase oxalates' power to crystalize and damage the kidneys and other tissues. Bicarbonate can also reduce tissue acidity and increase citrate excretion and urinary pH. Meanwhile, the liver turns some citrate into bicarbonate, which stimulates the kidney cells to release and excrete protective citrate into the urine.

Lemon Juice

Lemons, as citrus fruits, are an excellent source of citric acid and citrate. Several studies have demonstrated that about ½ cup of lemon juice daily is nearly as effective in reducing kidney-stone reoccurrence as potassium citrate treatment. Lemons are also very helpful in addressing the acidosis that accompanies oxalate clearing and other inflammatory states.

To use fresh lemons therapeutically, consume at least two per day. Take them straight—as a shot, or as hot lemonade (with hot water and an optional touch of sweetener), or as Alkalizing Lemon Fizz (see **Box 15.3**), which simply adds bicarbonate and water to lemon juice to create an even more alkalizing citrate drink. Enjoy the fizzy drink in the morning, the evening, or whenever you need a boost.

BOX 15.3: ALKALIZING LEMON FIZZ

¼ cup fresh lemon juice

⅛ teaspoon potassium bicarbonate

⅛ teaspoon potassium citrate

½ cup filtered water

In a tall glass, mix the lemon juice with the potassium bicarbonate and potassium citrate, and then allow to fizz for 1 to 2 minutes. Pour in the water and drink immediately.

Lemon juice is my favorite supplement, because it is so effective as first aid for any ailment! It is safe to consume lemon juice frequently. Although citrate has the power to strengthen teeth and improve mineralization, protect your teeth from the acid in lemon juice by sipping plain water afterward. Use your own saliva and tongue to wipe traces of the lemon away, then swallow. For your teeth's sake, avoid sipping acidified water all day. (That's one reason I recommend "shots.") As one client commented, "I've been drinking straight lemon juice 4 to 6 times a day for two years, and my teeth are great—not a single cavity!"

Citrate Supplements

Taking mineral supplements, citrate, and bicarbonate are proven ways to address your acidic conditions and, over time, to replenish critical nutrients to health-restoring levels. Most citrate supplements can achieve three goals simultaneously: (1) mineral supplementation; (2) citrate supplementation; and (3) alkalization of body tissues and urine. Potassium citrate is usually the preferential treatment for stones, although sodium citrate, calcium citrate, and potassium-magnesium citrate are commonly used. Citrate supplements come in many forms: bulk powder, tablets, capsules, and even in prescriptions. A combination of these forms is usually the most helpful and can be adjusted to suit individual needs and tolerance.

Although it does not provide minerals, a lesser-known citrate called hydroxycitrate also appears to be effective and may be a desirable option for kidney-stone formers who tend to have alkaline urine. Clinical studies of hydroxycitrate are limited. Though readily available as an OTC supplement, there have been some safety concerns with hydroxycitrate use, and if you have liver function issues, consult your doctor prior to and during use.

What If Citrate Doesn't Agree with Me?

While citrate is a valuable tool that works for many people, there is some evidence that, in a small fraction of susceptible people, repeated ingestion of manufactured citric acid may elicit low-grade inflammation and trigger sensitivity or allergic reactions. Manufactured citrate is not required for the low-oxalate diet to work. Additionally, all the mineral supplements are available in forms that do not include citrate, and the minerals themselves help alkalize body tissues. If you don't tolerate citrus fruit or manufactured citrate, possible alternatives include sodium bicarbonate or potassium bicarbonate. A scant ¼ teaspoon of sodium or potassium bicarbonate in water three times a day (between meals) can help address extracellular acid that goes with inflammation and oxalate illness, as well as increase urinary citrate. Coconut water is another option that has alkalizing effects and that can help raise citrate in the urine.

Table 15.5: Citrate and Mineral Supplement Suggestions

Supplement	Purpose	Amounts, Adults
Calcium citrate *without* vitamin D	Calcium binds oxalate, improving conditions for colonic excretion of oxalate. In this application, the goal is for Ca+ retention in the intestines.	800–1,400 mg, depending on calcium from dairy and food selections. Moderate use to avoid constipation.
Magnesium citrate	Prevents oxalate crystallization and may help break down existing crystals in the tissues. Can also help with constipation. Magnesium is important for cellular energy and thiamine activity. Magnesium deficiency is common.	300–1,600 mg per day with or without food, within bowel tolerance, meaning don't create diarrhea with an overdose.
Potassium citrate (K⁺Cit)	Helps prevent oxalate crystallization. Is a standard treatment for kidney stones. Restores depleted potassium levels in connective tissues and muscles. Improves muscle and nerve performance. Compensates for the effects of a low-carbohydrate diet or chronic inflammation.	99 mg tabs: 4 to 14 per day, spread throughout the day, taken with food. Or use the bulk powder in drinking water and sip all day long (¼ tsp. to 2 tsp./day). Or take in electrolyte drinks (see **Table 15.2**). *Persons with chronic kidney disease should consult a doctor.*

(table continues)

Supplement	Purpose	Amounts, Adults
Lemon and lime juice	Reduces crystal formation, protects the kidneys, supports digestion if taken with meals, and helps acute symptoms of any kind.	½ cup juice per day recommended for preventing kidney stones (1 to 4 lemons or 2 to 8 limes). Rinse teeth with water after consuming.
Trace-mineral complex	Important to have in small amounts	Use a combination of mineral-complex capsules and liquid forms.

Critical Vitamins

Certain essential vitamins play a role in oxalate toxicity and recovery. These include the B vitamins, vitamin C, and vitamin D. Vitamin D was discussed earlier (on page 238) and is best acquired through "Vitamin Sunlight," and vitamin C is only needed in small amounts.

So, let's begin with the B vitamins because these are so essential to health and they are depleted by excess oxalate. A deficiency in the B vitamins may increase the body's internal production of oxalates. Insufficient B vitamins and mineral deficiencies are not just related to oxalate toxicity, however. They accompany other hard-to-treat problems such as celiac disease, obesity, diabetes, and alcoholism. Getting adequate B vitamins can improve your state of mind, too. The capacity to mentally cope with chronic illness and stay on course with a program like low-oxalate eating may, in fact, depend on micronutrients at the cellular level!

Given that most of us are marginally malnourished, and oxalate toxicity promotes micronutrient deficiency, it's not surprising that the majority of my clients often also need B vitamin supplements to function as they recover from oxalate overload. Any deficiency will give the oxalate an upper hand, but three B vitamins are of particular concern: thiamin, biotin, and B_6 (P-5-P). These vitamins are especially critical to energy and oxalate metabolism. They are best taken in conjunction with a high-quality B-complex or desiccated liver supplement.

Thiamin (B_1)

Thiamin, also known as vitamin B_1, activates other B vitamins and is important to energy metabolism, heart health, and gut function, as well as the brain, nervous system, and overall psychological well-being. Thiamin has antioxidant properties and may have protective anti-aging effects. While thiamin deficiency increases the levels of glyoxylate and oxalic acid in the body, adequate thiamin restrains oxalate synthesis, which explains why thiamin can prevent kidney stones. In fact, supplementing thiamin is effective in alleviating a wide variety of chronic conditions.

Unfortunately, having a thiamin deficiency is common. Several foods contain factors that destroy thiamin (e.g., enzymes in raw fish, and tannic and caffeic acids found in coffee, tea, blueberries, black currants, Brussels sprouts, and red cabbage). Having low thiamin causes a variety of issues with neurological health (including Alzheimer's disease), interferes with glucose metabolism (leading to acidosis and low energy), and promotes the development of diabetes and related complications. Thiamin specialists also recommend thiamin supplementation for any condition involving depleted or damaged mitochondria.

I recommend thiamin especially when fatigue, pain, poor sleep, poor memory, mental fatigue, depression, diarrhea, or constipation are chronic. Correcting a thiamin deficiency takes time and consistent use of high-quality supplements, often at doses greater than 400 mg a day. It may take six months or more to see improvements. Fatigue may be relieved more quickly when higher doses are used. Ironically, fatigue is a likely response to thiamin supplements, possibly owing to the added energy demands of healing in the face of inadequate cellular enzymes.

This makes it hard to stay the course in taking thiamin supplements. A B-complex or multivitamin taken in addition to the thiamin may reduce those effects. According to the National Academy of Medicine in Washington, DC,* there is no determined tolerable upper intake level for thiamin. Supplements containing thiamin hydrochloride and thiamin mononitrate are not well absorbed into the cells and may be ineffective. Better cellular uptake and effectiveness may occur with the new forms of thiamin, such as benfotiamine, sulbutiamine, or lipothiamine.

Vitamin B$_6$

The active form of vitamin B$_6$, *pyridoxal-5'-phosphate* (abbreviated as P-5-P, or PLP), is an essential activator in over 150 enzymatic reactions. Inflammation consumes B$_6$ at a higher rate, and in people with inflammatory conditions (e.g., arthritis), blood plasma and liver levels of P-5-P are low. A vitamin B$_6$ deficiency delivers a three-stroke punch to an oxalate-overloaded body. The B$_6$ deficiency can (1) increase oxalate absorption; (2) elevate glycine levels, which can become glyoxylate, then oxalate, when in excess; and (3) lower citrate levels in the urine.

Additionally, a low plasma P-5-P increases the risk of cardiovascular disease and some cancers. A vitamin B$_6$ deficiency may trigger problems with production of the heme molecule that carries oxygen in the blood (in genetically inclined people). That may be one way deficiency contributes to fatigue.

When vitamin B$_6$ levels are deficient, increasing your vitamin B$_6$ intake (with food and supplements) improves some immune functions. However, the molecular form of vitamin B$_6$ that comes from plant foods, fortified foods, and most vitamin supplements, *pyridoxine HCl*, is a form

---

* National Academy of Medicine was formerly called the Institute of Medicine and is a component of the non-governmental, private institutions called the National Research Council and the National Academies of Sciences established in 1863.

that the body cannot use until it converts it to the biologically active P-5-P form. The conversion machinery in the intestines has very low capacity, and the unconverted pyridoxine can easily displace the P-5-P form required by B_6-dependent enzymes. Vitamin B_6 delivered as pyridoxine *can cause the symptoms of vitamin B_6 deficiency*, creating confusion about the source of the symptoms. As researchers have put it, *"even at relatively low dose, vitamin B_6 supplementation has given rise to complaints."*

The symptoms of a vitamin B_6 deficiency include weakness, numbness, and burning pain owing to nerve damage (demyelinating effects). These effects can cause pain and slurred speech, stumbling, falling, and lack of coordination. Also, a B_6 deficiency is associated with dry eyes and changes to tear secretions, as seen in arthritis and Sjögren's syndrome.

Distinguishing between the possible harms of pyridoxine and the potential therapeutic applications of P-5-P has yet to be put into consistent practice, in either research or medical care. Confusion over which forms are used may fuel the debate about a safe upper limit of B_6 intake. Based on neurological complaints occurring after taking 50 mg of pyridoxine per day, the European Food Safety Authority (EFSA) recently established an upper limit of 25 mg/day, which is one-fourth the previous upper limit of 100 mg/day indicated by the U.S. Department of Agriculture and other authorities. The appropriate dosage and timing of P-5-P supplements remains unstudied. Studies using P-5-P supplements for arthritis provide 100 mg doses and they have found it lowers inflammation.

Dosing: Start with a B-complex supplement containing 15 to 25 mg P-5-P. If you can tolerate that, you may later try adding an additional 15 mg (or up to 50 mg) of P-5-P, divided into two doses, with or without food. See if you feel calmer or have reduced pain after 6 to 10 weeks. Watch your reactions carefully, and consider gradually lowering your intake of the additional P-5-P for several weeks to compare how you feel with less, or even without it.

Biotin

Biotin (vitamin B_7) is essential for growth, development, and normal cell function, in part because it is required for five mitochondrial enzymes, the *carboxylases*. These enzymes do not work properly when oxalate gets into the mitochondria.

Suboptimal biotin levels also occur with long-term use of anticonvulsant drugs, parenteral nutrition, in chronic alcoholism, in people with inflammatory bowel disease, and during normal pregnancy. Having a biotin deficiency in pregnancy increases the risk of skeletal development birth defects, such as cleft palate. A deficiency of biotin has also been linked to blood sugar problems, increased inflammation, and epigenetic changes. On the other hand, taking biotin supplements has been shown to help enzymes work better and improves glucose tolerance.

Dosing: If you choose to take biotin supplements, I suggest 5 mg daily (5,000 mcg). Research suggests that 20 mg/day (or much more) is safe even in small children. A pilot trial program gave daily high-dose biotin (100–300 mg/day) to 23 patients with multiple sclerosis for several months; over 90 percent of the patients (21 of 23) had some degree of improvement.

B Vitamin Challenges

Some people appear to have trouble taking B vitamin supplements. There are various reasons that may happen. For example, we need balanced amounts of the B vitamins, so over-supplementing one without matching the others may sometimes be unhelpful. As a person recovers from oxalate overload, the body's needs for the B vitamins may change — what was too little or too much changes.

The other common problem is that the "stable" chemical forms used in the supplements are not the same as the biological forms needed by the body's cells. Recent research suggests that the use of some forms of B vitamins in supplements and in fortified foods—specifically niacin, B_6 (as *pyridoxine*), and folic acid—may be ineffective, or even toxic.

Similar to the problem with B_6 fortification, the folic acid used in fortified foods and in retail vitamin supplements requires conversion to the active form (*5-methyltetrahydrofolate*, or *5-methyl-THF*, or *L-5-MTHF*) by the intestinal cells. B-complex supplements may contain 100 or 200 times the amount of folic acid the body can convert to the useful form, and as a result, unmetabolized folic acid from fortified foods and supplements remains in the blood, where it may have detrimental effects, including possibly promoting cancer.

Unfortunately, most studies of vitamin supplementation, including human intervention trials and clinical case reports, have used the biologically inactive, interfering forms: pyridoxine and folic acid. No wonder researchers are getting mixed results. If you have had bad reactions to B vitamin supplements, it could be related to the wrong forms and combinations. However, supplements are available that contain B_6 in the P-5-P form and folate (5-MTHF), as well as more bioaccessible forms of thiamin (benfotiamine, sulbutiamine, allithiamine, or lipothiamine).

Multivitamin Supplements

The one-a-day combined supplement is a generally recommended practice, as it is seen as a safety-net precaution for filling in any nutrient gaps left by our diets. But the seemingly innocuous use of a basic, wide-spectrum supplement can easily fail to reach its intended goal of protecting the cells from vitamin deficiencies. Just because you might consume a multivitamin, that does not mean it is doing you any good.

The one-a-day approach requires that the B-complex vitamin supplements in it be well formulated, using the best forms such as P-5-P and folate (5-methyltetrahydrofolate), as well as have appropriate binders that facilitate a gradual but complete absorption into the bloodstream.

Even well-formulated multivitamin supplements may not meet specific, individual needs. Oxalate overload changes a person's nutrient needs. Those needs may also be affected by genetic and epigenetic differences, as well as by use of drugs, alcohol, smoking, and the consumption of excessive carbohydrates. What is safe and healthful for one person may be toxic for another, or simply inadequate for others.

Vitamin C: Less Is More

Vitamin C should not be viewed as a benign, water-soluble drug but rather as a drug that is potentially toxic, not only for diseased kidneys, but also for normal ones.

—S. Mashour et al., *Chest*

We need vitamin C—about 100 mg daily. It is best to get vitamin C from foods and it is important to limit any vitamin C supplements to amounts unlikely to raise oxalate levels (250 mg or less). That doesn't mean you can't ever supplement with vitamin C. Modest 50 to 100 mg doses of supplemental C can help reduce oxidative stress, when needed. If you are feeling ill and inflamed (possibly from oxalate clearing), a 100 mg dose of vitamin C taken up to three or four times a day may be reasonable. Taking more doesn't increase the benefits, and instead risks raising your oxalate levels; nor is it necessary to continue such a dose over a long period of time.

Table 15.6: Vitamin Supplement Suggestions

	Vitamin Supplement	Dosage (start with very low doses)
B-complex (containing bioactive forms)	Metabolic support.	Once daily.
Vitamin B_6 as P-5-P (alone or in B-complex)	Limits internal production of oxalate; to correct B_6 deficiency.	15–100 mg/day, split into 2 doses. Increase when dumping oxalate.
Thiamin supplement options: benfotiamine, sulbutiamine, lipothiamine, allithiamine	Assists energy metabolism and neurological function. Subclinical deficiency is common.	Can be taken in high doses, adjusted based on individual response.
Biotin	Helps reduce dumping side effects, including brain symptoms.	0.5–10 mg/day, divided in 2 doses. Increase when clearing symptoms are heavy, to as high as 100–200 mg, if needed.
Vitamin C	Prevent deficiency. Deficiency is not common.	Eat low-oxalate fresh foods such as lettuce. ¼ cup of lemon juice (1 large lemon) provides 25 to 30 mg. If additional C is needed, take 50–100 mg once or twice daily in supplement or C-enriched foods. Limit intake to 2 to 4 times the RDA to limit oxalate formation in the body.
Vitamin D	Prevent deficiency. Vitamin D deficiency is common.	Have your D levels checked to determine need. If needed, take 10,000 mg or more weekly or monthly, not daily.

Things You Probably Don't Need

As mentioned earlier, our modern notions of health are often driven by unreasonable expectations, myths, and just plain falsehoods. The same applies to certain things you might be tempted to do or to take to address oxalate overload. I am sad to say there are no magic bullets, and the idea of "superfoods" is just as wrong when applied to oxalate "cures" as it is to our diet in general.

Probiotics for Gut Health

As discussed earlier, trying to heal your gut with fiber may be counter-productive. Research further suggests that most probiotic products are ineffective, and can cause intestinal bacterial overgrowth, gas, bloating, lactic acidosis, and many other more serious harmful effects. When bacterial supplements are successful at colonizing the bowel, they may displace your native bacteria and make it harder for your gut to regulate its contents.

Don't fall for the myth that probiotics will protect you from the excessive oxalate you eat. While it is true that oxalate-eating gut bacteria do help the body get rid of some of the oxalate you previously absorbed, most people don't have these bacteria; repeated studies have shown that *Oxalobacter formigenes* cannot be reestablished through oral supplementation.

Antioxidants

You might be surprised to learn that research has found that long-term use of vitamin E and vitamin C supplements may shorten human life span. Apparently, when you routinely suppress cell-based oxidants with supplements, you disrupt the physiological balance and self-regulation in the cells. During acute oxalate-clearing episodes or during times of infectious illness, intermittent and light use of antioxidant supplements, such as vitamin E, N-acetyl cysteine (NAC), CoQ10, glutathione, and even low-dose vitamin C, may be beneficial. But as a rule, they probably should not be taken preemptively or daily over a long period because antioxidant supplements can inhibit the normal adaptive response to free radical stress. For example, they may even prevent the health-promoting effects of exercise. Thus routine use may create more problems than it solves.

Painkillers (NSAIDs)

When oxalate starts causing pain, doctors often send patients to non-steroidal anti-inflammatory drugs (NSAIDs), such as ibuprofen (Advil, Motrin, Brufen, and Nurofen), aspirin, celecoxib (Celebrex), naproxen (Aleve, Naprosyn), and others. Familiar and universally available, these drugs are easy to overuse. In the late 1990s, more than 30 million people worldwide were using these drugs every day, and today's numbers are probably higher.

In addressing the pain associated with oxalate overload and clearing, NSAIDs are both useless and may make matters worse. When people use drugs and supplements to suppress inflammation, they may impair the body's use of health-protecting, low-level inflammation while failing to support the body's ability to turn off the runaway inflammation. The short-term benefits may be offset as the underlying cause of inflammation does more damage. Anti-inflammatories may even shorten life. Studies suggest that the NSAIDs are ineffective for oxalate-related arthritis, for example. And, as noted earlier, NSAIDs also cause and aggravate gut inflammation; using them regularly is a significant risk factor for oxalate hyperabsorption (exposing your body to a much higher proportion of the oxalate in your food; see Chapter 8).

Pain medications have their place in palliative care and in very short-term acute situations. But it is important to keep the dangers and downsides of these medications in mind, and to approach the pain associated with oxalate overload and clearing with less damaging techniques, such as hot compresses, sauna, and the low-oxalate diet itself.

An Overview of Key Recovery Supports

There are four key categories of things you can do to aid your recovery from oxalate overload. And there's one category of things to avoid!

1. LIFESTYLE CHANGES

a. Get enough rest; this is critical to recovery.
b. Limit your toxic exposure.
c. Try heat therapies, such as sauna and hot packs, and cold showers and ice packs.
d. Get vitamin D from sunshine or supplements; it is an essential nutrient.
e. Use appropriate pain-management strategies (careful with pills!).

2. MINERAL SUPPLEMENTS

a. You need calcium to bind the oxalate in the gut and support the excretion of oxalate by way of the feces (and, with time, address any deficiencies you may have).
b. You need magnesium to bind the oxalate, address any deficiencies, restore enzyme function, and support bowel function.
c. You need potassium to replenish nutrients in the cells, and for protecting the health of bones, kidneys, and the heart, as well as for the alkalizing effects.
d. You need sodium from quality mineral salts—not refined salt—to keep electrolyte balance, support adrenal function, maintain cell energy, and improve exercise tolerance.

e. You need bioavailable sulfur to help oxalate handling in the body and overcome deficiency.

f. You need trace minerals to support enzyme function and tissue repair.

g. Purified drinking water should have nutritive minerals added.

h. Consider obtaining necessary minerals by using foot soaks and hot mineral baths.

3. CITRATES

Citrate, lemon juice, bicarbonate, and potassium are often needed to support kidney function, facilitate crystal removal from tissues, and keep your metabolic acid/base balance right (reducing *acidosis*).

4. B VITAMINS (AND NOT TOO MUCH VITAMIN C)

a. Vitamin B_1, B_6, and biotin (B_7) are especially important to support metabolic enzyme function and energy management in nerves, muscles, and connective tissues; to lower internal oxalate production; and for antioxidant and anti-inflammatory effects.

b. Vitamin C is an essential nutrient, but use of C supplements should be limited.

5. THINGS YOU DON'T NEED

a. Probiotics

b. Prolonged use of antioxidants

c. Painkillers (NSAIDs)

16

Unbroken

No written law has ever been more binding than unwritten custom supported by popular opinion.

—Carrie Chapman Catt (1900)

The case for low-oxalate eating is compelling, the success stories are inspiring, and the actual practice of lowering your oxalate consumption couldn't be easier. Having learned to change our diets, we deserve to experience fully the joy of healing and sharing it with others.

Changing to a low-oxalate diet does come with many challenges, not the least of which are our old beliefs, our resistance to change, and our need for support.

All you have learned about oxalates may have you feeling as if your world has been turned inside out. Your new knowledge may be at odds with what you and "everyone else" believe. That can be uncomfortably surreal and stressful. We are human beings, not just bodies. We have families. We live in a society. Along this astounding path to health and healing, some of you may find yourselves embroiled in skirmishes that are both social and deeply personal.

This book may help you resolve an annoying mystery ailment, perhaps quickly or maybe just a little bit at first. You may lift a heavy burden off your body and then, as you are feeling better, find that oxalate toxicity has left you a bit frayed, with a few symptoms to remind you of what you are leaving behind. It may take some time to rebuild your physical vitality. The social and emotional context of your life may add disorienting elements that intersect with the physical experience of oxalate overload. I'd like to add a few parting thoughts in hopes of supporting you in your journey along this strange and revealing path.

The Challenges Ahead

You can see from the cases I've shared in this book that oxalate overload causes many unique expressions of trouble, including "mental health" challenges and spiritual crises. Getting through the physical recovery symptoms can be emotionally challenging too. Beyond toughing it out, there are ways of living to meet the demands of recovery. Navigating the inevitable physical and mental setbacks need not kill your spirit.

Many people who adopt low-oxalate eating make big gains in emotional clarity, greater self-awareness, and lowered anxiety—increasing their capacity for emotional healing. And as you heal, it may be a good time to do some supportive reading and journaling, and to pursue other forms of spiritual and emotional growth. There are many layers to the process of reconciliation with yourself that can make you stronger. You're going to need that.

The experience of oxalate overload illness makes it obvious that our modern nutrition lore overflows with fanciful delusions. After millions of years during which people ate meat, how could it be true that avoiding animal foods and loading up on spinach, fiber, and chocolate leads to good health?

In our sell-sell-sell world, the profit motive behind today's nutrition hype should be obvious, but even those with oxalate problems get sucked into the symbolic powers of a good story. Nutrition myths and major cultural touchstones live large in our heads. Some of these myths were planted there before we could speak and are still reinforced every day.

Acknowledging our robust hunter past is a straightforward way to gain clarity and confidence in the face of the prevailing foolishness. The right mindset for maintaining solid health practices requires that you hold on to an ancestral perspective while living in a processed, plant-based, industrial-food-fueled social landscape.

The present food culture and oxalate overload obliviousness can make low-oxalate eating a lonely path. Few around you will know what you are up against in your healing. We lean on a crowd mentality for feelings of security, no matter how much they may pull us down in the end. You don't need the crowd. What you need is a healthy body, a healthy family, and a healthy future.

We all want to "look normal." Our culture uses food symbolically to create moments of happiness, celebration, and togetherness. Indeed, food rituals have been programmed into our nervous system and are hard to resist, but resist you must. You can do so by deciding to watch for and interrupt the impulse, and choose a different path. The evidence I've shared in this book about oxalate overload will give you the confidence to ignore the myths and misconceptions, and resist the temptations to stuff yourself with nuts, veggies, and "superfoods."

Remember, if you are ill with oxalate overload and are starting to benefit from low-oxalate eating, you don't have the luxury of "fitting in" or waiting for approval. Find your own truth, at your own pace. You can't depend on others to understand. You must take the necessary steps for yourself and stay focused on getting and staying well. Become a leader, not a follower.

It's gratifying to share and understand the common experience of recovering from oxalate overload, and to know that unpleasant aspects will fade with time. Chances are, you will have trouble sharing this message with others. Please don't spend too much energy on wishing your doctor and others in positions of authority would believe you, support your choices, and help you adopt and maintain low-oxalate eating. Most people are caught up in "modern" food practices and will question the benefits you enjoy from low-oxalate eating.

Indeed, friends and family members easily grow weary of hearing about other people's problems, especially their dietary solutions. Several of my clients have explained that, over the years, they repeatedly adopted the "diet du jour," convinced that it would provide the elusive answer — except it didn't. The last thing your loved ones want for you is more wasted effort. They have seen you head down this road before and have shared your disappointment. You are Peter, but you have cried "wolf" too many times. Indeed, when I began the low-oxalate diet for the second time and started to get better for good, I could sense my husband thinking, "Here we go again." Don't despair. Just get well. That's the best way to convince people that you've succeeded. My healing and the healing stories of my clients turned my husband into my most solid supporter.

Finding a safe social space doesn't require joining a club or adopting a group identity, or obtaining permission from an authority figure. Genuine success comes from developing a sense of purpose, setting and pursuing realistic goals, and holding a belief in personal responsibility. Groups are not necessarily a negative thing. If you can stay grounded, they are a way to learn from others and enjoy a healthy group creativity; and even find some inspiration. So, if you do join a group, take what you need and ignore the rest. Ultimately, you are the one who must decide what is right for you. Find the best ways you can to get the support you need, perhaps by enlisting a friend to try the low-oxalate diet with you. Stay in touch with people who have experience on this same path to help you read the signals your body gives you. Networks of support are emerging.

In short, be the right kind of friend for yourself—someone who is compassionate, understanding, and wise. That wise friend has a core of inner peace and confidence in life.

Daily Actions Will Get You There

Begin the low-oxalate diet honestly, carefully, and thoroughly. If you do that, you will learn the value of it for you. In times of doubt, you'll question yourself, but it's important that you be patient. Have faith that your biology will right itself in the context of sound nourishment, a safe pace of lowering your toxic burden, and adequate rest. Have faith that your consistent daily actions are adding up to a healthy future. Hand over the worry to God and trust your biology.

Remember, it's not just your body that needs time to heal but also your understanding of what you've endured, what you can overcome, and what is real. To be successful in reversing oxalate overload, you'll probably have to endure feelings of uncertainty, skepticism, or self-doubt. Somewhere along this path your life will begin anew, with strength springing up from within. That new life is the truer you, more solid and more kind. It's the new, better-informed you, who is also one tough cookie.

As mentioned, changing your own beliefs is not easy. Subconscious attitudes have the power to influence your behaviors, especially when you're under stress (for example, at a family event). Swimming against the tide risks emotional and spiritual fatigue; while uncritical compliance creates its own downward momentum. Emotional attachments to certain foods, striving for perfection, and full-blown eating disorders are real barriers to consistent follow-through on dietary best intentions.

My client Paulette was unwilling to give up potatoes, despite her many severe symptoms. What was it about her relationship with potatoes that they stood between her and her dire need to get out of pain? Was it an inability to make a real decision? Or was it a lack of social support? I bet both were at play. What exactly did eating potatoes provide for her emotionally? Understanding that dependency was her biggest challenge.

Emotional eating such as this is an insidious problem because it leads people to distrust and perhaps even to hate themselves. Watching ourselves make poor food choices can lead us to blame ourselves for our suffering. If you are driven by emotional eating, you may not be ready for any dietary restriction. First, you will need to repair your relationship with yourself. You must know who you are and what you want and need in life. Honor that knowledge directly, not with substitutes. Be it potatoes or chocolate, food will never fill the holes in a neglected soul. Trying to fill that emptiness with food will only create more emptiness. It is possible to overcome the tendency to use food to cope with stress, to feed emotional hungers, or to fit in socially. Start by creating a different set of symbols or, better yet, go for the real thing. Real togetherness and real joy don't require specific foods or food-based events! They do require that you strive for emotional honesty with yourself.

The emotional and physical aspects of low-oxalate eating can intersect in challenging ways. Odd swings in appetite are a common reaction, and that can be really unsettling. It's easy to worry that you're heading for binges. As has been shown in this book, there is a lot going on in the body. It takes patience, mindfulness, and self-compassion to sort it all out. Strong hunger is a possible sign that a big clearing episode may be starting. It might be time to increase your salt and mineral intake and resist the hunger, as a way to signal the body to slow down.

Just remember that your body is on your side, working for life itself, and it will reward you for looking out for it and freeing it from toxic stress.

The body heals most effectively when you're mentally and emotionally relaxed. Make inner peace the center of your daily intention. Find your own way to cultivate awareness and calm. A mindfulness practice focused on breathing can be helpful. Make time for creative activities that "feed" your soul and bring you contentment. Enjoy moderate physical activity, such as short hikes or yoga. Don't push yourself excessively. With daily practice, the centered, cared-for person you want to be will emerge. Growth and self-discovery are part of any healing journey. The challenges you face will eventually get you where you want to be. Not only will you restore your physical health, but you will gain hope, improve your mental outlook, and become strong at the core.

You will inevitably want to share your low-oxalate healing adventure with others. If you want to convince them with ideas, share this book. The most powerful truth, however, will shine from your own healed body.

Resources

Here are three tools to assist you through your oxalate-aware transition and beyond.

Self-Quiz: Risks, Symptoms, and Exposure
To help you determine if oxalate is already a factor in your health status and inspire insights and motivation for starting and maintaining oxalate-aware eating for the long-term.
The Swap Chart
Dosing Estimates for Selected High-Oxalate Foods

Self-Quiz: Risks, Symptoms, and Exposure

The inventory won't tell you conclusively if you have an oxalate problem, but if you are wavering about your need for a low-oxalate diet it may give you the nudge you need to try it.

Complete the three sections to identify (1) your major risk factors for oxalate toxicity; (2) symptoms you may have from chronic oxalate exposure; and (3) your major dietary sources of oxalate. Another feature of oxalate illness is that the symptoms may appear and disappear with no obvious trigger. Circle symptoms that you have only sometimes experienced.

Part 1. Risk Factors

Instructions: Check any rows that apply to you. Each factor increases the likelihood that your high-oxalate diet may be leading to oxalate overload.

☐	Dairy-free diet, low calcium intake, or low mineral levels
☐	Frequent prior or current use of gut-irritating foods (not necessarily high oxalate): beans, quinoa, bran, whole grains
☐	Lifetime history of repeated antibiotic or antifungal medications
☐	Prior or current use of nonsteroidal anti-inflammatory medications such as Motrin, Advil, Aleve, or aspirin
☐	Obesity, diabetes, or prediabetes
☐	Digestive issues such as Crohn's disease, IBS, leaky gut, food sensitivities, bariatric surgery, celiac disease, gut dysbiosis
☐	Frailty or other chronic non-oxalate illness
☐	Poor kidney health, history of kidney stones, family history of kidney disease

Part 2. Symptoms or Existing Diagnoses

Instructions: Circle all symptoms that you have experienced (not necessarily severely) either continuously or periodically over several months or more. No single symptom is indicative of oxalate overload. Symptoms often occur in different body systems, but some people experience only a limited number of problems unique to them.

Connective Tissue Problems

Joint pain, aching, or weakness	Arthritis or gout
Swelling or inflammation around joints	Tendinitis or joint weakness

Carpal tunnel pain impacting the wrist, elbow, or neck

Plantar fasciitis of the foot and heel

Cracking or noisy joints

Muscle knots, pain, aching, or weakness

Muscle or tendon stiffness or tenderness

Adhesions or fibrosis

Osteopenia or osteoporosis

Bone pain or fractures

Injury prone

Slow or incomplete healing

Tenderness at old injury sites

Low muscle mass

Dental cavities or loose teeth

Digestive Problems

Gastroenteritis

Bloating

Diarrhea and/or constipation

Reflux

Excessive belching

Rectal burning or pain

Calcifications

Dental tartar

Salivary stones

Thyroid stones

Bone spurs

Calcified arteries

Metabolic Problems

Generalized malaise

Chronic fatigue

Thyroid disease

Cold hands and feet

Yeast infections

Hormonal issues

Sugar "addiction"

Fainting or dizziness

Chemical sensitivity

Eye or Vision Problems

Red eyes

Dry eyes

Eye irritation

Watery eyes

Eye grit

Eye sties

Lost visual acuity

Cataracts

Neurological Issues

Mental fatigue

Insomnia or other sleep problems

Restless legs or aches in the legs or feet

Difficulty with concentration, memory, or decision-making

Brain fog

Attention problems or loss of organizational ability

Problems with your mood, including anxiety or irritability

Depression

Tooth sensitivity

Noise sensitivity

Eye pain or light sensitivity

Headaches

Ringing ears

Hiccups

Clumsiness, dropping things, bumping into things

Skin Problems

Dry skin, frail skin

Skin tags

Thin skin around the genitals or anus

Inflammatory Issues

Autoimmune disease

Mast cell activation syndrome

Grinding teeth, tension at the side of the face (TMJ)

Extensive allergies

Numerous food sensitivities

Autoimmune condition

Sinus pressure, sinus congestion

Rashes

Sarcoidosis (inflamed tissues)

Asthma, COPD, lung or breathing problems

Infertility or multiple miscarriages

Urinary Problems

Frequent urination

Urinary urgency

Kidney stones composed of calcium oxalate

Pelvic, urinary, or genital discomfort

Cloudy urine

Blood detected in urinalysis

Part 3. High-Oxalate Foods

Instructions: Check the appropriate box corresponding to how often you eat each of the foods listed here. Space is provided for counting up the total number of foods. This is not a complete list of high-oxalate foods, just common ones. It does not attempt to quantify your oxalate intake. Reliance even on just one very high-oxalate food can exceed your innate oxalate tolerance.

Food Item or Type	Eat Every Day	Eat Often (Now)	Eat Occasionally	Ate Frequently (Previously)
Beverages				
Black or green tea	☐	☐	☐	☐
Plant milk (carob or chocolate flavor)	☐	☐	☐	☐
Almond milk	☐	☐	☐	☐
Chocolate				
Cacao, cocoa nibs	☐	☐	☐	☐
Brownies, chocolate candies	☐	☐	☐	☐
Hot chocolate	☐	☐	☐	☐
Chocolate ice cream or cakes	☐	☐	☐	☐
Mocha beverages	☐	☐	☐	☐
Fruits				
Figs	☐	☐	☐	☐
Kiwifruit	☐	☐	☐	☐
Blackberries	☐	☐	☐	☐

(table continues)

Food Item or Type	Eat Every Day	Eat Often (Now)	Eat Occasionally	Ate Frequently (Previously)
Nuts, Seeds, and Products Containing Them				
Almonds	☐	☐	☐	☐
Cashews or other nuts	☐	☐	☐	☐
Chia seeds	☐	☐	☐	☐
Sesame seeds, tahini	☐	☐	☐	☐
Poppy seeds	☐	☐	☐	☐
Legumes				
Peanuts	☐	☐	☐	☐
Pinto beans	☐	☐	☐	☐
Black beans	☐	☐	☐	☐
Beans, other kinds	☐	☐	☐	☐
Soy flour or soy protein products	☐	☐	☐	☐
Vegetarian "meats"	☐	☐	☐	☐
Carob products	☐	☐	☐	☐
Whole Grains and Pseudo-Grains				
Bran cereals	☐	☐	☐	☐
Whole wheat or shredded wheat cereal	☐	☐	☐	☐
Quinoa	☐	☐	☐	☐
Buckwheat	☐	☐	☐	☐
Wheat germ	☐	☐	☐	☐

Food Item or Type	Eat Every Day	Eat Often (Now)	Eat Occasionally	Ate Frequently (Previously)
Vegetables				
Beets or beet greens	☐	☐	☐	☐
Carrots	☐	☐	☐	☐
Celery	☐	☐	☐	☐
Chard	☐	☐	☐	☐
Curly kale, collards, or dandelion greens	☐	☐	☐	☐
Okra	☐	☐	☐	☐
Plantain or plantain chips	☐	☐	☐	☐
Potatoes, chips, fries	☐	☐	☐	☐
Spinach	☐	☐	☐	☐
Sweet potatoes	☐	☐	☐	☐
"Exotic" vegetable chips	☐	☐	☐	☐
Spices				
Cinnamon	☐	☐	☐	☐
Cumin or curry powder	☐	☐	☐	☐
Turmeric	☐	☐	☐	☐
Supplements				
Milk thistle seed	☐	☐	☐	☐
Slippery elm bark	☐	☐	☐	☐
Vitamin C, 500 mg or higher per day	☐	☐	☐	☐

(table continues)

Food Item or Type	Eat Every Day	Eat Often (Now)	Eat Occasionally	Ate Frequently (Previously)
Count Checkmarks Down Each Column				
High-Oxalate Foods	————	————	————	————

Part 4. Assessment

The Inventory will show one of four results:

1. You've circled 4 or more symptoms, eat 3 or more servings of high-oxalate foods most days, or have several risk factors

If you're currently eating high-oxalate foods regularly and have several health concerns, you need a plan to transition your food choices with a deliberate, unhurried approach. A rush to "zero" could wake up your body's desire to unload before your kidneys are ready to handle it and potentially unleash debilitating symptoms. The secret to safe and successful oxalate release from your body is to lower intake gradually, a few foods at a time, and support your body with a few inexpensive mineral and B vitamins supplements. You can keep using the Inventory to track changes as you start cutting back. Learn to recognize clearing symptoms and how to employ supportive therapies (see Chapter 15) for limiting the damage that occurs when the body releases accumulated oxalate.

2. You have high intake of oxalates or several risk factors yet few symptoms.

What if you don't have serious or noteworthy symptoms? I've seen this with several spouses, parents, and children who joined in on the diet to be supportive of their family member. These companions were surprised to discover when they "tried" the diet, some significant annoyance that "wasn't really bothering them" got better.

For the lucky few who have been happily eating an indiscriminate high-oxalate diet and whose bodies haven't yet been overwhelmed, it is easy to try out the diet and then do the challenge test I describe on page 179. The experience might be your only option to determine if, for you, there is something to this oxalate business after all.

3. You have some symptoms but no history of eating high-oxalate foods.

Oxalate is not the only path to illness, but oxalate awareness may still support better health. Continue to avoid high-oxalate foods and improve your state of nutritional health and search for other toxic exposures that may be impacting your health.

4. You have no or few symptoms and low intake now and in the past.

Yay! You're one of the lucky ones. Now you have a list of some key foods to continue avoiding for the sake of your long-term well-being. Prevention is the best medicine.

The Swap Chart

High-Oxalate Food to Avoid . . .	Try Instead . . .
Greens (raw and cooked)	
Spinach Beet greens (Swiss) chard	Romaine, Bibb, butter, iceberg lettuce; pea greens, watercress, arugula; mâche Cabbage, bok choy, turnip or mustard greens, lacinato "dinosaur" kale (the lowest-oxalate variant; others are higher but still useful in moderation), capers, cilantro
Whole Fruits	
Apricots, blackberries, citrus peel, clementine, elderberries, figs, goji, kiwifruit, mulberries, tangerines	Apples, blueberries, dates, grapefruit (white), grapes (seedless), kumquat, mango, melons (cantaloupe, honeydew, watermelon), papaya, pineapple; juice (apple, lemon, lime, orange, pineapple), and raisins—in moderation
Grains and Seeds	
Bran, whole grains; most pseudo-grains (quinoa, amaranth, buckwheat); corn grits; thickeners: tapioca, arrowroot	White rice; white wheat flour (bleached or unbleached) contains moderate oxalate. For occasional use, blue corn chips cooked in organic coconut oil. Well-cooked winter squash, green peas, black-eyed peas, pearl barley, or coconut flour. Use potato starch as a thickener.
Sesame, chia, poppy, hemp seeds	Cellophane (mung bean) noodles, kelp noodles, shirataki "rice" or noodles
Roots and Tubers	
Beets, baking potatoes, sweet potatoes	Red new skinned potatoes (in ½-cup portions). Cauliflower, turnips, and celeriac (celery root) can be mashed like potatoes and are just as versatile. Rutabaga or celeriac can be steamed and mashed, alone or together. Starchy lower-oxalate vegetables include green peas, chestnuts, pumpkin, and winter squash.
Chocolate and Carob	
Chocolate, carob	Fresh fruit; ice cream, iced coconut milk; white chocolate; chocolate extract, chocolate liquor as a flavoring; herbal teas

High-Oxalate to Avoid . . .	Try Instead . . .
Tea	
Black tea, green tea	Many herbal teas: chamomile, lemon balm, mint, nettle, rooibos
	Coffee or coffee-like herbal drinks (e.g., Dandy Blend)
Nuts	
Peanuts (a legume), peanut butter, and most nuts and nut butters, especially almonds	Sprouted pumpkin seeds and pumpkin seed butter, sprouted sunflower seeds, or flax seeds (try "Go Raw" brand). Macadamia nuts (5 to 10 nuts), pistachios (20 nuts), walnuts (5 to 8 halves). Almond extract for flavoring. Quality raw-milk cheese; whole milk (fresh). Snack on bacon bits, coconut macaroons, coconut-based chips, plain yogurt.
Legumes	
Soy, soy products; black beans, white beans, and most other dried beans	Fresh or frozen green peas, cooked black-eyed peas, yellow or green split peas, mung beans, butter beans. Dried legumes must be soaked and drained before cooking at high heat to reduce phytates, lectins, soluble oxalate.
	Meats and small low-mercury fish from sustainable sources.
Vegetables	
Celery, carrots, artichoke hearts, okra	Red radishes, red bell pepper, chayote squash, kohlrabi, celery root. Cooked asparagus ($^1/_3$ cup or less), cooked turnips, cooked onions. Celery and carrot can be omitted in many recipes, but if small quantities of them are used in recipes, they are typically adding only low amounts of oxalate per serving.
Tomatoes	
Tomato sauce	Fresh tomatoes, in very small portions. Tomato paste used as a flavoring in dishes is usually low in oxalate.
Spices	
Black pepper, caraway seeds, parsley, poppy seeds, turmeric	White pepper, capers, chives (fresh), curcumin extract, dill, horseradish, marjoram, mustard, rosemary, sage, thyme; vanilla extract.

Dosing Estimates for Selected High-Oxalate Foods

This table provides *estimates* of the oxalate content of selected common high-oxalate foods (and in some cases, lower-oxalate counterparts). The estimates presented here are based on data published by reputable labs. Oxalate content of any given food varies from sample to sample and test to test. The extent of the variability in a given food is generally unknown in most foods due to limited testing. Where multiple tests are available, this table contains rounded estimates of oxalate content for evaluating or planning your diet: **All volumes and weights are rounded off.** Check my website (sallyknorton.com) for additional data resources.

Note on volume unit abbreviations: C = cup (8 fl. oz, or 240 ml); tsp = teaspoon (5 ml); Tbs = tablespoon (15 ml).

Note on selecting foods: Use caution when choosing foods with strong antinutrient or allergy potential, such as tomatoes, eggplant, chocolate, nuts, peanuts, or soy. Nuts and seeds contain several gut irritants, including phytates and lectins. I suggest avoiding nuts and seeds entirely if you have chronic digestive issues.

Leafy Green Vegetables

Item	Total mg / 100g	% Soluble	20 mg Oxalate		30 mg Oxalate	
			Weight	~ Size	Weight	~ Size
Beet greens (tops) or red stem chard, chopped						
raw	1,000	70%	2 g	2.5 tsp	3 g	4 tsp
steamed 12 min	1,000	60%	2 g	0.5 tsp	3 g	2 tsp
boiled 6 min	450	40%	4 g	1 tsp	7 g	2 tsp
Chard, green (white stem), chopped						
raw	900	70%	2 g	1.5 tsp	3 g	2 tsp
steamed 12 min	600	60%	3 g	1 tsp	5 g	1.5 tsp
boiled 6 min	300	40%	7 g	1.8 tsp	10 g	3 tsp
Dandelion greens, red rib, chopped						
raw	30	60%	65 g	1.2 C	110 g	2 C
boiled 15 min	15	60%	130 g	1.25 C	190 g	2 C
Spinach, chopped						
raw	1,000	75%	2 g	3 tsp	3 g	5 tsp
frozen	900	90%	2 g	3.5 tsp	3.3 g	5 tsp
steamed 12 min	700	60%	3 g	0.7 tsp	4.3 g	1 tsp
boiled 12 min	500	30%	4 g	1.2 tsp	6 g	2 tsp

Root Vegetables

Item	Total mg / 100g	% Soluble	20 mg Oxalate		30 mg Oxalate	
			Weight	~ Size	Weight	~ Size
Beets, red						
raw	65	75%	30 g	0.2 C	45 g	0.33 C
sliced, steamed	60	75%	30 g	0.2 C	50 g	0.25 C
boiled 12 min	50	70%	40 g	0.25 C	60 g	0.4 C
Beets, golden						
boiled 40 min	95	85%	20 g	1.6 Tbs	30 g	3.2 Tbs
Carrot, sliced						
raw	45	70%	45 g	0.34 C	65 g	0.5 C
steamed 12 min	20	70%	100 g	0.7 C	150 g	1 C
boiled	20	70%	100 g	0.7 C	150 g	1 C
Potato						
red, new, boiled 30 min, with skin	20	90%	100 g	0.6 C	150 g	1 C
Russet, Burbank, or Idaho, baked, flesh only	50	70%	40 g	2.2 Tbs	60 g	3.3 Tbs
Russet, Burbank, or Idaho, baked, skin only	400	60%	5 g	0.6 skin	8 g	0.8 skin
instant, white, dry	100	85%	20 g	0.3 C	30 g	0.5 C
Sweet potato or yam						
orange, without skin, raw	50	79%	42 g	3 Tbs	64 g	4.5 Tbs
orange, with skin, baked 1 hour at 400°F	100	35%	20 g	1 Tbs	30 g	1.5 Tbs
orange, without skin, baked 1 hour at 400°F	60	29%	32 g	1.5 Tbs	49 g	2.5 Tbs
Stokes purple, without skin, baked 1 hour at 400°F	170	50%	12 g	1.75 tsp	18 g	2.5 tsp

(table continues)

Other Vegetables

Item	Total mg / 100g	% Soluble	20 mg Oxalate Weight	20 mg Oxalate ~ Size	30 mg Oxalate Weight	30 mg Oxalate ~ Size
Artichoke hearts						
fresh boiled 30 min	35	57%	60 g	0.36 C	90 g	0.5 C
canned in water, drained (Kroger)	30	40%	70 g	2.3 pieces	100 g	3.5 pieces
Asparagus, boiled or steamed, 10 min	10	29%	190 g	1.1 C	290 g	1.6 C
Bamboo shoots, cultivated, boiled, drained	95	55%	22 g	0.76 wt. oz	30 g	1.14 wt. oz
Broccolini, chopped, steamed	14	41%	152 g	1 C	230 g	1.5 C
Cactus (nopal), boiled 30 min	350	39%	6 g	1.8 tsp	9 g	2.7 tsp
Celery stalk, raw, diced	25	90%	80 g	0.7 C	120 g	1 C
Eggplant, purple, Chinese, raw (limited data)	18	NA	110 g	0.8 C	170 g	1.2 C
Eggplant, white, sliced, baked 30 min at 350°F	45	75%	45 g	0.3 C	70 g	0.5 C
Hearts of palm (Haddon House), whole, canned	60	8%	35 g	3 Tbs	50 g	5 Tbs
Okra (Melissa's Produce), boiled 5 min	130	6%	15 g	2.5 Tbs	23 g	3 Tbs
Pepper, bell, raw						
green	10	95%	110 g	4 wt. oz	170 g	6 wt. oz
yellow	25	0%	75 g	2.7 wt. oz	110 g	4 wt. oz
purple	30	99%	65 g	2.3 wt. oz	100 g	3.5 wt. oz
Rhubarb stalk, diced						
raw	530	42%	3.8 g	1.5 tsp	6 g	2.3 tsp
steamed	500	42%	4 g	0.8 tsp	6 g	1 tsp
boiled 12 min	310	28%	6 g	1.3 tsp	10 g	2 tsp (scant)
Tomato sauce (Hunt's), canned, with 2% oregano, garlic, salt, basil, "spice"	24	46%	80 g	0.33 C	120 g	0.5 C

Nuts and Seeds

Item	Total mg / 100g	% Soluble	20 mg Oxalate		30 mg Oxalate	
			Weight	~ Size	Weight	~ Size
Macadamia nuts						
raw	40	54%	50 g	23 nuts	75 g	34 nuts
dry-roasted	45	75%	40 g	18 nuts	65 g	26 nuts
Peanuts						
butter (Skippy, Super Chunk)	170	80%	12 g	2.2 tsp	18 g	3.3 tsp
roasted	160	68%	12 g	12 nuts	19 g	18 nuts
Walnuts						
raw, halves	75	75%	25 g	12 halves	40 g	19 halves
roasted, halves	50	51%	40 g	18 halves	60 g	26 halves

Grains / Grain Products

Item	Total mg / 100g	% Soluble	20 mg Oxalate		30 mg Oxalate	
			Weight	~ Size	Weight	~ Size
Buckwheat, boiled	130	43%	15 g	1.4 Tbs	23 g	2 Tbs
Cornmeal (Bob's Red Mill)	45	96%	45 g	0.4 C	70 g	0.6 C
Corn tortilla (Mission)	25	87%	80 g	3 tortillas	120 g	4.5 tortillas
Cream of Wheat cereal (Nabisco), dry	30	42%	70 g	0.4 C	100 g	0.6 C
Millet (Arrowhead Mills)	30	100%	75 g	0.4 C	110 g	0.6 C
Oats, rolled, dry	25	40%	75 g	1 C	110 g	1.42 C
Oats, rolled, prepared	11	80%	180 g	0.75 C	270 g	1.15 C
Quinoa, cooked	60	79%	35 g	3 Tbs	50 g	0.25 C
Rice, black, cooked 30 minutes	17	39%	110 g	0.8 C	170 g	1.2 C
Rice, brown, boiled	12	88%	160 g	0.8 C	240 g	1.25 C
Teff, brown (Maskal)	220	41%	9 g	1 Tbs	14 g	1.5 Tbs

(table continues)

Fruits

Item	Total mg / 100g	% Soluble	20 mg Oxalate		30 mg Oxalate	
			Weight	~ Size	Weight	~ Size
Apricots						
Raw, variety unspecified, sliced	35	43%	55 g	0.34 C	85 g	0.5 C
dried (Mariani Ultimate)	90	16%	22 g	6 halves	35 g	9 halves
Berries, black raspberries / blackberries, raw	50	34%	40 g	1.4 wt. oz	60 g	2 wt. oz
Citrus						
Orange, clementine, raw, medium	30	11%	70 g	1 orange	110 g	1.4 oranges
Orange marmalade (Smucker's)	50	32%	40 g	2 Tbs	60 g	3 Tbs
Orange, tangelo, raw, medium (2½")	40	17%	50 g	0.5 fruit	80 g	0.75 fruit
Figs (Mission, Sun-Maid)	80	16%	25 g	2.5 figs	40 g	4 figs (¼ C)
Kiwifruit, raw, peeled (1 kiwi = 0.5 C)	30	18%	55 g	0.33 C	80 g	0.5 C
Olives, black						
canned (brand and variety not specified)	25	NA	75 g	19 olives	110 g	29 olives
canned (Albertsons)	50	36%	40 g	16 olives	60 g	23 olives
Olives, green						
canned (no prep specified)	45	3%	45 g	12 olives	65 g	18 olives
Spanish, w/ pimiento, Manzanilla	55	26%	40 g	13 olives	55 g	19 olives
Plantain, ripe, slices sautéed in butter + olive oil	110	100%	18 g	1.8 Tbs	25 g	2.7 Tbs
Prunes, pitted (Sunsweet)	30	35%	65 g	8 prunes	95 g	12 prunes

Breads

Item	Total mg / 100g	% Soluble	20 mg Oxalate		30 mg Oxalate	
			Weight	~ Size	Weight	~ Size
Bagel						
cinnamon raisin (Thomas')	30	30%	70 g	0.75 bagel	110 g	1.1 bagels
whole grain, plain (Sara Lee Soft Smooth)	30	39%	70 g	1.25 bagels	100 g	1.9 bagels
Bread slices, wheat or rye						
rye, 100% (Sunflower, Rye-Ola, Rubschlager)	35	48%	60 g	1.4 slices	85 g	2.1 slices
pumpernickel (Pepperidge Farm)	60	46%	35 g	1 slice	50 g	1.5 slices
sourdough, round (Francisco International)	25	55%	75 g	1.75 slices	110 g	2.6 slices
whole wheat (Arnold 100% Natural)	35	36%	55 g	1.5 slices	85 g	2.25 slices
wheat (Arnold Country Oatmeal)	40	41%	50 g	1.1 slices	70 g	1.75 slices
wheat, farmhouse style (Pepperidge Farm)	25	35%	75 g	3 slices	110 g	4.5 slices
wheat, light (Wonder)	30	34%	65 g	1.7 slices	95 g	2.5 slices
wheat, light white (Wonder)	25	44%	75 g	2 slices	110 g	3 slices
wheat, whole grain (Sara Lee Country)	25	32%	75 g	2 slices	110 g	3 slices
Whole Grain White (Wonder)	30	36%	65 g	1.7 slices	95 g	2.5 slices
whole wheat, 100% (Pepperidge Farm)	35	38%	55 g	2.2 slices	80 g	3.25 slices

(table continues)

Beverages

Item	Total mg / 100g	% Soluble	20 mg Oxalate		30 mg Oxalate	
			Weight	~ Size	Weight	~ Size
Almond milk						
various brands	11	100%	200 g	0.75 C	300 g	1.1 C
Coffee, flavored						
Starbucks Latte, Dark Chocolate Mocha	20	30%	100 g	3.3 fl. oz	150 g	5 fl. oz
Tea (weight for dry tea, oxalate as brewed)						
black tea, steeped 5 min	12	100%	2.6 g	1.3 teabags	4 g	2 teabags
Constant Comment (Bigelow), steeped 1 min	11	100%	1.6 g	0.8 teabag	2.2 g	1.1 teabags
Earl Grey (Bigelow), steeped 1 min	10	100%	1.6 g	0.8 teabag	2.5 g	1.25 teabags
White tea (Pai Mu Tan, Bigelow), steeped 4 min	8	100%	2.2 g	1.1 teabags	3.4 g	1.7 teabags
Yerba maté tea (no prep specified)	2.9	NA	6 g	3 teabags	9 g	4.5 teabags

Chocolate and Carob

Item	Total mg / 100g	% Soluble	20 mg Oxalate		30 mg Oxalate	
			Weight	~ Size	Weight	~ Size
Carob						
chips	150	40%	14 g	1.4 Tbs	21 g	2 Tbs
powder	460	6%	4 g	0.6 Tbs	6 g	0.9 Tbs
Dark chocolate bars						
Green & Black (70%)	210	85%	10 g	0.33 wt. oz	15 g	0.5 wt. oz
Scharffen Berger, Extra Dark Chocolate (82%)	250	76%	8 g	0.3 wt. oz	12 g	0.4 wt. oz
Lindt, Excellence Bitter (99%)	480	71%	4.2 g	0.15 wt. oz	6 g	0.2 wt. oz
Milk chocolate						
M&M's	70	48%	28 g	30 pieces	43 g	46 pieces
Hershey bar	75	42%	28 g	⅔ bar	42 g	1 bar
Chocolate chips						
semi-sweet	160	86%	12 g	0.8 Tbs	18 g	1.2 Tbs
milk chocolate (Hershey's)	110	48%	19 g	2.5 Tbs	30 g	3.75 Tbs
Cocoa powder						
Mean of 15 brands purchased worldwide	690	64%	2.9 g	0.5 Tbs	4.3 g	0.8 Tbs

(table continues)

Chips and Cookie Snacks

Item	Total mg / 100g	% Soluble	20 mg Oxalate		30 mg Oxalate	
			Weight	~ Size	Weight	~ Size
Chips						
plantain chips (Inka Crops)	140	95%	14 g	10 chips	21 g	15 chips
potato chips (Lay's Regular)	75	94%	25 g	13 chips	40 g	20 chips
potato chips (Ruffles)	85	91%	23 g	11.5 chips	35 g	17 chips
sweet potato (Terra)	220	36%	9 g	0.3 wt. oz	14 g	0.5 wt. oz
Cookies						
chocolate chip (Pamela's Gluten Free)	40	38%	45 g	2 cookies	70 g	3 cookies
Fig Newton (Nabisco)	60	26%	30 g	2.2 cookies	50 g	3.3 cookies
Milano Double Chocolate (Pepperidge Farm)	80	68%	25 g	1.75 cookies	40 g	2.75 cookies
Milano Mint (Pepperidge Farm)	45	64%	45 g	3.5 cookies	65 g	5.25 cookies
Crackers						
wheat, sesame crispbread (Wasa)	210	10%	10 g	0.7 slice	14 g	1 slice

Seasonings

Item	Total mg / 100g	% Soluble	20 mg Oxalate		30 mg Oxalate	
			Weight	~ Size	Weight	~ Size
Allspice, ground (McCormick)	1,080	10%	2 g	1 tsp	2.8 g	1.5 tsp
Basil, raw	130	22%	15 g	2.4 Tbs	23 g	3.6 Tbs
Chili powder: pepper/garlic/ spices (McCormick)	310	26%	6 g	2.5 tsp	10 g	3.7 tsp
Cinnamon, ground	1,790	6%	1.1 g	0.33 tsp	1.7 g	0.5 tsp
Citrus peel, dried	750	10%	2.7 g	1.3 tsp	4 g	2 tsp
Cloves, ground (McCormick)	2,000	52%	1 g	0.5 tsp	1.5 g	0.7 tsp
Coriander seeds (McCormick)	1,030	18%	1.9 g	1.1 tsp	2.9 g	1.6 tsp
Cumin seeds (Schilling)	1,110	18%	1.8 g	0.9 tsp	2.7 g	1.3 tsp
Curry powder: coriander, fenugreek, turmeric, cumin, black pepper (McCormick)	1,200	42%	1.7 g	0.8 tsp	2.5 g	1.25 tsp
Ginger						
raw, grated	240	100%	8 g	1.4 Tbs	12 g	2 Tbs
ground	960	75%	2.1 g	1.2 tsp	3.1 g	1.7 tsp
Parsley leaves, raw	140	56%	15 g	3.3 Tbs	22 g	5 Tbs
Turmeric, ground	2,180	94%	0.9 g	0.4 tsp	1.4 g	0.6 tsp

Peer-to-Peer Oxalate Education Organizations

VP Foundation: http://thevpfoundation.org

Autism Oxalate Project / Trying Low Oxalates:
http://www.lowoxalate.info (Information site);
https://www.facebook.com/groups/TryingLowOxalates (Public Facebook)

Sally K. Norton Website: https://sallyknorton.com

Suggested Reading

Buxton, Jayne. *The Great Plant-Based Con: Why Eating a Plants-Only Diet Won't Improve Your Health or Save the Planet.* London: Piatkus, 2023.

Harris, Richard. *Rigor Mortis: How Sloppy Science Creates Worthless Cures, Crushes Hope, and Wastes Billions.* New York: Basic Books, 2017.

Lierre, Keith. *The Vegetarian Myth: Food, Justice, and Sustainability.* Crescent City, CA: Flashpoint Press, 2009.

Niman, Nicolette Hahn. *Defending Beef: The Case for Sustainable Meat Production.* White River Junction, VT: Chelsea Green Publishing, 2014.

Rodgers, Diana, and Robb Wolf. *Sacred Cow: The Case for (Better) Meat.* Dallas: BenBella Books, 2020.

Roth, Geneen. *Breaking Free from Emotional Eating.* New York: Plume, 2004.

Roth, Geneen. *Women, Food and God: An Unexpected Path to Almost Everything.* New York: Scribner, 2010.

Saladino, Paul. *The Carnivore Code: Unlocking the Secrets to Optimal Health by Returning to Our Ancestral Diet.* New York: HarperCollins, 2020.

Schindler, Bill. *Eat Like a Human: Nourishing Foods and Ancient Ways of Cooking to Revolutionize Your Health.* Boston: Little, Brown Spark, 2021.

Taleb, Nassim Nicholas. *Antifragile: Things That Gain from Disorder.* New York: Random House, 2012.

Teicholz, Nina. *The Big Fat Surprise: Why Butter, Meat and Cheese Belong in a Healthy Diet.* New York: Simon & Schuster, 2014.

Endnotes

vii   **[W]e often let many things slip away from us**
Robert Hooke, *Micrographia*, 1664.

Introduction

1   **Despite the fact**
P. Sanz and R. Reig, "Clinical and Pathological Findings in Fatal Plant Oxalosis. A Review," *The American Journal of Forensic Medicine and Pathology* 13, no. 4 (December 1992): 342–45.

Chapter 1

9   **The greatest obstacle**
Daniel Joseph Boorstin, *The Discoverers* (New York: Vintage Books, 1985).

9   **I was feeling really low and lethargic**
Lauren Williamson, "Liam Hemsworth Says He Was Forced to Stop Vegan Diet After Health Scare," *Australian Men's Health*, May 2020, https://www.menshealth.com.au/liam-hemsworth-quit-vegan-diet.

9   **I had to completely rethink what I was putting into my body**
Scott Henderson, "Liam Hemsworth Is Back in Action," *Men's Health*, April 13, 2020; Williamson, "Liam Hemsworth Says He Was Forced to Stop Vegan Diet After Health Scare."

10   **Eighty percent of them are formed from oxalate**
Eric N. Taylor and Gary C. Curhan, "Oxalate Intake and the Risk for Nephrolithiasis," *Journal of the American Society of Nephrology* 18, no. 7 (July 1, 2007): 2198–2204, https://doi.org/10.1681/ASN.2007020219.

10   **a 10-day "green smoothie cleanse"**
Swetha Makkapati, Vivette D. D'Agati, and Leah Balsam, " 'Green Smoothie Cleanse'

Causing Acute Oxalate Nephropathy," *American Journal of Kidney Diseases* 71, no. 2 (February 1, 2018): 281–86, https://doi.org/10.1053/j.ajkd.2017.08.002.

10   months for his kidney function to improve

Jane E. Getting et al., "Oxalate Nephropathy Due to 'Juicing': Case Report and Review," *The American Journal of Medicine* 126, no. 9 (September 2013): 768–72, https://doi .org/10.1016/j.amjmed.2013.03.019.

11   Parkinson's disease and dementia disorders

Adam Heller and Sheryl S. Coffman, "Submicron Crystals of the Parkinson's Disease Substantia Nigra: Calcium Oxalate, Titanium Dioxide and Iron Oxide," *BioRxiv*, January 17, 2019, 523878, https://doi.org/10.1101/523878; Adam Heller, Sheryl S. Coffman, and Karalee Jarvis, "Potentially Pathogenic Calcium Oxalate Dihydrate and Titanium Dioxide Crystals in the Alzheimer's Disease Entorhinal Cortex," *Journal of Alzheimer's Disease: JAD* 77, no. 2 (2020): 547–50, https://doi.org/10.3233/JAD-200535.

12   Frequent use of gut-irritating foods

Quinoa is not only high in oxalate but also contains a toxin with the power of soap.

15   Crystal-laden urine is a risk factor

Simona Verdesca et al., "Crystalluria: Prevalence, Different Types of Crystals and the Role of Infrared Spectroscopy," *Clinical Chemistry and Laboratory Medicine* 49, no. 3 (2011): 515–20.

15   two hallmarks of gout

Erick Prado de Oliveira and Roberto Carlos Burini, "High Plasma Uric Acid Concentration: Causes and Consequences," *Diabetology & Metabolic Syndrome* 4 (April 4, 2012): 12, https://doi.org/10.1186/1758-5996-4-12.

15   now called "pseudo-gout"

More updated and comprehensive understanding of gout is that it is an expression of a generalized inflammatory and metabolic disorder and not confined to the joints. For example, see Georgiana Cabău et al., "Urate-Induced Immune Programming: Consequences for Gouty Arthritis and Hyperuricemia," *Immunological Reviews* 294, no. 1 (March 2020): 92–105, https://doi.org/10.1111/imr.12833.

Chapter 2

19   Feed a man pulverized glass

B. G. R. Williams and E. M. Williams, "Observations upon Some Laboratory Features of Painful Oxaluria," *The Archives of Diagnosis* VI (1913): 263–76.

19   oxalic acid's toxic powers

Vincent R. Franceschi and Paul A. Nakata, "Calcium Oxalate in Plants: Formation and Function," *Annual Review of Plant Biology* 56 (2005): 41–71, https://doi.org/10.1146/ annurev.arplant.56.032604.144106.

19   very toxic to honeybee larvae

Bethany Terpin et al., "A Scientific Note on the Effect of Oxalic Acid on Honey Bee Larvae," *Apidologie* 50, no. 3 (July 1, 2019): 363–68, https://doi.org/10.1007/s13592-019 -00650-7.

20   the oxalate content of honey

Eva Rademacher and Marika Harz, "Oxalic Acid for the Control of Varroosis in Honey Bee Colonies—a Review," *Apidologie* 37, no. 1 (2006): 98–120. They observe that "[t]he oxalic acid content in plants is much higher than in honey," and "The oxalic acid content of honey from treated colonies is only slightly increased. Even the highest levels found after spring treatment did not exceed the naturally occurring oxalic acid content of honey from various botanical origins." Citing Jean-Daniel Charrière and Anton Imdorf, "Oxalic Acid Treatment by Trickling against Varroa Destructor: Recommendations for Use in Central Europe and under Temperate Climate Conditions," *Bee World* 83, no. 2 (January 1, 2002): 51–60, https://doi.org/10.1080/00057 72X.2002.11099541.

The US Environmental Protection Agency eliminated the need to establish a maximum permissible level of oxalic acid residues of oxalic acid in honey, ruling that oxalate exposure from honey is "indistinguishable from background levels of oxalic acid" and that normal use is unlikely to result in short-term, long-term, prenatal developmental, mutagenic, or other toxic effects; see "Oxalic Acid; Exemption from the Requirement of a Tolerance," *Federal Register*, February 23, 2021, https://www.federalregister.gov/documents/2021/02/23/2021-03256/oxalic-acid-exemption-from-the-requirement-of-a-tolerance.

20   oxalic acid in the tree sap

Y. N. Singh and W. F. Dryden, "Muscle Paralyzing Effect of the Juice from the Trunk of the Banana Tree," *Toxicon: Official Journal of the International Society on Toxinology* 23, no. 6 (1985): 973–81, https://doi.org/10.1016/0041-0101(85)90390-3; M. A. Benitez et al., "Pharmacological Study of the Muscle Paralyzing Activity of the Juice of the Banana Trunk," *Toxicon: Official Journal of the International Society on Toxinology* 29, no. 4–5 (1991): 511–15, https://doi.org/10.1016/0041-0101(91)90025-m.

20   The shapes of these creations

Xingxiang Li et al., "Isolation of a Crystal Matrix Protein Associated with Calcium Oxalate Precipitation in Vacuoles of Specialized Cells," *Plant Physiology* 133, no. 2 (October 2003): 549–59, https://doi.org/10.1104/pp.103.023556; Franceschi and Nakata, "Calcium Oxalate in Plants"; G. M. Volk et al., "The Role of Druse and Raphide Calcium Oxalate Crystals in Tissue Calcium Regulation in Pistia Stratiotes Leaves," *Plant Biology* 4, no. 1 (January 1, 2002): 34–45, https://doi.org/10.1055/s-2002-20434.

20   needle shapes are called *raphides*

Dietrich Frohne and Jurgen Pfander, *Poisonous Plants: A Handbook for Doctors, Pharmacists, Toxicologists, Biologists and Veterinarians*, 2nd ed. (Portland, Oregon: Timber Press, Inc., 2005).

20   wound, stun, and paralyze

Robert L. Harrison and Bryony C. Bonning, "Proteases as Insecticidal Agents," *Toxins* 2, no. 5 (May 2010): 935–53, https://doi.org/10.3390/toxins2050935.

20   arrows "dipped" in natural toxins

Kotaro Konno, Takashi A. Inoue, and Masatoshi Nakamura, "Synergistic Defensive Function of Raphides and Protease through the Needle Effect," *PloS One* 9, no. 3 (2014): e91341, https://doi.org/10.1371/journal.pone.0091341.

20   The inedible houseplant *Dieffenbachia*

Frohne and Pfander, *Poisonous Plants*.

22   couldn't finish the salad

TreeOfLife, "Kiwi's: Yay or Nay? - Food Preparation Discussions on The Community
Forum," The Rawtarian Community Forum, accessed April 13, 2016, https://www
.therawtarian.com/community/f/discussion/7396/kiwi-s-yay-or-nay.

22   located adjacent to the seeds

Conrad O. Perera et al., "Calcium Oxalate Crystals: The Irritant Factor in Kiwifruit,"
JFDS Journal of Food Science 55, no. 4 (1990): 1066–69.

23   the oxalate in almond beverages

Demetrius Ellis and Jessica Lieb, "Hyperoxaluria and Genitourinary Disorders in
Children Ingesting Almond Milk Products," *The Journal of Pediatrics* 167, no. 5
(November 2015): 1155–58, https://doi.org/10.1016/j.jpeds.2015.08.029.

23   oxalate bound to calcium enters the blood intact

Denise A. Hanes et al., "Absorption of Calcium Oxalate Does Not Require Dissociation
in Rats," *The Journal of Nutrition* 129, no. 1 (January 1999): 170–73.

23   the more dilute the oxalate

Robert Christison and Charles Coindet, "An Experimental Inquiry on Poisoning by
Oxalic Acid," *Edinburgh Medical and Surgical Journal: Exhibiting a Concise View of the
Latest and Most Important Discoveries in Medicine, Surgery, and Pharmacy* 19, no. 75
(1823): 163–99.

23   workers on agave plantations

M. L. Salinas, T. Ogura, and L. Soffchi, "Irritant Contact Dermatitis Caused by
Needle-like Calcium Oxalate Crystals, Raphides, in Agave Tequilana among Workers in
Tequila Distilleries and Agave Plantations," *Contact Dermatitis* 44, no. 2 (February
2001): 94–96.

23   invaluable tools for plant self-defense

Franceschi and Nakata, "Calcium Oxalate in Plants."

23   smoke, soot, and ash

Russ Crutcher and Heidie Crutcher, "Calcium Oxalate Phytoliths in Environmental
Samples," *The Microscope* 67 (2019): 3–11.

23   fruits defend their seeds

Franceschi and Nakata, "Calcium Oxalate in Plants."

24   releasing free oxalic acid

H. Ilarslan, R. G. Palmer, and H. T. Horner, "Calcium Oxalate Crystals in Developing
Seeds of Soybean," *Annals of Botany* 88, no. 2 (August 1, 2001): 243–57, https://doi
.org/10.1006/anbo.2001.1453.

Tests of soaked nuts prior to dehydration demonstrating an increase amount of soluble
oxalate were published by the VP Foundation. Research confirming these preliminary
findings has not been done.

25   manage and excrete calcium

P. C. Nagajyoti, K. D. Lee, and T. V. M. Sreekanth, "Heavy Metals, Occurrence and
Toxicity for Plants: A Review," *Environmental Chemistry Letters* 8, no. 3 (2010): 199–216.

25 **the crystals can damage cell structures**

C. De Kreij et al., "The Incidence of Calcium Oxalate Crystals in Fruit Walls of Tomato (*Lycopersicon esculentum* Mill.) as Affected by Humidity, Phosphate and Calcium Supply," *Journal of Horticultural Science* 67, no. 1 (January 1, 1992): 45–50, https://doi .org/10.1080/00221589.1992.11516219.

25 **desert plants use oxalate crystals**

Georgia Tooulakou et al., "Alarm Photosynthesis: Calcium Oxalate Crystals as an Internal CO2 Source in Plants," *Plant Physiology* 171, no. 4 (August 2016): 2577–85, https://doi.org/10.1104/pp.16.00111; Elder Antônio Sousa Paiva, "Are Calcium Oxalate Crystals a Dynamic Calcium Store in Plants?," *New Phytologist* 223, no. 4 (2019): 1707–11, https://doi.org/10.1111/nph.15912.

25 **seven times as much**

"The Low Oxalate Diet Addendum, 2018 Winter, Numerical Values Table," *The VP Foundation Newsletter*, no. 46 (February 2018): 46.

26 **highest when the beans are immature**

Ilarslan, Palmer, and Horner, "Calcium Oxalate Crystals in Developing Seeds of Soybean."

28 **knowing the plant family**

Roswitha Siener et al., "Oxalate Contents of Species of the Polygonaceae, Amaranthaceae and Chenopodiaceae Families," *Food Chemistry* 98, no. 2 (January 1, 2006): 220–24, https://doi.org/10.1016/j.foodchem.2005.05.059.

29 **contamination by oxalate-producing molds**

Darina Pickova, Vladimir Ostry, and Frantisek Malir, "A Recent Overview of Producers and Important Dietary Sources of Aflatoxins," *Toxins* 13, no. 3 (March 3, 2021): 186, https://doi.org/10.3390/toxins13030186.

Nouara Aït Mimoune et al., "Fungal Contamination and Mycotoxin Production by *Aspergillus* Spp. in Nuts and Sesame Seeds," *Journal of Microbiology, Biotechnology and Food Sciences* 4, no. 5 (February 2016): 301–5.

Wenxiao Jiao et al., "Organic Acid, a Virulence Factor for Pathogenic Fungi, Causing Postharvest Decay in Fruits," *Molecular Plant Pathology* 23, no. 2 (February 2022): 304–12, https://doi.org/10.1111/mpp.13159.

29 **common fungal contaminants in wheat flours**

M. Weidenbörner et al., "Whole Wheat and White Wheat Flour—the Mycobiota and Potential Mycotoxins," *Food Microbiology* 17, no. 1 (February 1, 2000): 103–7, https:// doi.org/10.1006/fmic.1999.0279.

29 **use of oxalic acid to slow yellowing**

Maria Cefola and Bernardo Pace, "Application of Oxalic Acid to Preserve the Overall Quality of Rocket and Baby Spinach Leaves During Storage," *JFPP Journal of Food Processing and Preservation* 39, no. 6 (2015): 2523–32.

Chapter 3

30 **"No, I'll look first"**

Lewis Carroll, *Alice's Adventures in Wonderland* (S.I.: Duke Classics, 1865), https://api .overdrive.com/v1/collections/v1L1BmUAAAA2X/products/6b5bbcfb-6533-41f4-95da

-5d2303e7e0f0. Before and during the years of debate that led to the Pharmacy Act of 1868, Carroll wrote this scene of a child encountering a bottle of medicine marked "poison." That was a cute way of teaching about the recent innovation of the poison symbol and "poison bottle" designs developed in the era of accidental deaths in the 1800s. W. A. Campbell, "Oxalic Acid, Epsom Salt and the Poison Bottle," *Human Toxicology* 1, no. 2 (March 1982): 187–93.

30   **oxalate killed all of them**

E. I. Robertson, M. Brin, and L. C. Norris, "The Use of Dehydrated Beet Leaves in Chick Rations," *Poultry Science* 26, no. 6 (1947): 582–87, https://doi.org/10.3382/ps.0260582.

30   **When horses consume high-oxalate forages**

S. Groenendyk and A. A. Seawright, "Osteodystrophia Fibrosa in Horses Grazing *Setaria sphacelata*," *Australian Veterinary Journal* 50, no. 3 (1974): 131–32, https://doi.org/10.1111/j.1751-0813.1974.tb05286.x; R. A. McKenzie et al., "Control of Nutritional Secondary Hyperparathyroidism in Grazing Horses with Calcium plus Phosphorus Supplementation," *Australian Veterinary Journal* 57, no. 12 (December 1981): 554–57, https://doi.org/10.1111/j.1751-0813.1981.tb00433.x; B. J. Blaney, R. J. W. Gartner, and R. A. McKenzie, "The Effects of Oxalate in Some Tropical Grasses on the Availability to Horses of Calcium, Phosphorus and Magnesium," *The Journal of Agricultural Science* 97, no. 3 (December 1981): 507–14, https://doi.org/10.1017/S0021859600036820.

31   **disorganized scar tissue takes over**

Groenendyk and Seawright, "Osteodystrophia Fibrosa in Horses Grazing *Setaria sphacelata*." "Big head" is also known medically as "osteodystrophia fibrosa" or "nutritional secondary hyperparathyroidism."

Collagen production and removal is a dynamic balance that determines tissue architecture. Disruption of this homeostasis can lead to tissue destruction or fibrosis. Kamran Atabai, Christopher D. Yang, and Michael J Podolsky, "You Say You Want a Resolution (of Fibrosis)," *American Journal of Respiratory Cell and Molecular Biology* 63, no. 4 (July 2020): 424–35, https://doi.org/10.1165/rcmb.2020-0182TR.

31   **sheep, unlike horses, are ruminants**

Sabry El-Khodery et al., "Hypocalcaemia in Ossimi Sheep Associated with Feeding on Beet Tops (*Beta vulgaris*)," *Turkish Journal of Veterinary and Animal Sciences* 32, no. 3 (May 26, 2008): 199–205; M. M. Rahman, R. B. Abdullah, and W. E. Wan Khadijah, "A Review of Oxalate Poisoning in Domestic Animals: Tolerance and Performance Aspects," *Journal of Animal Physiology and Animal Nutrition* 97, no. 4 (2013): 605–14, https://doi.org/10.1111/j.1439-0396.2012.01309.x; Marnie R. Robinson et al., "Urolithiasis: Not Just a 2-Legged Animal Disease," *The Journal of Urology* 179, no. 1 (January 2008): 46–52, https://doi.org/10.1016/j.juro.2007.08.123.

31   **a flock of Egyptian sheep**

El-Khodery et al., "Hypocalcaemia in Ossimi Sheep Associated with Feeding on Beet Tops (*Beta vulgaris*)."

31   **within the range of 150 to 200 mg a day**

A. M. Duce et al., "Intestinal Absorption of Oxalic Acid in Ileostomized Patients," *Acta Chirurgica Scandinavica* 154, no. 4 (April 1988): 297–99; R. P. Holmes, H. O. Goodman, and D. G. Assimos, "Dietary Oxalate and Its Intestinal Absorption," *Scanning Microscopy* 9, no. 4 (1995): 1109–18; discussion 1118–20.

31 defined as 250 mg or more per day

Joseph J. Crivelli et al., "Contribution of Dietary Oxalate and Oxalate Precursors to Urinary Oxalate Excretion," *Nutrients* 13, no. 1 (January 2021): 62, https://doi .org/10.3390/nu13010062; Tanecia Mitchell et al., "Dietary Oxalate and Kidney Stone Formation," *American Journal of Physiology. Renal Physiology* 316, no. 3 (2019): F409–13, https://doi.org/10.1152/ajprenal.00373.2018.

31 over 600 mg a day are considered "extremely high"

Diana J. Zimmermann, Albrecht Hesse, and Gerd E. von Unruh, "Influence of a High-Oxalate Diet on Intestinal Oxalate Absorption," *World Journal of Urology* 23, no. 5 (November 5, 2005): 324–29, https://doi.org/10.1007/s00345-005-0028-0.

36 a small 1.4-ounce dark chocolate bar

Theresa Schroder, Leo Vanhanen, and Geoffrey P. Savage, "Oxalate Content in Commercially Produced Cocoa and Dark Chocolate," *Journal of Food Composition and Analysis* 24, no. 7 (November 1, 2011): 916–22, https://doi.org/10.1016/j.jfca.2011.03.008.

41 under 100 mg/day is the goal

Ross P. Holmes, John Knight, and Dean G. Assimos, "Lowering Urinary Oxalate Excretion to Decrease Calcium Oxalate Stone Disease," *Urolithiasis* 44, no. 1 (February 2016): 27–32, https://doi.org/10.1007/s00240-015-0839-4; Ross P. Holmes, John Knight, and Dean G. Assimos. "Origin of Urinary Oxalate," vol. 900 (Renal Stone Disease: 1st Annual International Urolithiasis Research Symposium, American Institute of Physics, 2007), 176–82.

42 oxalate can enable and amplify the effects of other toxins

Chien-Liang Chen et al., "Neurotoxic Effects of Carambola in Rats: The Role of Oxalate," *Journal of the Formosan Medical Association = Taiwan Yi Zhi* 101, no. 5 (May 2002): 337–41.

42 neurodegenerative diseases and gut dysfunction

Stephen J. Genuis and Kasie L. Kelln, "Toxicant Exposure and Bioaccumulation: A Common and Potentially Reversible Cause of Cognitive Dysfunction and Dementia," *Behavioural Neurology* 2015 (2015): 620143, https://doi.org/10.1155/2015/620143; Rajnish K. Chaturvedi and M. Flint Beal, "Mitochondrial Approaches for Neuroprotection," *Annals of the New York Academy of Sciences* 1147 (December 2008): 395–412, https://doi.org/10.1196/annals.1427.027; Zeynep Celebi Sözener et al., "Environmental Factors in Epithelial Barrier Dysfunction," *Journal of Allergy and Clinical Immunology* 145, no. 6 (June 1, 2020): 1517–28, https://doi.org/10.1016/ j.jaci.2020.04.024.

42 Exposure to lead, thallium, or mercury

Walter F. Stewart and Brian S. Schwartz, "Effects of Lead on the Adult Brain: A 15-Year Exploration," *American Journal of Industrial Medicine* 50, no. 10 (2007): 729–39, https:// doi.org/10.1002/ajim.20434.

Chapter 4

44 Salad gluttons, defined as people

Jeffrey Steingarten, *The Man Who Ate Everything: And Other Gastronomic Feats, Disputes, and Pleasurable Pursuits* (New York: Vintage Books, 1998).

45   the crops with the highest increases in acreage

Carol Miller, "Sweet Potatoes and Spinach Lead List of Most Acreage Increases [2017 Census of Agriculture]," *Growing Produce* (blog), April 17, 2019, https://www .growingproduce.com/vegetables/sweet-potatoes-and-spinach-lead-list-of-most-acreage -increases-2017-census-of-agriculture/.

45   marketed as nature's nutritional "gifts"

P. Dasgupta, P. Chakraborty, and N. N. Bala, "Averrhoa Carambola: An Updated Review," *International Journal of Pharma Research & Review* 2, no. 7 (July 2013): 54–63. Stating, "So from the current review of the literature [. . .] it may thus be considered an important gift from nature to mankind" (p. 61).

45   percentage of adults who snack

Carmen Piernas and Barry M. Popkin, "Snacking Increased among U.S. Adults between 1977 and 2006," *The Journal of Nutrition* 140, no. 2 (February 2010): 325–32, https://doi .org/10.3945/jn.109.112763.

47   U.S. soymilk sales alone generated about $881 million

"U.S. Soy Milk Sales 2015-2020," Statista, accessed February 4, 2022, https://www .statista.com/statistics/552967/us-soy-milk-sales/.

47   U.S. almond milk sales soared to $1.3 billion

Anna Aleena Paul et al., "Milk Analog: Plant Based Alternatives to Conventional Milk, Production, Potential and Health Concerns," *Critical Reviews in Food Science and Nutrition* 60, no. 18 (2020): 1–19, https://doi.org/10.1080/10408398.2019.1674243; "Milk Alternatives: Dollar Sales by Type in U.S. 2019," Statista, accessed May 20, 2020, https://www.statista.com/statistics/932707/sales-milk-dairy-free-alternatives-us/; "Sales of the Leading Almond Milk Brands in the U.S. 2021," Statista, accessed February 4, 2022, https://www.statista.com/statistics/417533/leading-almond-milk-vendors-in-the-us-based -on-sales/.

48   Manufacturing "veggie milks" involves

Sai Kranthi Vanga and Vijaya Raghavan, "How Well Do Plant Based Alternatives Fare Nutritionally Compared to Cow's Milk?," *Journal of Food Science and Technology* 55, no. 1 (January 2018): 10–20, https://doi.org/10.1007/s13197-017-2915-y; David Julian McClements, "Development of Next-Generation Nutritionally Fortified Plant-Based Milk Substitutes: Structural Design Principles," *Foods* 9, no. 4 (April 2020): 421, https:// doi.org/10.3390/foods9040421.

48   these products have very high oxalate content

James F. Borin et al., "Plant-Based Milk Alternatives and Risk Factors for Kidney Stones and Chronic Kidney Disease," *Journal of Renal Nutrition* 32, no. 3 (May 2021): 363–65, https://doi.org/10.1053/j.jrn.2021.03.011.

49   much of that calcium is not even consumed

Sebastian Chalupa-Krebzdak, Chloe J. Long, and Benjamin M. Bohrer, "Nutrient Density and Nutritional Value of Milk and Plant-Based Milk Alternatives," *International Dairy Journal* 87 (December 1, 2018): 84–92, https://doi.org/10.1016/j.idairyj.2018.07 .018.

49   reduced protein digestibility and lower nutritional utility

Furong Hou et al., "Alkali Solution Extraction of Rice Residue Protein Isolates: Influence of Alkali Concentration on Protein Functional, Structural Properties and

Lysinoalanine Formation," *Food Chemistry* 218 (March 1, 2017): 207–15, https://doi
.org/10.1016/j.foodchem.2016.09.064. "To date, people have not paid sufficient attention
to the nutrient [sic] and safety of alkali extraction of protein, in spite of the fact that this
method has been widely employed in the protein extraction industry."

50   **more than 80 percent of Americans consume a diet deficient in vitamins**

Bruce N. Ames, Hani Atamna, and David W. Killilea, "Mineral and Vitamin
Deficiencies Can Accelerate the Mitochondrial Decay of Aging," *Molecular Aspects of
Medicine* 26, no. 4–5 (October 2005): 363–78, https://doi.org/10.1016/j.mam
.2005.07.007.

National Research Council (US) Committee on Diet and Health, *Diet and Health:
Implications for Reducing Chronic Disease Risk* (Washington (DC): National Academies
Press (US), 1989, http://www.ncbi.nlm.nih.gov/books/NBK218743/.

50   **weakness, and muscle atrophy**

Peter S. Spencer and Valerie S. Palmer, "Interrelationships of Undernutrition and
Neurotoxicity: Food for Thought and Research Attention," *NeuroToxicology*, Special
Review Section, 33, no. 3 (June 2012): 605–16, https://doi.org/10.1016/j.neuro
.2012.02.015.

50   **predispose us to injury**

A. Rashid Qureshi et al., "Inflammation, Malnutrition, and Cardiac Disease as
Predictors of Mortality in Hemodialysis Patients," *Journal of the American Society of
Nephrology: JASN* 13, Suppl 1 (January 2002): S28-36.

50   **contribution of oxalates to deficiencies**

At the cellular level especially, oxalate ions cause (often transitory) shortages in
magnesium, calcium, and other mineral ions that seriously disrupt vital cell functions.
Other mechanisms are also discussed here.

50   **Maternal malnutrition impairs fetal and early life**

Ryan James Wood-Bradley et al., "Understanding the Role of Maternal Diet on Kidney
Development; an Opportunity to Improve Cardiovascular and Renal Health for Future
Generations," *Nutrients* 7, no. 3 (March 12, 2015): 1881–1905, https://doi.org/10.3390/
nu7031881.

50   **a high-oxalate diet is inherently mineral deficient**

R. P. Heaney and C. M. Weaver, "Oxalate: Effect on Calcium Absorbability," *The
American Journal of Clinical Nutrition* 50, no. 4 (October 1989): 830–32.

A. A. Hoover and N. C. Karunairatnam, "Oxalate Content of Some Leafy Green
Vegetables and Its Relation to Oxaluria and Calcium Utilization," *The Biochemical
Journal* 39, no. 3 (1945): 237, https://doi.org/10.1042/bj0390237.

51   **phytic acid (or phytate) also interferes with macronutrient**

G. Sarwar Gilani, Kevin A. Cockell, and Estatira Sepehr, "Effects of Antinutritional
Factors on Protein Digestibility and Amino Acid Availability in Foods," *Journal of AOAC
International* 88, no. 3 (June 2005): 967–87; Margie Profet, "The Function of Allergy:
Immunological Defense Against Toxins," *The Quarterly Review of Biology* 66, no. 1
(March 1, 1991): 23–62, https://doi.org/10.1086/417049.

51   **the calcium [and magnesium] content of food**

P. M. Zarembski and A. Hodgkinson, "The Oxalic Acid Content of English Diets,"

British Journal of Nutrition 16, no. 1 (February 1962): p. 627, https://doi.org/10.1079/ BJN19620061.

51   foods that bind nutrients and obstruct digestion alter

Augustine Amalraj and Anitha Pius, "Bioavailability of Calcium and Its Absorption Inhibitors in Raw and Cooked Green Leafy Vegetables Commonly Consumed in India—an in Vitro Study," *Food Chemistry* 170 (March 1, 2015): 430–36, https://doi .org/10.1016/j.foodchem.2014.08.031; T. C. Mosha et al., "Effect of Blanching on the Content of Antinutritional Factors in Selected Vegetables," *Plant Foods for Human Nutrition (Dordrecht, Netherlands)* 47, no. 4 (June 1995): 361–67, https://doi .org/10.1007/BF01088275.

Lectins in Many Foods

Ilka M. Vasconcelos and José Tadeu A. Oliveira, "Antinutritional Properties of Plant Lectins," *Toxicon* 44, no. 4 (September 15, 2004): 385–403, https://doi.org/10.1016/j .toxicon.2004.05.005; Loren Cordain et al., "Modulation of Immune Function by Dietary Lectins in Rheumatoid Arthritis," *British Journal of Nutrition* 83, no. 3 (March 2000): 207–17, https://doi.org/10.1017/S0007114500000271; Arpad Pusztai and Susan Bardocz, eds., *Lectins: Biomedical Perspectives* (London: Taylor & Francis, 1995).

J. T. A. de Oliveira, A. Pusztai, and G. Grant, "Changes in Organs and Tissues Induced by Feeding of Purified Kidney Bean (*Phaseolus vulgaris*) Lectins," *Nutrition Research* 8, no. 8 (August 1, 1988): 943–47, https://doi.org/10.1016/S0271-5317(88)80133-7; Jose T. A. Oliveira et al., "*Canavalia brasiliensis* Seeds. Protein Quality and Nutritional Implications of Dietary Lectin," *Journal of the Science of Food and Agriculture* 64, no. 4 (April 1, 1994): 417–24, https://doi.org/10.1002/jsfa.2740640405; Pusztai and Bardocz, *Lectins*; A. Pusztai et al., "Antinutritive Effects of Wheat-Germ Agglutinin and Other N-Acetylglucosamine-Specific Lectins," *British Journal of Nutrition* 70, no. 1 (July 1993): 313–21, https://doi.org/10.1079/BJN19930124; Helmut Haas et al., "Dietary Lectins Can Induce in Vitro Release of IL-4 and IL-13 from Human Basophils," *European Journal of Immunology* 29, no. 3 (1999): 918–27, https://doi.org/ 10.1002/(SICI)1521-4141(199903) 29:03<918::AID-IMMU918>3.0.CO;2-T.

Tannins in Foods

L. Hallberg and L. Hulthén, "Prediction of Dietary Iron Absorption: An Algorithm for Calculating Absorption and Bioavailability of Dietary Iron," *The American Journal of Clinical Nutrition* 71, no. 5 (May 2000): 1147–60, https://doi.org/10.1093/ajcn/ 71.5.1147.

Theobromine Toxicity

M. U. Eteng et al., "Recent Advances in Caffeine and Theobromine Toxicities: A Review," *Plant Foods for Human Nutrition* 51, no. 3 (October 1, 1997): 231–43, https:// doi.org/10.1023/A:1007976831684; M. Rusconi and A. Conti, "Theobroma Cacao L., the Food of the Gods: A Scientific Approach beyond Myths and Claims," *Pharmacological Research* 61, no. 1 (January 1, 2010): 5–13, https://doi.org/10.1016/ j.phrs.2009.08.008.

51   low nutrient content makes that a fallacy

For example, to consume 100 percent of needed selenium and 50 percent of recommended levels of calcium from peanut butter, you would need to eat 7,800 calories.

52   5 out of 12 rats who were fed spinach died

E. F. Kohman, "Oxalic Acid in Foods and Its Behavior and Fate in the Diet," *The Journal of Nutrition* 18, no. 3 (September 1939): 233–46, https://doi.org/10.1093/jn/18.3.233.

52   feeding spinach to human infants depletes them of calcium and iron

Council on Foods, "The Nutritional Value of Spinach," *Journal of the American Medical Association* 109, no. 23 (December 4, 1937): 1907–9, https://doi.org/10.1001/jama.1937.02780490045014; Genevieve Stearns and Dorothy Stinger, "Iron Retention in Infancy: Four Figures," *The Journal of Nutrition* 13, no. 2 (February 1, 1937): 127–41, https://doi.org/10.1093/jn/13.2.127.

52   some researchers were dismissive

Council on Foods, "The Nutritional Value of Spinach."

52   1968 study using rhubarb

Iancu Gontzea et al., *Natural Antinutritive Substances in Foodstuffs and Forages* (Basel; New York: S. Karger, 1968).

52   1988 study feeding spinach to humans

R. P. Heaney, C. M. Weaver, and R. R. Recker, "Calcium Absorbability from Spinach," *The American Journal of Clinical Nutrition* 47, no. 4 (April 1988): 707–9, https://doi.org/10.1093/ajcn/47.4.707.

52   "spinach not only has poorly bioavailable calcium

A. G. Poneros-Schneier and J. W. Erdman, "Bioavailability of Calcium from Sesame Seeds, Almond Powder, Whole Wheat Bread, Spinach and Nonfat Dry Milk in Rats," *Journal of Food Science* 54, no. 1 (January 1989): 150–53, https://doi.org/10.1111/j.1365-2621.1989.tb08589.x.

52   "kale, mustard greens and collards, markedly improve growth

Kohman, "Oxalic Acid in Foods and Its Behavior and Fate in the Diet."

52   Growing children have a harder time excreting oxalate

Tadeusz Porowski et al., "Reference Values of Plasma Oxalate in Children and Adolescents," *Pediatric Nephrology* (Berlin, Germany) 23, no. 10 (October 2008): 1787–94, https://doi.org/10.1007/s00467-008-0889-8.

53   usable information about the quantities and implications of compounds

Hallberg and Hulthén, "Prediction of Dietary Iron Absorption."

54   claims that eating 9 cups of vegetables a day will reverse

Terry L. Wahls and Eve Adamson, *The Wahls Protocol: A Radical New Way to Treat All Chronic Autoimmune Conditions Using Paleo Principles* (New York: Avery, 2014).

57   the Mediterranean diet has mistakenly been characterized

Nina Teicholz, *The Big Fat Surprise: Why Butter, Meat, and Cheese Belong in a Healthy Diet* (New York: Simon & Schuster, 2014).

60   amplifies the power of certain flavonoids

Amar K. Chandra and Neela De, "Goitrogenic/Antithyroidal Potential of Green Tea Extract in Relation to Catechin in Rats," *Food and Chemical Toxicology* 48, no. 8 (August 1, 2010): 2304–11, https://doi.org/10.1016/j.fct.2010.05.064; Amar K. Chandra et al., "Synergic Actions of Polyphenols and Cyanogens of Peanut Seed Coat (*Arachis hypogaea*) on Cytological, Biochemical and Functional Changes in Thyroid," *Indian Journal of Experimental Biology* 53, no. 3 (March 2015): 143–51.

Miren García-Cortés et al., "Hepatotoxicity by Dietary Supplements: A Tabular Listing and Clinical Characteristics," *International Journal of Molecular Sciences* 17, no. 4 (April 9, 2016): 537, https://doi.org/10.3390/ijms17040537.

60   **supplement that disrupts cell membranes**

Jonathan Bisson et al., "Can Invalid Bioactives Undermine Natural Product-Based Drug Discovery?," *Journal of Medicinal Chemistry* 59, no. 5 (March 10, 2016): 1671–90, https://doi.org/10.1021/acs.jmedchem.5b01009.

60   **"No double-blinded, placebo controlled clinical trial of curcumin**

Kathryn M. Nelson et al., "The Essential Medicinal Chemistry of Curcumin," *Journal of Medicinal Chemistry* 60, no. 5 (March 9, 2017): 1620–37, https://doi.org/10.1021/acs.jmedchem.6b00975.

61   **"not enough to prove its safety**

Estefanía Burgos-Morón et al., "The Dark Side of Curcumin," *International Journal of Cancer* 126, no. 7 (April 1, 2010): 1771–75, https://doi.org/10.1002/ijc.24967.

61   **The body limits curcumin absorption**

Savita Bisht and Anirban Maitra, "Systemic Delivery of Curcumin: 21st Century Solutions for an Ancient Conundrum," *Current Drug Discovery Technologies* 6, no. 3 (September 2009): 192–99, https://doi.org/10.2174/157016309789054933.

61   **curcumin otherwise would likely cause DNA damage**

Burgos-Morón et al., "The Dark Side of Curcumin"; Rajesh K. Naz, "Can Curcumin Provide an Ideal Contraceptive?," *Molecular Reproduction and Development* 78, no. 2 (February 2011): 116–23, https://doi.org/10.1002/mrd.21276.

"Curcumin not only affected sperm motility and function in vitro, but also inhibited in vivo fertility in female mice when delivered i.v. There was no effect of curcumin when administered orally a delivery method where 60% of the curcumin is absorbed and is subsequently excreted as glucuronide and sulfate conjugate in urine (Bisht and Maitra, 2009). It is interesting that when curcumin is taken orally with piperine, a major component of black pepper that inhibits hepatic and intestinal glucuronidation, the curcumin bioavailability increases by 2,000% (Anand et al., 2007). It is envisaged that after intravaginal administration, curcumin in DMSO is absorbed quickly by the vaginal epithelium."—Rajesh K. Naz, "Can Curcumin Provide an Ideal Contraceptive?" *Molecular Reproduction and Development* 78, no. 2 (February 2011): 121. https://doi.org/10.1002/mrd.21276.

61   **10-week period without dietary fruits and vegetables**

J. F. Young et al., "Green Tea Extract Only Affects Markers of Oxidative Status Postprandially: Lasting Antioxidant Effect of Flavonoid-Free Diet," *The British Journal of Nutrition* 87, no. 4 (April 2002): 343–55.

61   *no beneficial effects* **on oxidative DNA damage**

Peter Møller et al., "No Effect of 600 Grams Fruit and Vegetables Per Day on Oxidative DNA Damage and Repair in Healthy Nonsmokers," *Cancer Epidemiology and Prevention Biomarkers* 12, no. 10 (October 1, 2003): 1016–22.

62   antioxidant supplements have found harmful effects

Ralf Henkel and Ashok Agarwal, "Harmful Effects of Antioxidant Therapy," in *Male Infertility: Contemporary Clinical Approaches, Andrology, ART and Antioxidants*, 2nd ed., eds. Sijo J. Parekattil, Sandro C. Esteves, and Ashok Agarwal (Cham: Springer International Publishing, 2020), 845–54, https://doi.org/10.1007/978-3-030-32300-4_68.

62   "There is no good evidence in human populations

Barry Halliwell, "The Antioxidant Paradox: Less Paradoxical Now?," *British Journal of Clinical Pharmacology* 75, no. 3 (March 2012): 637–44, https://doi.org/10.1111/j.1365-2125.2012.04272.x.

62   "[I]t is premature to use polyphenolic compounds

Daniele Del Rio et al., "Dietary (Poly)Phenolics in Human Health: Structures, Bioavailability, and Evidence of Protective Effects Against Chronic Diseases," *Antioxidants & Redox Signaling* 18, no. 14 (July 15, 2012): 1818–92, https://doi.org/10.1089/ars.2012.4581.

62   directly protects cells from oxidation

Flore Depeint et al., "Mitochondrial Function and Toxicity: Role of the B Vitamin Family on Mitochondrial Energy Metabolism," *Chemico-Biological Interactions* 163, no. 1–2 (October 27, 2006): 94–112, https://doi.org/10.1016/j.cbi.2006.04.014.

62   the best source of B_1, while consuming tea

Laura L. Frank, "Thiamin in Clinical Practice," *JPEN. Journal of Parenteral and Enteral Nutrition* 39, no. 5 (July 2015): 503–20, https://doi.org/10.1177/0148607114565245.

63   "accurate measures of the prevailing bias"

John P. A. Ioannidis, "Why Most Published Research Findings Are False," *PLoS Medicine* 2, no. 8 (August 2005): e124, https://doi.org/10.1371/journal.pmed.0020124.

63   "[the] neurotoxicity provoked by the ingestion of the fruit

Miguel Moyses Neto et al., "Star Fruit: Simultaneous Neurotoxic and Nephrotoxic Effects in People with Previously Normal Renal Function," *NDT Plus* 2, no. 6 (December 2009): 485–88, https://doi.org/10.1093/ndtplus/sfp108.

63   "an important gift from nature

Dasgupta, Chakraborty, and Bala, "Averrhoa carambola: An Updated Review."

64   Tannins, for example, are made by plants

Tannins got their name from their use in "tanning," the process of converting animal hides into leather.

64   bitter-tasting polyphenols are abundant

Hallberg and Hulthén, "Prediction of Dietary Iron Absorption," has a long list of tannins with foods.

64   cause metabolic problems and liver damage

K. T. Chung et al., "Tannins and Human Health: A Review," *Critical Reviews in Food Science and Nutrition* 38, no. 6 (August 1998): 421–64, https://doi.org/10.1080/10408699891274273.

64   *Tannins are considered nutritionally undesirable*

King-Thom Chung, Cheng-I Wei, and Michael G Johnson, "Are Tannins a Double-Edged

Sword in Biology and Health?," *Trends in Food Science & Technology* 9, no. 4 (April 1, 1998): 168–75, https://doi.org/10.1016/S0924-2244(98)00028-4.

64 human saliva has proteins that disarm tannins

Anders Bennick, "Interaction of Plant Polyphenols with Salivary Proteins," *Critical Reviews in Oral Biology and Medicine: An Official Publication of the American Association of Oral Biologists* 13, no. 2 (2002): 184–96, https://doi.org/10.1177/154411130201300208.

65 the "right" gut bacteria and the "right" genetics

Alan Crozier, Indu B. Jaganath, and Michael N. Clifford, "Dietary Phenolics: Chemistry, Bioavailability and Effects on Health," *Natural Product Reports* 26, no. 8 (2009): 1001–43, https://doi.org/10.1039/b802662a.

66 "A . . . serious drawback of increasing the fiber

Jane E Brody, *Jane Brody's Good Food Book: Living the High-Carbohydrate Way* (New York: Norton, 1985), p. 26.

67 a high-fiber, low-purine, low animal-protein diet

R. A. Hiatt et al., "Randomized Controlled Trial of a Low Animal Protein, High Fiber Diet in the Prevention of Recurrent Calcium Oxalate Kidney Stones," *American Journal of Epidemiology* 144, no. 1 (July 1, 1996): 25–33.

70 so damaged by ibuprofen, lectins, and oxalates

When I was a vegan, I ate improperly cooked beans prepared using a slow cooker. My frequent consumption of lectins explains a sudden and debilitating outbreak of irritable bowel syndrome in 1990, with effects lasting to this day.

71 "The first two years [of my vegan diet] I felt great

Lauren Williamson, "Liam Hemsworth Says He Was Forced to Stop Vegan Diet After Health Scare," *Australian Men's Health*, May 2020, https://www.menshealth.com.au/liam-hemsworth-quit-vegan-diet.

71 his veggie diet landed him in the hospital

Scott Henderson, "Liam Hemsworth Is Back in Action," *Men's Health*, April 13, 2020, s.

72 "keep doing it" (a vegan diet) until "you're not feeling great"

Williamson, "Liam Hemsworth Says He Was Forced to Stop Vegan Diet After Health Scare."

Chapter 5

76 "Salts of lemons"

J. Clendinning, "Observation on the History of Oxalic Acid as a Poison," *The London Medical and Surgical Journal* 3, no. 53 (1833).

Fannie Merritt Farmer, *Selections from the Original 1896 Boston Cooking-School Cook Book* (New York, N.Y.: Penguin Books, 1995), p. 46. "Helpful Hints to the Young Housekeeper."

78   in 1632, oxalic acid was fittingly referred to as "tartar"

Albert Hodgkinson, *Oxalic Acid in Biology and Medicine* (London; New York: Academic Press, 1977).

78   used industrially since the 1780s

Jay M. Arena, *Poisoning : Toxicology, Symptoms, Treatments*, 4th ed. (Springfield, IL: Charles C. Thomas, 1979), https://www.worldcat.org/title/poisoning-toxicology -symptoms-treatments/oclc/476721515?referer=br&ht=edition.

R. A. Witthaus and Tracy C. Becker, *Medical Jurisprudence, Forensic Medicine and Toxicology* (USA: William Wood and Company, 1896).

J. Keith Schreiber, "Potassium Oxalate Developer," accessed August 31, 2022, https:// jkschreiber.wordpress.com/platinumpalladium-notes/potassium-oxalate-developer/

78   led to a rash of accidental fatalities in England

Epsom salts being the standard home remedy for stomach ailments and constipation.

78   1823 Scottish publication of a major experimental toxicology study

Robert Christison and Charles Coindet, "An Experimental Inquiry on Poisoning by Oxalic Acid," *Edinburgh Medical and Surgical Journal: Exhibiting a Concise View of the Latest and Most Important Discoveries in Medicine, Surgery, and Pharmacy* 19, no. 75 (1823): 163–99.

79   "Since 1814, [oxalic acid] has fully vindicated its dignity

Clendinning, "Observation on the History of Oxalic Acid as a Poison."

79   the problems arising from skin absorption

Arena, *Poisoning: Toxicology, Symptoms, Treatments*, p. 229.

79   ground banana peels to snatch toxic heavy metals

Muhammad Aqeel Ashraf et al., "Low Cost Biosorbent Banana Peel (*Musa sapientum*) for the Removal of Heavy Metals," *Sci. Res. Essays* 6, no. 19 (2011): 4055–64.

80   *free oxalic acid* ions can take two different forms

Sorrel salt is potassium oxalate—a soluble oxalate which easily dissolves in water into reactive charged particles (oxalic acid ions). The "ate" portion of the name "oxalate" identifies the compound as a "salt" with the potential to dissolve in water.

Chemically salts work like this: Molecules (ions) with positive and negative charges (cations and anions) strongly interact with each other through intense electrostatic forces, which generate bonds. The resulting compounds have bounds of varying strengths determining their relative ability to come apart in solution. The pH of the solution affects the ion form: The single charge anion tends to dominate in blood and body solutions where the pH is neutral or moderately acidic. When pH is basic, it favors the two-anion form, which is more likely to form crystals.

80   Oxalate ions readily attract minerals from the blood plasma

Other minerals that bond to oxalic acid include potassium, lithium, calcium, magnesium, iron, aluminum, manganese, copper, and cadmium.

81   oxalate crystals produce enough membrane damage

J. G. Elferink, "The Mechanism of Calcium Oxalate Crystal-Induced Haemolysis of Human Erythrocytes.," *British Journal of Experimental Pathology* 68, no. 4 (August 1987): 551–57; J. G. Elferink and M. Deierkauf, "Enzyme Release from

Polymorphonuclear Leukocytes during Interaction with Calcium Oxalate Microcrystals," *The Journal of Urology* 138, no. 1 (July 1987): 164–67.

81   **used when testing blood glucose levels**

R. Astles, C. P. Williams, and F. Sedor, "Stability of Plasma Lactate in Vitro in the Presence of Antiglycolytic Agents," *Clinical Chemistry* 40, no. 7, pt 1 (July 1994): 1327–30.

82   **The report in the *Lancet* medical journal**

"*The N.E.J.M.* and *The Lancet* are among the oldest, most respected and most widely read medical journals in the world. They were established in 1821 and 1823 and are ranked often first and second among general-interest medical journals by their 'impact factor,' the frequency with which their studies are cited in other research." Roni Caryn Rabin, "The Pandemic Claims New Victims: Prestigious Medical Journals," *The New York Times*, June 14, 2020, https://www.nytimes.com/2020/06/14/health/virus-journals .html.

82   *"impairment of consciousness soon after the ingestion of a vegetable soup*

Merce Farre et al., "Fatal Oxalic Acid Poisoning from Sorrel Soup," *The Lancet* 334, no. 8678–8679 (December 1989): 1524, https://doi.org/10.1016/S0140-6736(89)92967-X.

82   **"Plants containing oxalic acid are used in cooking**

Farre et al., "Fatal Oxalic Acid Poisoning."

82   **sorrel is considered a health food**

E. Kaegi, "Unconventional Therapies for Cancer: 1. Essiac. The Task Force on Alternative Therapies of the Canadian Breast Cancer Research Initiative," *CMAJ: Canadian Medical Association Journal = Journal de l'Association Medicale Canadienne* 158, no. 7 (April 7, 1998): 897–902.

Chapter 6

84   **Prevention of dietary hyperoxaluria**

Yijuan Sun et al., "Chronic Nephropathy from Dietary Hyperoxaluria: Sustained Improvement of Renal Function after Dietary Intervention," *Cureus* 9, no. 3 (March 20, 2017): e1105, https://doi.org/10.7759/cureus.1105.

84   **emerged as a medical condition associated with diet**

James Begbie, "On Stomach and Nervous Disorder, as Connected with the Oxalic Diathesis," *Monthly Journal of Medical Science* 9 (1849): 943.

Wilson, H., "On the Influence of the Rhubarb Plant in Producing Oxalate of Lime in Urine," *Provincial Medical & Surgical Journal* 10, no. 35 (1846): 413–15.

85   **"oxalate of lime . . . merits special attention . . .**

Golding Bird, *Urinary Deposits: Their Diagnosis, Pathology and Therapeutical Indications*, 5th ed., 1 vol. (London: John Churchill, New Burlington Street, 1857), http://collections.nlm.nih.gov/ext/mhlf/101504251/PDF/101504251.pdf.

85   **in England, rhubarb was wildly popular and was strictly a seasonal treat**

Danny L. Barney and Kim E. Hummer, "Rhubarb: Botany, Horticulture, and Genetic Resources," in *Horticultural Reviews*, Vol. 40 (John Wiley & Sons, Ltd, 2012), 147–82, https://doi.org/10.1002/9781118351871.ch4; Thomas Watson, "Lectures on the

Principles and Practice of Physic (Jaundice, Nephritis Different Kinds of Gravel),"
London Medical Gazette 30, no. Friday, June 3, 1842 (1842): 369–78.

85   **By 1933, the disease was called the *oxalic acid syndrome***

Carl E. Burkland, "Etiology and Prevention of Oxalate Calculi in the Urinary Tract: A
Plan of Therapy," *The Journal of Urology* 46, no. 1 (1941): 82–88., citing a 1933 article
written in French.

85   **"many patients suffering from oxalate stones are nervous**

Burkland, "Etiology and Prevention of Oxalate."

85   **exhaustion of the central nervous system's energy reserves**

Burkland, "Etiology and Prevention of Oxalate." Others have described neurasthenia is
an "imbalance" of the autonomic nervous system (calling it dysautonomia).

86   **"seems now to run some risk of being tossed aside**

Bird, *Urinary Deposits*, 217.

86   **Flexner Report laid out a program**

Thomas P. Duffy, "The Flexner Report—100 Years Later," *The Yale Journal of Biology
and Medicine* 84, no. 3 (September 2011): 269–76.

Note that Dr. Flexner's older brother, Simon, was the first president of the Rockefeller
Institute for Medical Research.

87   **Flexner, lead author of the 1910 report**

Paul Starr and American Council of Learned Societies, *The Social Transformation of
American Medicine* (New York: Basic Books, 1982).

87   **conferences on oxalate held since 1986**

Saeed Khan, PhD, co-chaired the first and organized successive oxalate conferences.

87   **displaced by corporate ownership**

Starr and American Council of Learned Societies; Starr and American Council of
Learned Societies.

89   **"For many years, oxalate has been viewed**

Susan R. Marengo and Andrea M. P. Romani, "Oxalate in Renal Stone Disease: The
Terminal Metabolite That Just Won't Go Away," *Nature Clinical Practice. Nephrology* 4,
no. 7 (July 2008): 368–77, https://doi.org/10.1038/ncpneph0845.

89   **"Excessive consumption of oxalic acid by human beings deserves**

P. P. Singh et al., "Nutritional Value of Foods in Relation to Their Oxalic Acid Content,"
The American Journal of Clinical Nutrition 25, no. 11 (November 1, 1972): 1147–52.

89   **Wilbur Atwater (1844–1907) established the fundamental concepts**

W. O. (Wilbur Olin) Atwater, "Principles of Nutrition and Nutritive Value of Food,"
Bulletin (Washington, DC: U.S. Department of Agriculture, 1902).

90   **remarkable analytical chemist, Ellen Swallow Richards**

Hamilton Cravens, "Establishing the Science of Nutrition at the USDA: Ellen Swallow
Richards and Her Allies," *Agricultural History* 64, no. 2 (1990): 122–33. Mrs. Richards
was a consulting chemist for the Massachusetts State Board of Health from 1872 to 1875,
and the Commonwealth's official water analyst from 1887 until 1897. She also served as
nutrition expert for the US Department of Agriculture. —Wikipedia, accessed May 2021.

90   spread the gospel of New Nutrition

H. Levenstein, "The New England Kitchen and the Origins of Modern American Eating Habits," *American Quarterly* 32, no. 4 (1980): 369–86.

91   vegetarian and strong adherent to Adventist beliefs

M. I. Barber, "Lenna Frances COOPER, February 25, 1875 February 23, 1961," *Journal of the American Dietetic Association* 38 (May 1961): 458.

91   founding 1928 dietetic textbook

Linnea Anderson and Lenna Frances Cooper, *Nutrition in Health and Disease* (Philadelphia: Lippincott, 1982).

92   "It would seem to require a rather improbable combination

David W. Fassett, "Oxalates," in *Toxicants Occurring Naturally in Foods*, 2nd ed. (Washington, DC: National Academy of Sciences, 1973), 346–62, http://www.worldcat .org/title/toxicants-occurring-naturally-in-foods/oclc/650653&referer=brief_results.

Chapter 7

93   It appears that

Robert Christison, "On the Properties of the Ordeal-Bean of Old Calabar, Western Africa," *Monthly Journal of Medicine* 20, no. 3 (March 1855): 199.

94   Every time we pee, we're removing oxalate

Major forms of oxalate in urine are oxalate ions (2-) and Mg-Oxalate. Major forms of calcium in urine are Ca-Cit and Ca++.

Jaroslav Streit, Lan-Chi Tran-Ho, and Erich Königsberger, "Solubility of the Three Calcium Oxalate Hydrates in Sodium Chloride Solutions and Urine-Like Liquors," *Monatshefte Für Chemie / Chemical Monthly* 129, no. 12 (December 1, 1998): 1225–36, https://doi.org/10.1007/PL00010134.

94   unavoidably generate roughly 12 mg of oxalate every day

Ohana, 2013 citing Aronson, 2006. Fargue et al., 2018, "Hydroxyproline Metabolism."

Ehud Ohana et al., "SLC26A6 and NaDC-1 Transporters Interact to Regulate Oxalate and Citrate Homeostasis," *Journal of the American Society of Nephrology* 24, no. 10 (October 1, 2013): 1617–26, https://doi.org/10.1681/ASN.2013010080; Sonia Fargue et al., "Hydroxyproline Metabolism and Oxalate Synthesis in Primary Hyperoxaluria," *Journal of the American Society of Nephrology: JASN* 29, no. 6 (June 2018): 1615–23, https://doi.org/10.1681/ASN.2017040390.

94   total urinary oxalate traffic leaving the body

Hyperoxaluria is often clinically defined as >40 mg in 24 hours. "Normal" levels of oxalate in the urine average 26 mg/ 24 hours. Recent research now suggests a range with an upper limit of 25 mg/ day.

94   The urine oxalate threshold at which hyperoxaluria is identified

Stef Robijn et al., "Hyperoxaluria: A Gut-Kidney Axis?," *Kidney International* 80, no. 11 (December 2011): 1146–58, https://doi.org/10.1038/ki.2011.287.

94   25 mg of oxalate per day in our urine

Ross P. Holmes, Walter T. Ambrosius, and Dean G. Assimos, "Dietary Oxalate Loads and Renal Oxalate Handling," *The Journal of Urology* 174, no. 3 (September 2005): 943–47; discussion 947, https://doi.org/10.1097/01.ju.0000169476.85935.e2;

John Knight, Ross P. Holmes, and Dean G. Assimos, "Intestinal and Renal Handling of Oxalate Loads in Normal Individuals and Stone Formers," *Urological Research* 35, no. 3 (June 2007): 111–17, https://doi.org/10.1007/s00240-007-0090-8;

Tanecia Mitchell et al., "Dietary Oxalate and Kidney Stone Formation," *American Journal of Physiology. Renal Physiology* 316, no. 3 (01 2019): F409–13, https://doi .org/10.1152/ajprenal.00373.2018;

Parveen Kumar et al., "Dietary Oxalate Induces Urinary Nanocrystals in Humans," *Kidney International Reports*, 2020, https://doi.org/10.1016/j.ekir.2020.04.029.

95   **the surfaces of the tubules are built to repel crystals**

Anja Verhulst et al., "Crystal Retention Capacity of Cells in the Human Nephron: Involvement of CD44 and Its Ligands Hyaluronic Acid and Osteopontin in the Transition of a Crystal Binding—into a Nonadherent Epithelium," *Journal of the American Society of Nephrology: JASN* 14, no. 1 (January 2003): 107–15.

95   **stone-resistant kidneys can dilate**

Jacob A. Torres et al., "Crystal Deposition Triggers Tubule Dilation That Accelerates Cystogenesis in Polycystic Kidney Disease," *The Journal of Clinical Investigation* 130 (July 30, 2019), https://doi.org/10.1172/JCI128503.

95   **giving our kidneys a surprisingly high tolerance**

Knight, Holmes, and Assimos, "Intestinal and Renal Handling of Oxalate Loads in Normal Individuals and Stone Formers"; B. Pinto et al., "Patterns of Oxalate Metabolism in Recurrent Oxalate Stone Formers," *Kidney International* 5, no. 4 (April 1, 1974): 285–91, https://doi.org/10.1038/ki.1974.38.

95   **oxalate intake and excretion don't, by themselves, reliably predict**

Knight, Holmes, and Assimos, "Intestinal and Renal Handling of Oxalate Loads in Normal Individuals and Stone Formers"; Pinto et al., "Patterns of Oxalate Metabolism in Recurrent Oxalate Stone Formers."

96   **rare genetic disorders called *primary hyperoxaluria***

PH is believed to affect fewer than three people per million. "Primary" is a term used in medicine to refer to "genetic" or "epi-genetic" causes.

98   **accurate measurement of blood and urine**

Pinto et al., "Patterns of Oxalate Metabolism."

98   **excretion will *increase* after intake goes *down***

M. Hatch et al., "Effect of Megadoses of Ascorbic Acid on Serum and Urinary Oxalate," *European Urology* 6, no. 3 (1980): 166–69.

99   **There are daily rhythms**

P. M. Zarembski and A. Hodgkinson, "Some Factors Influencing the Urinary Excretion of Oxalic Acid in Man," *Clinica Chimica Acta; International Journal of Clinical Chemistry* 25, no. 1 (July 1969): 1–10.

99   **the urine of nearly 4,000 women**

Joanne Yount and Annie Gottlieb, *The Low Oxalate Cookbook, Book Two* (Graham, NC: Vulvar Pain Foundation, 2005), 3–5, 11.

99   followed 13 volunteers in the UK over a full year

W. G. Robertson, A. Hodgkinson, and D. H. Marshall, "Seasonal Variations in the Composition of Urine from Normal Subjects: A Longitudinal Study," *Clinica Chimica Acta; International Journal of Clinical Chemistry* 80, no. 2 (October 15, 1977): 347–53, https://doi.org/10.1016/0009-8981(77)90043-2.

100   you'd need *nine* 24-hour urinalyses

Pallavoor S. Anandaram et al., "Problems in the Metabolic Evaluation of Renal Stone Disease: Audit of Intra-Individual Variation in Urine Metabolites," *Urological Research* 34, no. 4 (August 2006): 249–54, https://doi.org/10.1007/s00240-006-0053-5; Joan H. Parks et al., "A Single 24-Hour Urine Collection Is Inadequate for the Medical Evaluation of Nephrolithiasis," *The Journal of Urology* 167, no. 4 (April 2002): 1607–12; Madhur Nayan, Mohamed A. Elkoushy, and Sero Andonian, "Variations between Two 24-Hour Urine Collections in Patients Presenting to a Tertiary Stone Clinic," *Canadian Urological Association Journal* 6, no. 1 (February 2012): 30–33, https://doi.org/10.5489/cuaj.11131; Abdulrahman F. Alruwaily et al., "How Much Information Is Lost When You Only Collect One 24-Hour Urine Sample during the Initial Metabolic Evaluation?," *The Journal of Urology* 196, no. 4 (October 2016): 1143–48, https://doi.org/10.1016/j.juro.2016.04.074.

R. P. Holmes et al., "Relationship of Protein Intake to Urinary Oxalate and Glycolate Excretion," *Kidney International* 44, no. 2 (August 1993): 366–72.

100   averages are not a useful indicator of oxalate-related problems

Yount and Gottlieb, *The Low Oxalate Cookbook, Book Two*, 4.

100   kidneys are overwhelmed and damaged

Shrikant R. Mulay and Hans-Joachim Anders, "Crystal Nephropathies: Mechanisms of Crystal-Induced Kidney Injury," *Nature Reviews Nephrology* 13, no. 4 (April 2017): 226–40, https://doi.org/10.1038/nrneph.2017.10.

100   "a selective sponge that [retains] most of the oxalates"

W. E. Blackburn et al., "Severe Vascular Complications in Oxalosis after Bilateral Nephrectomy," *Annals of Internal Medicine* 82, no. 1 (January 1975): 44–46, https://doi.org/10.7326/0003-4819-82-1-44.

100   patient's "serum [blood] oxalate level was undetectable"

Gebran Khneizer et al., "Chronic Dietary Oxalate Nephropathy after Intensive Dietary Weight Loss Regimen," *Journal of Nephropathology* 6, no. 3 (July 2017): 126–29, https://doi.org/10.15171/jnp.2017.21.

101   "plasma oxalate measurement is of little diagnostic benefit"

Bernd Hoppe, Bodo B. Beck, and Dawn S. Milliner, "The Primary Hyperoxalurias," *Kidney International* 75, no. 12 (February 18, 2009): 1264–71, https://doi.org/10.1038/ki.2009.32.

102   Box 7.2: Clinical Indicators of Oxalate Overload

Aman Kumar, Prateek Kinra, and A. W. Kashif, "Autopsy Finding in an Infant with Primary Hyperoxaluria (Type-1)," *Annals of Pathology and Laboratory Medicine* 7, no. 12 (December 2020): C-178–82; J. J. Kuiper, "Initial Manifestation of Primary

Hyperoxaluria Type I in Adults—Recognition, Diagnosis, and Management.," *Western Journal of Medicine* 164, no. 1 (January 1996): 42–53.

103 **invaluable information about the effects of high oxalate loads**

H. Pfeiffer et al., "Fatal Cerebro-Renal Oxalosis after Appendectomy," *International Journal of Legal Medicine* 118, no. 2 (April 2004): 98–100, https://doi.org/10.1007/s00414-003-0414-3.

103 **toxicity of xylitol infusions**

Joseph J. Crivelli et al., "Contribution of Dietary Oxalate and Oxalate Precursors to Urinary Oxalate Excretion," *Nutrients* 13, no. 1 (January 2021): 62, https://doi.org/10.3390/nu13010062.

103 **People with PH suffer greatly from various combinations**

Shatha Murad and Yuval Eisenberg, "Endocrine Manifestations of Primary Hyperoxaluria," *Endocrine Practice* 23, no. 12 (November 16, 2017): 1414–24, https://doi.org/10.4158/EP-2017-0029; U. Saatçi et al., "Late Cardiac and Vascular Complications of Primary Hyperoxaluria in Childhood," *Pediatric Nephrology* (Berlin, Germany) 10, no. 5 (October 1996): 677–78, https://doi.org/10.1007/BF03035426; Panagiotis G. Theodossiadis et al., "Choroidal Neovascularization in Primary Hyperoxaluria," *American Journal of Ophthalmology* 134, no. 1 (July 1, 2002): 134–37, https://doi.org/10.1016/S0002-9394(02)01458-7; Neal M. Rao et al., "Stroke in Primary Hyperoxaluria Type I," *Journal of Neuroimaging : Official Journal of the American Society of Neuroimaging* 24, no. 4 (2014): 411–13, https://doi.org/10.1111/jon.12020; Sarah E. Berini et al., "Progressive Polyradiculoneuropathy Due to Intraneural Oxalate Deposition in Type 1 Primary Hyperoxaluria," *Muscle & Nerve* 51, no. 3 (March 2015): 449–54, https://doi.org/10.1002/mus.24495; John Farrell et al., "Primary Hyperoxaluria in an Adult with Renal Failure, Livedo Reticularis, Retinopathy, and Peripheral Neuropathy," *American Journal of Kidney Diseases* 29, no. 6 (June 1, 1997): 947–52, https://doi.org/10.1016/S0272-6386(97)90471-6.

104 **"produces a *confusing multitude of symptoms***

Hoppe, Beck, and Milliner, "The Primary Hyperoxalurias," 1266.

104 **leads to poisoning through accidental ingestion**

Uditha Dassanayake and Christeine Ariaranee Gnanathasan, "Acute Renal Failure Following Oxalic Acid Poisoning: A Case Report," *Journal of Occupational Medicine and Toxicology* (London, England) 7, no. 1 (2012): 17, https://doi.org/10.1186/1745-6673-7-17.

104 **researchers who use EG to create oxalate toxicity**

In rat studies, using 0.75 percent ethylene glycol in drinking water for 28 days is one of the standard techniques used by researchers create high oxalate.

104 **despite relatively normal-looking CT scans**

Bryan M. Freilich et al., "Neuropsychological Sequelae of Ethylene Glycol Intoxication: A Case Study," *Applied Neuropsychology* 14, no. 1 (2007): 56–61, https://doi.org/10.1080/09084280701280494; Majed Mark Samarneh et al., "Severe Oxalosis with Systemic Manifestations," *Journal of Clinical Medicine Research* 4, no. 1 (February 2012): 56–60, https://doi.org/10.4021/jocmr525w; Nandi J. Reddy, Madhuri Sudini, and Lionel D. Lewis, "Delayed Neurological Sequelae from Ethylene Glycol, Diethylene Glycol and Methanol Poisonings," *Clinical Toxicology* 48, no. 10 (December 2010): 967–73, https://doi.org/10.3109/15563650.2010.532803.

Chapter 8

106   **The truth of the ancient adage**

James Begbie, "On Stomach and Nervous Disorder, as Connected with the Oxalic Diathesis," *Monthly Journal of Medical Science* 9 (1849): 943.

106   **50 percent of total body oxalate arrives directly**

R. P. Holmes, H. O. Goodman, and D. G. Assimos, "Contribution of Dietary Oxalate to Urinary Oxalate Excretion," *Kidney International* 59, no. 1 (January 2001): 270–76, https://doi.org/10.1046/j.1523-1755.2001.00488.x.

106   **The remainder (~12 mg) forms inside the body**

J. Knight et al., "Hydroxyproline Ingestion and Urinary Oxalate and Glycolate Excretion," *Kidney International* 70, no. 11 (December 2006): 1929–34, https://doi.org/10.1038/sj.ki.5001906.

107   **Red blood cells also produce low levels**

Ehud Ohana et al., "SLC26A6 and NaDC-1 Transporters Interact to Regulate Oxalate and Citrate Homeostasis," *Journal of the American Society of Nephrology* 24, no. 10 (October 1, 2013): 1617–26, https://doi.org/10.1681/ASN.2013010080; Peter S. Aronson, "Role of SLC26-Mediated Cl-/Base Exchange in Proximal Tubule NaCl Transport," in *Epithelial Anion Transport in Health and Disease: The Role of the SLC26 Transporters Family*, ed. Derek J. Chadwick and Jamie Goode (John Wiley & Sons, Ltd, 2006), 148–63, https://doi.org/10.1002/0470029579.ch10; Joseph J. Crivelli et al., "Contribution of Dietary Oxalate and Oxalate Precursors to Urinary Oxalate Excretion," *Nutrients* 13, no. 1 (January 2021): 62, https://doi.org/10.3390/nu13010062.

109   **"It is frightening to see any glyphosate**

Zen Honeycutt, "Glyphosate Test Results," Moms Across America, accessed February 5, 2022, https://www.momsacrossamerica.com/glyphosate_testing_results.

110   **the excess increases oxalate in the body**

John Knight et al., "Ascorbic Acid Intake and Oxalate Synthesis," *Urolithiasis*, March 22, 2016, https://doi.org/10.1007/s00240-016-0868-7; Holmes, Goodman, and Assimos, "Contribution of Dietary Oxalate to Urinary Oxalate Excretion."

110   **has been shown to increase internal oxalate**

M. Hatch et al., "Effect of Megadoses of Ascorbic Acid on Serum and Urinary Oxalate," *European Urology* 6, no. 3 (1980): 166–69; S. Mashour, J. F. Turner, and R. Merrell, "Acute Renal Failure, Oxalosis, and Vitamin C Supplementation - A Case Report and Review of the Literature," *Chest* 118, no. 2 (August 2000): 561–63, https://doi.org/10.1378/chest.118.2.561; G. J. Mchugh, M. L. Graber, and R. C. Freebairn, "Fatal Vitamin C-Associated Acute Renal Failure," *Anaesthesia and Intensive Care* 36, no. 4 (July 2008): 585–88, https://doi.org/10.1177/0310057X0803600413; Jessica N. Lange et al., "Glyoxal Formation and Its Role in Endogenous Oxalate Synthesis," *Advances in Urology* 2012 (2012), https://doi.org/10.1155/2012/819202.

111   **"misguided use of [IV] vitamin C**

Sofia Marques et al., "A Case of Oxalate Nephropathy: When a Single Cause Is Not Crystal Clear," *American Journal of Kidney Diseases: The Official Journal of the National*

Kidney Foundation 70, no. 5 (November 2017): 722–24, https://doi.org/10 .1053/j.ajkd.2017.05.022.

111   high animal-protein intake in humans lowered oxalate

John Knight et al., "Increased Protein Intake on Controlled Oxalate Diets Does Not Increase Urinary Oxalate Excretion," *Urological Research* 37, no. 2 (April 2009): 63–68, https://doi.org/10.1007/s00240-009-0170-z.

111   feeding meat to rats lowered their oxalate production

P. W. Baker, R. Bais, and A. M. Rofe, "Formation of the L-Cysteine-Glyoxylate Adduct Is the Mechanism by Which L-Cysteine Decreases Oxalate Production from Glycollate in Rat Hepatocytes," *The Biochemical Journal* 302 (Pt 3) (September 15, 1994): 753–57; Paul R. S. Baker et al., "Glycolate and Glyoxylate Metabolism in HepG2 Cells," *American Journal of Physiology—Cell Physiology* 287, no. 5 (November 1, 2004): C1359–65, https://doi.org/10.1152/ajpcell.00238.2004.

112   "the intake of meat proteins may maintain a more balanced

Yingying Zhu et al., "Meat, Dairy and Plant Proteins Alter Bacterial Composition of Rat Gut Bacteria," *Scientific Reports* 5 (October 14, 2015): 15220, https://doi.org/10.1038/ srep15220.

112   Heavy use of gelatin or collagen supplements

Eric N. Taylor and Gary C. Curhan, "Oxalate Intake and the Risk for Nephrolithiasis," *Journal of the American Society of Nephrology* 18, no. 7 (July 1, 2007): 2198–2204, https://doi.org/10.1681/ASN.2007020219; Knight et al., "Hydroxyproline Ingestion and Urinary Oxalate and Glycolate Excretion."

112   suspicion that a high-carb diet contributed directly

J. Knight et al., "Metabolism of Fructose to Oxalate and Glycolate," *Hormone and Metabolic Research = Hormon- Und Stoffwechselforschung = Hormones Et Métabolisme* 42, no. 12 (November 2010): 868–73, https://doi.org/10.1055/s-0030-1265145.

112   diabetes and insulin resistance may be powered by oxalate damage

Tonya N. Zeczycki, Martin St Maurice, and Paul V. Attwood, "Inhibitors of Pyruvate Carboxylase," *The Open Enzyme Inhibition Journal* 3 (2010): 8–26, https://doi.org/10.217 4/1874940201003010008; Urmila P. Kodavanti et al., "Early and Delayed Effects of Naturally Occurring Asbestos on Serum Biomarkers of Inflammation and Metabolism," *Journal of Toxicology and Environmental Health. Part A* 77, no. 17 (2014): 1024–39, https://doi.org/10.1080/15287394.2014.899171.

112   an ultra-low-carbohydrate diet increases production

David J. Sas, Peter C. Harris, and Dawn S. Milliner, "Recent Advances in the Identification and Management of Inherited Hyperoxalurias," *Urolithiasis* 47, no. 1 (February 1, 2019): 79–89, https://doi.org/10.1007/s00240-018-1093-3.

113   human liver cells produce more oxalate when deprived of sugar

Knight et al., "Metabolism of Fructose to Oxalate and Glycolate."

113   include animal-sourced foods

R. A. Hiatt et al., "Randomized Controlled Trial of a Low Animal Protein, High Fiber Diet in the Prevention of Recurrent Calcium Oxalate Kidney Stones," *American Journal of Epidemiology* 144, no. 1 (July 1, 1996): 25–33.

113   **When a person absorbs more than 15 percent**

Ross P. Holmes and Martha Kennedy, "Estimation of the Oxalate Content of Foods and Daily Oxalate Intake," *Kidney International* 57, no. 4 (April 2000): 1662–67, https://doi .org/10.1046/j.1523-1755.2000.00010.x.

114   **the proportion of oxalate getting into the blood can be dramatically higher**

Holmes and Kennedy, "Estimation of the Oxalate Content."

114   **often shared by family members**

M. Peeters, B. Geypens, D. Claus, H. Nevens, Y. Ghoos, G. Verbeke, F. Baert, S. Vermeire, R. Vlietinck, and P. Rutgeerts. "Clustering of Increased Small Intestinal Permeability in Families with Crohn's Disease." *Gastroenterology* 113, no. 3 (September 1997): 802–7. https://doi.org/10.1016/s0016-5085(97)70174-4.

114   **a fact of life for those with gastrointestinal inflammation**

Mohamed Bashir et al., "Enhanced Gastrointestinal Passive Paracellular Permeability Contributes to the Obesity-Associated Hyperoxaluria," *American Journal of Physiology. Gastrointestinal and Liver Physiology* 316, no. 1 (01 2019): G1–14, https://doi.org/ 10.1152/ajpgi.00266.2018. This experiment with rats demonstrated that in obesity there is much higher oxalate absorption and permeability along the entire digestive tract.

114   **a 10-day "green smoothie cleanse"**

Swetha Makkapati, Vivette D. D'Agati, and Leah Balsam, " 'Green Smoothie Cleanse' Causing Acute Oxalate Nephropathy," *American Journal of Kidney Diseases* 71, no. 2 (February 1, 2018): 281–86, https://doi.org/10.1053/j.ajkd.2017.08.002.

114   **Nonsteroidal anti-inflammatory drugs**

Angel Lanas et al., "Prescription Patterns and Appropriateness of NSAID Therapy According to Gastrointestinal Risk and Cardiovascular History in Patients with Diagnoses of Osteoarthritis," *BMC Medicine* 9 (April 14, 2011): 38, https://doi.org/10.1186/1741 -7015-9-38.

115   **60 to 70 percent of NSAID users have gut inflammation**

Carlos Sostres, Carla J. Gargallo, and Angel Lanas, "Nonsteroidal Anti-Inflammatory Drugs and Upper and Lower Gastrointestinal Mucosal Damage," *Arthritis Research & Therapy* 15, no. Suppl 3 (2013): S3, https://doi.org/10.1186/ar4175.

115   **Over a third of NSAID users have intestinal ulcerations**

Sostres, Gargallo, and Lanas, "Nonsteroidal Anti-Inflammatory Drugs."

115   **Oxalate ions and molecules enter the bloodstream**

A. Hesse et al., "Intestinal Hyperabsorption of Oxalate in Calcium Oxalate Stone Formers: Application of a New Test with [13C2]Oxalate," *Journal of the American Society of Nephrology: JASN* 10 Suppl 14 (November 1999): S329-333; Roswitha Siener et al., "Dietary Risk Factors for Hyperoxaluria in Calcium Oxalate Stone Formers," *Kidney International* 63, no. 3 (March 2003): 1037–43, https://doi.org/10.1046/ j.1523-1755.2003.00807.x; Hatim A. Hassan, Ming Cheng, and Peter S. Aronson, "Cholinergic Signaling Inhibits Oxalate Transport by Human Intestinal T84 Cells," *American Journal of Physiology—Cell Physiology* 302, no. 1 (January 1, 2012): C46–58, https://doi.org/10.1152/ajpcell.00075.2011.

115   **membrane *oxalate ion transporters***

These transporters exchange one ion type for another. Like revolving doors, they send one passenger out while pulling a different one into the cell.

115   **fewer active oxalate transporters**

Ruhul Amin et al., "Reduced Active Transcellular Intestinal Oxalate Secretion Contributes to the Pathogenesis of Obesity-Associated Hyperoxaluria," *Kidney International* 93, no. 5 (May 1, 2018): 1098–1107, https://doi.org/10.1016/j.kint.2017.11.011.

115   **when our meals contain gut irritants, lack calcium**

S. Sharma et al., "Comparative Studies on the Effect of Vitamin A, B_1 and B_6 Deficiency on Oxalate Metabolism in Male Rats," *Annals of Nutrition & Metabolism* 34, no. 2 (1990): 104–11, https://doi.org/10.1159/000177576; S. Farooqui et al., "Effect of Pyridoxine Deficiency on Intestinal Absorption of Calcium and Oxalate: Chemical Composition of Brush Border Membranes in Rats," *Biochemical Medicine* 32, no. 1 (August 1984): 34–42.

117   **Blood and urine oxalate levels will already be elevated**

S. B. Erickson et al., "Oxalate Absorption and Postprandial Urine Supersaturation in an Experimental Human Model of Absorptive Hypercalciuria," *Clinical Science* (London, England: 1979) 67, no. 1 (July 1984): 131–38.

117   **man who assiduously followed an antioxidant-rich diet for years**

Barbara Clark, Mohammad Wisam Baqdunes, and Gregory M. Kunkel, "Diet-Induced Oxalate Nephropathy," *BMJ Case Reports* 12, no. 9 (September 16, 2019), https://doi.org/10.1136/bcr-2019-231284.

118   **encourage the colon to excrete more oxalate**

M. Hatch et al., "*Oxalobacter* Sp. Reduces Urinary Oxalate Excretion by Promoting Enteric Oxalate Secretion," *Kidney International* 69, no. 4 (February 2006): 691–98, https://doi.org/10.1038/sj.ki.5000162; Donna Arvans et al., "Oxalobacter Formigenes–Derived Bioactive Factors Stimulate Oxalate Transport by Intestinal Epithelial Cells," *Journal of the American Society of Nephrology* 28, no. 3 (2017): 876–87, https://doi.org/10.1681/ASN.2016020132.

119   **Fewer than one-third of healthy American adults have detectable colonies**

Clea Barnett et al., "The Presence of *Oxalobacter Formigenes* in the Microbiome of Healthy Young Adults," *The Journal of Urology* 195, no. 2 (February 2016): 499–506, https://doi.org/10.1016/j.juro.2015.08.070.

119   **The oxalate in foods enters the blood from**

Z. Chen et al., "Clinical Investigation on Gastric Oxalate Absorption," *Chinese Medical Journal* 116, no. 11 (November 2003): 1749–51.

119   **40 minutes after a healthy person eats spinach**

Parveen Kumar et al., "Dietary Oxalate Loading Impacts Monocyte Metabolism and Inflammatory Signaling in Humans," *Frontiers in Immunology* (2021), https://doi.org/10.3389/fimmu.2021.617508.

Chapter 9

120   **It is fair to assume**

Rostyslav Bilyy et al., "Neutrophils as Main Players of Immune Response towards Nondegradable Nanoparticles," *Nanomaterials* 10, no. 7 (June 29, 2020), https://doi.org/10.3390/nano10071273.

121 "pre-existent calcium-oxalate crystals adherent to tissue(s)

P. O. Schwelle responding to this study:

R. P. Holmes, H. O. Goodman, and D. G. Assimos, "Dietary Oxalate and Its Intestinal Absorption," *Scanning Microscopy* 9, no. 4 (1995): 1109–18; discussion 1118–20. In short-term studies, with a few male participants, normally eating only 200 mg oxalate, an decrease in oxalate excretion often occurs (as Holmes et al., 1995, noted).

123 moderate-oxalate diet becomes an oxalate-depositing diet

C. W. Vermeulen et al., "The Renal Papilla and Calculogenesis.," *J. Urol* 97 (1967): 573–82. They created a spike in oxalate levels by feeding a dose of 1.2 gm per 100 gm of food for 4 days. This was the "trigger" that generates oxalate stones in rats' kidneys. Following the trigger dose, a moderate oxalate intake (0.3 gm oxamide/100 g food) prevented the rats' bodies from clearing the crystals. Thus, the combination of a high dose for 4 days followed by a moderate dose for 24 days created stone disease in every rat. Without the moderate dose following the 4 days of trigger, the initial deposits were cleared. Without a trigger dose, the maintenance diet created stones in only one of twenty rats.

123 tested Dr. Vermeulen's trigger-maintenance theory

Susan Ruth Marengo et al., "The Trigger-Maintenance Model of Persistent Mild to Moderate Hyperoxaluria Induces Oxalate Accumulation in Non-Renal Tissues," *Urolithiasis* 41, no. 6 (November 1, 2013): 455–66, https://doi.org/10.1007/s00240-013-0584-5.

124 In a similar rat study in 1986

M. J. Blumenfrucht, C. Cheeks, and R. P. Wedeen, "Multiorgan Crystal Deposition Following Intravenous Oxalate Infusion in Rat," *The Journal of Urology* 135, no. 6 (June 1986): 1274–79.

125 When they increased their intake to 600 mg

Diana J. Zimmermann, Albrecht Hesse, and Gerd E. von Unruh, "Influence of a High-Oxalate Diet on Intestinal Oxalate Absorption," *World Journal of Urology* 23, no. 5 (November 5, 2005): 324–29, https://doi.org/10.1007/s00345-005-0028-0.

125 eating just 1.6 ounces (50 grams) of milk chocolate

P. Balcke et al., "Transient Hyperoxaluria after Ingestion of Chocolate as a High Risk Factor for Calcium Oxalate Calculi," *Nephron* 51, no. 1 (1989): 32–34.

126 detection requires careful preparation and polarized light microscopy

Blumenfrucht, Cheeks, and Wedeen, "Multiorgan Crystal Deposition Following Intravenous Oxalate Infusion in Rat."

126 can still easily be mistaken for other non-oxalate crystals

A. J. Reginato and B. Kurnik, "Calcium Oxalate and Other Crystals Associated with Kidney Diseases and Arthritis," *Seminars in Arthritis and Rheumatism* 18, no. 3 (February 1989): 198–224.

126 easy to miss or destroy oxalate crystals

C. J. D'Orsi et al., "Is Calcium Oxalate an Adequate Explanation for Nonvisualization of Breast Specimen Calcifications?," *Radiology* 182, no. 3 (March 1992): 801–3, https://doi.org/10.1148/radiology.182.3.1535898; P. J. Symmans, K. Brady, and C. E. Keen, "Calcium Oxalate Crystal Deposition in Epithelioid Histiocytes of Granulomatous Lymphadenitis: Analysis by Light and Electronmicroscopy," *Histopathology* 27, no. 5

(November 1995): 423–29; R. Katoh et al., "Nature and Significance of Calcium Oxalate Crystals in Normal Human Thyroid Gland. A Clinicopathological and Immunohistochemical Study," *Virchows Archiv. A, Pathological Anatomy and Histopathology* 422, no. 4 (1993): 301–6.

Research using electron scanning microscopes has captured images of previously invisible nano-sized oxalate crystals. However, the electron beam destroys the crystals after just a couple of minutes. L. de Meis, W. Hasselbach, and R. D. Machado, "Characterization of Calcium Oxalate and Calcium Phosphate Deposits in Sarcoplasmic Reticulum Vesicles," *The Journal of Cell Biology* 62, no. 2 (August 1, 1974): 505–9.

126   **Oxalate lipids have been found in liver**

P. M. Zarembski and A. Hodgkinson, "Plasma Oxalic Acid and Calcium Levels in Oxalate Poisoning," *Journal of Clinical Pathology* 20, no. 3 (May 1967): 283–85; Reginato and Kurnik, "Calcium Oxalate and Other Crystals Associated with Kidney Diseases and Arthritis"; P. A. Schlesinger, M. T. Stillman, and L. Peterson, "Polyarthritis with Birefringent Lipid within Synovial Fluid Macrophages: Case Report and Ultrastructural Study," *Arthritis and Rheumatism* 25, no. 11 (November 1982): 1365–68.

126   **scans used in clinical diagnosis cannot reliably see oxalate crystals**

L. D. Lewis, B. W. Smith, and A. C. Mamourian, "Delayed Sequelae after Acute Overdoses or Poisonings: Cranial Neuropathy Related to Ethylene Glycol Ingestion," *Clinical Pharmacology and Therapeutics* 61, no. 6 (June 1997): 692–99, https://doi.org/10.1016/S0009-9236(97)90105-3.

127   **from ingestion of ethylene glycol**

Ethylene glycol (coolant chemical) ingestion causes poisoning because it gets transformed into oxalate inside the body. Ethylene glycol does not easily enter by skin or inhalation, but when ingested orally, it can cause serious oxalate poisoning.

127   **CT scans of the head on the day**

Bryan M. Freilich et al., "Neuropsychological Sequelae of Ethylene Glycol Intoxication: A Case Study," *Applied Neuropsychology* 14, no. 1 (2007): 56–61, https://doi.org/10.1080/09084280701280494.

127   **Oxalate crystals have been found in tissues**

S. Bischetti et al., "Carotid Plaque Instability Is Not Related to Quantity but to Elemental Composition of Calcification," *Nutrition, Metabolism, and Cardiovascular Diseases: NMCD* 27, no. 9 (September 2017): 768–74, https://doi.org/10.1016/j.numecd.2017.05.006; Zarembski and Hodgkinson, "Plasma Oxalic Acid and Calcium Levels in Oxalate Poisoning."

127   **crystal accumulation, which can lead to tissue degeneration**

K. W. Small, J. Scheinman, and G. K. Klintworth, "A Clinicopathological Study of Ocular Involvement in Primary Hyperoxaluria Type I.," *The British Journal of Ophthalmology* 76, no. 1 (January 1992): 54–57; C. G. Wells et al., "Retinal Oxalosis— a Clinicopathologic Report," *Archives of Ophthalmology* 107, no. 11 (November 1989): 1638–43.

127   **Oxalate deposits are found in the arteries and in calcified arterial plaques**

Gregory A. Fishbein and Michael C. Fishbein, "Arteriosclerosis: Rethinking the Current Classification," *Archives of Pathology & Laboratory Medicine* 133, no. 8 (August 2009): 1309–16, https://doi.org/10.1043/1543-2165-133.8.1309.

127   Oxalate crystals are associated with blood vessel weakness

Neal M. Rao et al., "Stroke in Primary Hyperoxaluria Type I," *Journal of Neuroimaging: Official Journal of the American Society of Neuroimaging* 24, no. 4 (2014): 411–13, https://doi.org/10.1111/jon.12020; Paniz Fathi et al., "An Unusual Presentation of a Child with Hyperoxaluria," *Archives of Pediatric Infectious Diseases* 7, no. 1 (2019): 1–4, https://doi.org/10.5812/pedinfect.67357.

127   unexplained oxalate deposits in the eyelids

I. Pecorella et al., "Histological Study of Oxalosis in the Eye and Adnexa of AIDS Patients," *Histopathology* 27, no. 5 (November 1995): 431–38; I Pecorella et al., "Postmortem Histological Survey of the Ocular Lesions in a British Population of AIDS Patients," *The British Journal of Ophthalmology* 84, no. 11 (November 2000): 1275–81, https://doi.org/10.1136/bjo.84.11.1275.

127   photoreceptor neurons at the back of the eyes

F. Ungar, I. Piscopo, and E. Holtzman, "Calcium Accumulation in Intracellular Compartments of Frog Retinal Rod Photoreceptors," *Brain Research* 205, no. 1 (January 26, 1981): 200–206, https://doi.org/10.1016/0006-8993(81)90733-2.

128   "Deposition of calcium oxalate crystals in the eye

A. Garner, "Retinal Oxalosis," *The British Journal of Ophthalmology* 58, no. 6 (June 1974): 613–19.

128   Over 70 percent of normal thyroids show oxalate accumulation

Katoh et al., "Nature and Significance of Calcium Oxalate Crystals in Normal Human Thyroid Gland. A Clinicopathological and Immunohistochemical Study"; R. Wahl, R. Fuchs, and E. Kallee, "Oxalate in the Human Thyroid Gland," *European Journal of Clinical Chemistry and Clinical Biochemistry: Journal of the Forum of European Clinical Chemistry Societies* 31, no. 9 (September 1993): 559–65.

128   oxalic acid or oxalate crystal deposits in breasts

Andrés M. Castellaro et al., "Oxalate Induces Breast Cancer," *BMC Cancer* 15 (2015): 761, https://doi.org/10.1186/s12885-015-1747-2; Manuel Scimeca et al., "Microcalcifications Drive Breast Cancer Occurrence and Development by Macrophage-Mediated Epithelial to Mesenchymal Transition," *International Journal of Molecular Sciences* 20, no. 22 (November 11, 2019): 5633, https://doi.org/10.3390/ijms20225633.

128   teeth, bones, bone marrow, ligaments, and joint spaces

L. Pijnenburg et al., "Type 1 Primary Hyperoxaluria: A Case Report and Focus on Bone Impairment of Systemic Oxalosis," *Morphologie* 102, no. 336 (March 1, 2018): 48–53, https://doi.org/10.1016/j.morpho.2017.09.004; Justine Bacchetta et al., "Bone Metabolism in Oxalosis: A Single-Center Study Using New Imaging Techniques and Biomarkers," *Pediatric Nephrology* 25, no. 6 (June 1, 2010): 1081–89, https://doi.org/10.1007/s00467-010-1453-x; R. W. McKenna and L. P. Dehner, "Oxalosis. An Unusual Cause of Myelophthisis in Childhood," *American Journal of Clinical Pathology* 66, no. 6 (December 1976): 991–97, https://doi.org/10.1093/ajcp/66.6.991; Fathi et al., "An Unusual Presentation of a Child with Hyperoxaluria."

128   "The incidence of [bone oxalosis] may be underestimated

Eun Ji Choi et al., "Bone Oxaloma—a Localized Manifestation of Bone Oxalosis," *Skeletal Radiology* 49, no. 4 (2020): 651–55, https://doi.org/10.1007/s00256-019-03348-0.

128 connective tissues that maintain the spine's structure

Helen E. Gruber et al., "Crystal Deposits in the Human Intervertebral Disc: Implications for Disc Degeneration," *The Spine Journal: Official Journal of the North American Spine Society* 7, no. 4 (August 2007): 444–50, https://doi.org/10.1016/j.spinee.2006.08.015.

128 varied oxalate crystals found in and around the joint spaces

P. A. Simkin, "Towards a Coherent Terminology of Gout," *Annals of the Rheumatic Diseases* 52, no. 9 (September 1993): 693–94.

128 oxalate in the painful knee of a patient

H. R. Schumacher, A. J. Reginato, and S. Pullman, "Synovial Fluid Oxalate Deposition Complicating Rheumatoid Arthritis with Amyloidosis and Renal Failure. Demonstration of Intracellular Oxalate Crystals," *The Journal of Rheumatology* 14, no. 2 (April 1987): 361–66.

128 Oxalate accumulation is associated with Parkinson's disease

Sarah E. Berini et al., "Progressive Polyradiculoneuropathy Due to Intraneural Oxalate Deposition in Type 1 Primary Hyperoxaluria," *Muscle & Nerve* 51, no. 3 (March 2015): 449–54, https://doi.org/10.1002/mus.24495; Adam Heller and Sheryl S. Coffman, "Submicron Crystals of the Parkinson's Disease Substantia Nigra: Calcium Oxalate, Titanium Dioxide and Iron Oxide," *BioRxiv*, January 17, 2019, 523878, https://doi.org/10.1101/523878.

129 far more likely to rebuff crystal attachment

C. F. Verkoelen, "Crystal Retention in Renal Stone Disease: A Crucial Role for the Glycosaminoglycan Hyaluronan?," *Journal of the American Society of Nephrology* 17, no. 6 (June 2006): 1673–87, https://doi.org/10.1681/ASN.2006010088.

129 inflammation, low oxygen levels, and low pH (acidity) interfere

Ruhul Amin et al., "Extracellular Nucleotides Inhibit Oxalate Transport by Human Intestinal Caco-2-BBe Cells through PKC-δ Activation," *American Journal of Physiology—Cell Physiology* 305, no. 1 (July 1, 2013): C78–89, https://doi.org/10.1152/ajpcell.00339.2012.

129 cling to the membrane fragments of struggling cells

Garner, "Retinal Oxalosis"; M. Asselman et al., "Calcium Oxalate Crystal Adherence to Hyaluronan-, Osteopontin-, and CD44-Expressing Injured/Regenerating Tubular Epithelial Cells in Rat Kidneys.," *Journal of the American Society of Nephrology: JASN* 14, no. 12 (2003): 3155; Charles M. Brown, Farah Novin, and Daniel L. Purich, "Calcium Oxalate Crystal Morphology: Influence of Phospholipid Micelles with Compositions Based on Each Leaflet of the Erythrocyte Membrane," *Journal of Crystal Growth* 135, no. 3 (February 1, 1994): 523–32, https://doi.org/10.1016/0022-0248(94)90143-0.

130 tissues with transporters include

Seth L. Alper and Alok K. Sharma, "The SLC26 Gene Family of Anion Transporters and Channels," *Molecular Aspects of Medicine* 34, no. 2–3 (April 2013): 494–515, https://doi.org/10.1016/j.mam.2012.07.009.

Feyemi et. al. (1979) observed *"that under certain physiologic and pathologic conditions the thyroid may actively transport oxalate and maintain a concentration gradient over the plasma levels."* A. O. Fayemi, M. Ali, and E. V. Braun, "Oxalosis in Hemodialysis

Patients: A Pathologic Study of 80 Cases," *Archives of Pathology & Laboratory Medicine* 103, no. 2 (February 1979): 58–62.

Membrane transporters exchange chloride/bicarbonate ions in the salivary and pancreatic duct. In their daily work of managing ions, tissues may develop oxalate-related stress and oxalate accumulation problems. Ehud Ohana et al., "SLC26A6 and NaDC-1 Transporters Interact to Regulate Oxalate and Citrate Homeostasis," *Journal of the American Society of Nephrology* 24, no. 10 (October 1, 2013): 1617–26, https://doi .org/10.1681/ASN.2013010080.

130   **Salivary glands concentrate the oxalate**

Miroslav Mydlík and Katarína Derzsiová, "Oxalic Acid as a Uremic Toxin," *Journal of Renal Nutrition: The Official Journal of the Council on Renal Nutrition of the National Kidney Foundation* 18, no. 1 (January 2008): 33–39, https://doi.org/10.1053/j.jrn.2007.10 .008.

130   **oxalate may contribute to salivary stone formation**

Min Goo Lee et al., "Molecular Mechanism of Pancreatic and Salivary Glands Fluid and HCO3– Secretion," *Physiological Reviews* 92, no. 1 (January 2012): 39–74, https:// doi.org/10.1152/physrev.00011.2011; H. Yamamoto et al., "Weddellite in Submandibular Gland Calculus," *Journal of Dental Research* 62, no. 1 (January 1983): 16–19, https://doi .org/10.1177/00220345830620010301; A. T. Jensen and M. Danø, "Crystallography of Dental Calculus and the Precipitation of Certain Calcium Phosphates," *Journal of Dental Research* 33, no. 6 (December 1954): 741–50, https://doi.org/10.1177/002203455 40330060201.

131   **oxalate crystal deposits can provoke chronic inflammatory disease**

J. G. Elferink, "The Mechanism of Calcium Oxalate Crystal-Induced Haemolysis of Human Erythrocytes.," *British Journal of Experimental Pathology* 68, no. 4 (August 1987): 551–57; Benjamin A. Vervaet et al., "An Active Renal Crystal Clearance Mechanism in Rat and Man," *Kidney International* 75, no. 1 (January 2009): 41–51, https://doi.org/10.1038/ki.2008.450; Benjamin A. Vervaet et al., "Response to 'Active Renal Crystal Clearance in Rats and Humans,'" *Kidney International* 75, no. 12 (June 2, 2009): 1357–58, https://doi.org/10.1038/ki.2009.118.

131   **The stealthier nanocrystals are especially destructive**

R. J. Riese et al., "Cell Polarity and Calcium Oxalate Crystal Adherence to Cultured Collecting Duct Cells," *American Journal of Physiology - Renal Physiology* 262, no. 2 (February 1, 1992): F177–84; Xin-Yuan Sun et al., "Size-Dependent Toxicity and Interactions of Calcium Oxalate Dihydrate Crystals on Vero Renal Epithelial Cells," *Journal of Materials Chemistry B* 3, no. 9 (February 18, 2015): 1864–78, https://doi.org/ 10.1039/C4TB01626B.

131   **Oxalate-induced inflammation can occur anywhere**

Tohru Umekawa, Nasser Chegini, and Saeed R. Khan, "Oxalate Ions and Calcium Oxalate Crystals Stimulate MCP-1 Expression by Renal Epithelial Cells," *Kidney International* 61, no. 1 (January 1, 2002): 105–12, https://doi.org/10.1046/j.1523-1755 .2002.00106.x.

131   **"a prime candidate to contribute to the progression of CKD**

T. Ermer et al., "Oxalate, Inflammasome, and Progression of Kidney Disease," *Current Opinion Nephrol Hypertens* 25, no. 4 (July 2016): 363–71.

131 **alarms that may rally more immune cells to gather and clump**

Yale Rosen, "Pathology of Sarcoidosis," *Seminars in Respiratory and Critical Care Medicine* 28, no. 1 (February 2007): 36–52, https://doi.org/10.1055/s-2007-970332.

131 **These compact tumors are called *granulomas***

D. James, "A Clinicopathological Classification of Granulomatous Disorders," *Postgraduate Medical Journal* 76, no. 898 (August 2000): 457–65, https://doi.org/10.1136/pmj.76.898.457.

131 **clustered immune cells become a crystal-containment device**

Shrikant R. Mulay and Hans-Joachim Anders, "Crystallopathies," *New England Journal of Medicine* 374, no. 25 (2016): 2465–76.

131 **"buried" crystals may be accompanied by dormant viruses and bacteria**

Mihail-Alexandru Badea et al., "The Value of Histopathological Diagnosis in the Elderly Patients with Granulomatous Dermatoses. Case Series," *Romanian Journal of Morphology and Embryology* 57, no. 2 (2016): 525–29.

132 **Oxalate-containing granulomas are often asymptomatic**

In some susceptible people, the immune system has trouble switching to cloaking and containment and continues attacking crystals, which encourages additional granuloma formation elsewhere. Multiorgan (non-infectious) granuloma disease is called sarcoidosis and can occur in any organ or tissue. A research pathologist explains: "Granulomas in sarcoidosis develop as a response to the presence of a persistent and poorly degradable antigen" and oxalate is the most common inclusion. Rosen, "Pathology of Sarcoidosis." J. Andrew Carlson and Ko-Ron Chen, "Cutaneous Vasculitis Update: Neutrophilic Muscular Vessel and Eosinophilic, Granulomatous, and Lymphocytic Vasculitis Syndromes," *The American Journal of Dermatopathology* 29, no. 1 (February 2007): 32–43, https://doi.org/10.1097/01.dad.0000245198.80847.ff; J. D. Reid and M. E. Andersen, "Calcium Oxalate in Sarcoid Granulomas. With Particular Reference to the Small Ovoid Body and a Note on the Finding of Dolomite," *American Journal of Clinical Pathology* 90, no. 5 (November 1988): 545–58; Shrikant R. Mulay and Hans-Joachim Anders, "Crystallopathies," *New England Journal of Medicine* 374, no. 25 (2016): 2465–76; J. S. Campbell et al., "Mineral Oil Granulomas of the Uterus and Parametrium and Five Cases Granulomatous Salpingitis with Schaumann Bodies and Oxalate Deposits (of the Uterus, Oviducts, Overies) Were Encountered in the Surgical Pathology Services of the Ottawa General Hospital from 1957 to 1962," *Fertility and Sterility* 15 (June 1964): 278–89, https://doi.org/10.1016/s0015-0282(16)35224-4; J. Coyne et al., "Secondary Oxalosis and Sperm Granuloma of the Epididymis," *Journal of Clinical Pathology* 47, no. 5 (May 1994): 470–71; Naciye Sinem Gezer et al., "Abdominal Sarcoidosis: Cross-Sectional Imaging Findings," *Diagnostic and Interventional Radiology* (Ankara, Turkey) 21, no. 2 (April 2015): 111–17, https://doi.org/10.5152/dir.2014.14210; K. F. Pearce and T. E. Nolan, "Endometrial Sarcoidosis as a Cause of Postmenopausal Bleeding. A Case Report," *The Journal of Reproductive Medicine* 41, no. 11 (November 1996): 878–80.

132 **lead to a condition called *sarcoidosis***

Reid and Andersen, "Calcium Oxalate in Sarcoid Granulomas. With Particular Reference to the Small Ovoid Body and a Note on the Finding of Dolomite."

This study, despite technical challenges, found oxalate deposits in 86 percent of lymph node tissue samples taken from patients with sarcoidosis.

Pathologists have called artery wall plaques (atherosclerosis, hardened arteries) "inside-out granulomas." Antonio J. Pagán and Lalita Ramakrishnan, "The Formation and Function of Granulomas," *Annual Review of Immunology* 36, no. 1 (2018): 639–65, https://doi.org/10.1146/annurev-immunol-032712-100022.

Another study found oxalate crystals in 40 percent of the arterial plaques examined. Fishbein and Fishbein, "Arteriosclerosis."

132   another method for shielding surrounding tissues from oxalate crystals

Esther Fousert, René Toes, and Jyaysi Desai, "Neutrophil Extracellular Traps (NETs) Take the Central Stage in Driving Autoimmune Responses," *Cells* 9, no. 4 (April 8, 2020), https://doi.org/10.3390/cells9040915; Venizelos Papayannopoulos, "Neutrophil Extracellular Traps in Immunity and Disease," *Nature Reviews Immunology* 18, no. 2 (February 2018): 134–47, https://doi.org/10.1038/nri.2017.105; Shrikant R. Mulay and Hans-Joachim Anders, "Neutrophils and Neutrophil Extracellular Traps Regulate Immune Responses in Health and Disease," *Cells* 9, no. 9 (September 20, 2020), https://doi.org/10.3390/cells9092130.

132   oxalates may contribute to gallstones

Bilyy et al., "Neutrophils as Main Players of Immune Response towards Nondegradable Nanoparticles."

Chapter 10

133   With stockpiled toxicants

Stephen J. Genuis and Kasie L. Kelln, "Toxicant Exposure and Bioaccumulation: A Common and Potentially Reversible Cause of Cognitive Dysfunction and Dementia," *Behavioural Neurology* 2015 (2015): 620143, https://doi.org/10.1155/2015/620143.

133   a condition called *oxidative stress*

Kenneth E. McMartin and Kendall B. Wallace, "Calcium Oxalate Monohydrate, a Metabolite of Ethylene Glycol, Is Toxic for Rat Renal Mitochondrial Function," *Toxicological Sciences: An Official Journal of the Society of Toxicology* 84, no. 1 (March 2005): 195–200, https://doi.org/10.1093/toxsci/kfi062.

134   *chronic immune activation* and related damage control

Rostyslav Bilyy et al., "Neutrophils as Main Players of Immune Response towards Nondegradable Nanoparticles," *Nanomaterials* 10, no. 7 (June 29, 2020), https://doi.org/10.3390/nano10071273.

134   lead to insulin resistance, neurological troubles

Ruslan Medzhitov, "Origin and Physiological Roles of Inflammation," *Nature* 454, no. 7203 (July 24, 2008): 428–35, https://doi.org/10.1038/nature07201.

135   They are deficient in needed lipids and glucose

Hélène A. Buc et al., "Metabolic Consequences of Pyruvate Kinase Inhibition by Oxalate in Intact Rat Hepatocytes," *Biochimie* 63, no. 7 (July 20, 1981): 595–602, https://doi.org/10.1016/S0300-9084(81)80057-0.

135   **Their protein production slows down**

W. R. McClure et al., "Rat Liver Pyruvate Carboxylase. II. Kinetic Studies of the Forward Reaction," *The Journal of Biological Chemistry* 246, no. 11 (June 10, 1971): 3579–83.

135   **difficulties with tissue healing, nerve function**

Hélène Buc, France Demaugre, and Jean-Paul Leroux, "The Kinetic Effects of Oxalate on Liver and Erythrocyte Pyruvate Kinases," *Biochemical and Biophysical Research Communications* 85, no. 2 (November 29, 1978): 774–79, https://doi.org/10.1016/0006 -291X(78)91228-7; R. I. Levin, P. W. Kantoff, and E. A. Jaffe, "Uremic Levels of Oxalic Acid Suppress Replication and Migration of Human Endothelial Cells.," *Arteriosclerosis, Thrombosis, and Vascular Biology* 10, no. 2 (March 1, 1990): 198–207, https://doi.org/10 .1161/01.ATV.10.2.198.

135   **reliance on inefficient anaerobic energy production**

Buc, Demaugre, and Leroux, "The Kinetic Effects of Oxalate on Liver and Erythrocyte Pyruvate Kinases"; Buc et al., "Metabolic Consequences of Pyruvate Kinase Inhibition by Oxalate in Intact Rat Hepatocytes."

Oxalate Lowers ATP in RBCs Due to Inhibition of Enzymes

W. B. Novoa et al., "Lactic Dehydrogenase. V. Inhibition by Oxamate and by Oxalate," *The Journal of Biological Chemistry* 234, no. 5 (May 1959): 1143–48; A. S. Mildvan and M. Cohn, "Kinetic and Magnetic Resonance Studies of the Pyruvate Kinase Reaction. II. Complexes of Enzyme, Metal, and Substrates," *The Journal of Biological Chemistry* 241, no. 5 (March 10, 1966): 1178–93; D. B. Northrop and H. G. Wood, "Transcarboxylase. VII. Exchange Reactions and Kinetics of Oxalate Inhibition," *The Journal of Biological Chemistry* 244, no. 21 (November 10, 1969): 5820–27; George H. Reed and Susan D. Morgan, "Kinetic and Magnetic Resonance Studies of the Interaction of Oxalate with Pyruvate Kinase," *Biochemistry* 13, no. 17 (August 1, 1974): 3537–41, https://doi.org/10.1021/bi00714a020; G. Michaels, Y. Milner, and G. H. Reed, "Magnetic Resonance and Kinetic Studies of Pyruvate, Phosphate Dikinase. Interaction of Oxalate with the Phosphorylated Form of the Enzyme," *Biochemistry* 14, no. 14 (July 15, 1975): 3213–19, https://doi.org/10.1021/bi00685a028; Buc et al., "Metabolic Consequences of Pyruvate Kinase Inhibition by Oxalate in Intact Rat Hepatocytes"; D. T. Lodato and G. H. Reed, "Structure of the Oxalate-ATP Complex with Pyruvate Kinase: ATP as a Bridging Ligand for the Two Divalent Cations," *Biochemistry* 26, no. 8 (April 21, 1987): 2243–50, https://doi.org/10.1021/bi00382a026; T. M. Larsen et al., "Structure of the Bis(Mg2+)-ATP-Oxalate Complex of the Rabbit Muscle Pyruvate Kinase at 2.1 A Resolution: ATP Binding over a Barrel," *Biochemistry* 37, no. 18 (May 5, 1998): 6247–55, https://doi.org/10.1021/bi980243s; Jesús Oria-Hernández et al., "Pyruvate Kinase Revisited: The Activating Effect of K+," *The Journal of Biological Chemistry* 280, no. 45 (November 11, 2005): 37924–29, https://doi.org/10.1074/jbc .M508490200.

Oxalate quickly enters cells and penetrates the mitochondria, where it strongly inhibits enzymes needed for glucose generation (pyruvate carboxylase, pyruvate kinase, and lactate dehydrogenase). Compensations such as decreased peripheral use of glucose do not influence glucose release from glycogen.

Emily A. Yount and Robert A. Harris, "Studies on the Inhibition of Gluconeogenesis by Oxalate," *Biochimica et Biophysica Acta (BBA) - General Subjects* 633, no. 1 (November 17, 1980): 122–33, https://doi.org/10.1016/0304-4165(80)90044-6.

135 **Injured mitochondria are a likely factor**

Thomas N. Seyfried, "Ketone Strong: Emerging Evidence for a Therapeutic Role of Ketone Bodies in Neurological and Neurodegenerative Diseases," *Journal of Lipid Research* 55, no. 9 (September 2014): 1815–17, https://doi.org/10.1194/jlr.E052944; Thomas N. Seyfried and Leanne C. Huysentruyt, "On the Origin of Cancer Metastasis," *Critical Reviews in Oncogenesis* 18, no. 1–2 (2013): 43–73; Ann Gardner and Richard G. Boles, "Beyond the Serotonin Hypothesis: Mitochondria, Inflammation and Neurodegeneration in Major Depression and Affective Spectrum Disorders," *Progress in Neuro-Psychopharmacology & Biological Psychiatry* 35, no. 3 (April 29, 2011): 730–43, https://doi.org/10.1016/j.pnpbp.2010.07.030.

135 **mitochondria are unable to generate sufficient energy**

Gardner and Boles, "Beyond the Serotonin Hypothesis."

135 **Circulatory problems, vascular diseases, and**

Levin, Kantoff, and Jaffe, "Uremic Levels of Oxalic Acid Suppress Replication and Migration of Human Endothelial Cells."

135 **Critical tissues with high energy needs**

Frédéric Sedel et al., "Targeting Demyelination and Virtual Hypoxia with High-Dose Biotin as a Treatment for Progressive Multiple Sclerosis," *Neuropharmacology* 110, no. Pt B (November 2016): 644–53, https://doi.org/10.1016/j.neuropharm.2015.08.028; Bruce D. Trapp and Peter K. Stys, "Virtual Hypoxia and Chronic Necrosis of Demyelinated Axons in Multiple Sclerosis," *The Lancet Neurology* 8, no. 3 (March 1, 2009): 280–91, https://doi.org/10.1016/S1474-4422(09)70043-2. Nerve cell distress contributes to muscle weakness, fatigue, poor physical coordination, abdominal pain, twitches and muscle spasms, headaches, memory problems, irritability, and dementia.

136 **the adult human brain requires energy**

A. D. Purdon et al., "Energy Consumption by Phospholipid Metabolism in Mammalian Brain," *Neurochemical Research* 27, no. 12 (December 1, 2002): 1641–47, https://doi.org/10.1023/A:1021635027211.

136 **Oxalate also interferes with the enzymes that replenish**

Yount and Harris, "Studies on the Inhibition of Gluconeogenesis by Oxalate"; F. Demaugre, C. Cepanec, and J. P. Leroux, "Characterization of Oxalate as a Catabolite of Dichloroacetate Responsible for the Inhibition of Gluconeogenesis and Pyruvate Carboxylation in Rat Liver Cells," *Biochemical and Biophysical Research Communications* 85, no. 3 (December 14, 1978): 1180–85, https://doi.org/10.1016/0006-291x(78)90666-6.

136 **diets high in oxalic acid caused hypothyroidism**

M. Goldman and G. J. Doering, "The Effect of Dietary Ingestion of Oxalic Acid on Thyroid Function in Male and Female Long-Evans Rats," *Toxicology and Applied Pharmacology* 48, no. 3 (May 1979): 409–14.

136 **Oxalate in the bone marrow injures the immature blood cells**

Justine Bacchetta et al., "Bone Impairment in Oxalosis: An Ultrastructural Bone Analysis," *Bone* 81 (December 2015): 161–67, https://doi.org/10.1016/j.bone.2015.07.010.

136 **"oxalate-rich meals could cause inflammation**

Mikita Patel et al., "Oxalate Induces Mitochondrial Dysfunction and Disrupts Redox Homeostasis in a Human Monocyte Derived Cell Line," *Redox Biology* 15 (2018): 207–15, https://doi.org/10.1016/j.redox.2017.12.003.

137 Immune responses to oxalates generate additional biochemical

Bernardo S. Franklin, Matthew S. Mangan, and Eicke Latz, "Crystal Formation in Inflammation," *Annual Review of Immunology* 34, no. 1 (2016): 173–202, https://doi.org/ 10.1146/annurev-immunol-041015-055539; Shrikant R. Mulay et al., "Cytotoxicity of Crystals Involves RIPK3-MLKL-Mediated Necroptosis," *Nature Communications* 7 (January 28, 2016): 10274, https://doi.org/10.1038/ncomms10274.

137 gout attacks stop when the body's own enzymes

Christine Schauer et al., "Aggregated Neutrophil Extracellular Traps Limit Inflammation by Degrading Cytokines and Chemokines," *Nature Medicine* 20, no. 5 (May 2014): 511–17, https://doi.org/10.1038/nm.3547.

138 granulomas around crystals may create long-term changes

Marc Hilhorst et al., "T Cell–Macrophage Interactions and Granuloma Formation in Vasculitis," *Frontiers in Immunology* 5 (September 12, 2014), https://doi.org/10.3389/ fimmu.2014.00432; Jean C. Pfau, "Immunotoxicity of Asbestos," *Current Opinion in Toxicology*, Systems Toxicology: *Immunotoxicity* 10 (August 1, 2018): 1–7, https://doi .org/10.1016/j.cotox.2017.11.005.

138 "chronic autoaggression seen in autoimmune disease

P. Matzinger, "Tolerance, Danger, and the Extended Family," *Annual Review of Immunology* 12 (1994): 991–1045, https://doi.org/10.1146/annurev.iy.12.040194.005015. "[The] primary driving force [of the immune system] is the need to detect and protect against danger, and that it does not do the job alone, but receives positive and negative communications from an extended network of other bodily tissues."

138 Such "autoimmunity" is a factor in dozens of illnesses

Mariele De Paola et al., "Granuloma Annulare, Autoimmune Thyroiditis, and Lichen Sclerosus in a Woman: Randomness or Significant Association?," *Case Reports in Dermatological Medicine* 2013 (May 7, 2013): e289084, https://doi.org/10.1155/2013/ 289084.

139 When protecting the kidneys from stones

Kanu Priya Aggarwal et al., "Nephrolithiasis: Molecular Mechanism of Renal Stone Formation and the Critical Role Played by Modulators," *BioMed Research International* 2013 (2013), https://doi.org/10.1155/2013/292953; Saeed R. Khan et al., "Regulation of Macromolecular Modulators of Urinary Stone Formation by Reactive Oxygen Species: Transcriptional Study in an Animal Model of Hyperoxaluria," *American Journal of Physiology - Renal Physiology* 306, no. 11 (June 1, 2014): F1285–95, https://doi.org/ 10.1152/ajprenal.00057.2014; J. C. Lieske et al., "Renal Cell Osteopontin Production Is Stimulated by Calcium Oxalate Monohydrate Crystals," *Kidney International* 51, no. 3 (March 1997): 679–86, https://doi.org/10.1038/ki.1997.98.

Osteopontin is needed for bone metabolism and immune functions and is produced in non-kidney tissues (glands, lungs, GI tract).

139 chronic production of OPN fosters crystal retention

Khan et al., "Regulation of Macromolecular Modulators of Urinary Stone Formation by Reactive Oxygen Species"; Felix Grases et al., "Characterization of Deposits in Patients with Calcific Tendinopathy of the Supraspinatus. Role of Phytate and Osteopontin," *Journal of Orthopaedic Research: Official Publication of the Orthopaedic Research Society* 33, no. 4 (April 2015): 475–82, https://doi.org/10.1002/jor.22801.

139 **periodic spikes in serum osteopontin may be a sign**

Claudia Chiodoni, Mario P. Colombo, and Sabina Sangaletti, "Matricellular Proteins: From Homeostasis to Inflammation, Cancer, and Metastasis," *Cancer and Metastasis Reviews* 29, no. 2 (2010): 295–307; Rasheed Ahmad et al., "Interaction of Osteopontin with IL-18 in Obese Individuals: Implications for Insulin Resistance," *PloS One* 8, no. 5 (2013): e63944, https://doi.org/10.1371/journal.pone.0063944; Urmila P. Kodavanti et al., "Early and Delayed Effects of Naturally Occurring Asbestos on Serum Biomarkers of Inflammation and Metabolism," *Journal of Toxicology and Environmental Health. Part A* 77, no. 17 (2014): 1024–39, https://doi.org/10.1080/15287394.2014.899171.

139 **Serum osteopontin is elevated in people with muscle-pain**

Chiodoni, Colombo, and Sangaletti, "Matricellular Proteins: From Homeostasis to Inflammation, Cancer, and Metastasis."

139 **and other inflammatory diseases such as Crohn's disease**

J. Agnholt et al., "Osteopontin, a Protein with Cytokine-like Properties, Is Associated with Inflammation in Crohn's Disease," *Scandinavian Journal of Immunology* 65, no. 5 (May 2007): 453–60, https://doi.org/10.1111/j.1365-3083.2007.01908.x; Mohamed K. El-Tanani et al., "The Regulation and Role of Osteopontin in Malignant Transformation and Cancer," *Cytokine & Growth Factor Reviews* 17, no. 6 (December 2006): 463–74, https://doi.org/10.1016/j.cytogfr.2006.09.010; Jonathan Golledge et al., "Association between Osteopontin and Human Abdominal Aortic Aneurysm," *Arteriosclerosis, Thrombosis, and Vascular Biology* 27, no. 3 (March 2007): 655–60, https://doi.org/10.1161/01.ATV.0000255560.49503.4e; S. N. Kariuki et al., "Age- and Gender-Specific Modulation of Serum Osteopontin and Interferon-Alpha by Osteopontin Genotype in Systemic Lupus Erythematosus," *Genes and Immunity* 10, no. 5 (July 2009): 487–94, https://doi.org/10.1038/gene.2009.15; Manuel Comabella et al., "Plasma Osteopontin Levels in Multiple Sclerosis," *Journal of Neuroimmunology* 158, no. 1–2 (January 2005): 231–39, https://doi.org/10.1016/j.jneuroim.2004.09.004; Hp Sennels et al., "Circulating Levels of Osteopontin, Osteoprotegerin, Total Soluble Receptor Activator of Nuclear Factor-Kappa B Ligand, and High-Sensitivity C-Reactive Protein in Patients with Active Rheumatoid Arthritis Randomized to Etanercept Alone or in Combination with Methotrexate," *Scandinavian Journal of Rheumatology* 37, no. 4 (August 2008): 241–47, https://doi.org/10.1080/03009740801910320; Susan Amanda Lund, Cecilia M. Giachelli, and Marta Scatena, "The Role of Osteopontin in Inflammatory Processes," *Journal of Cell Communication and Signaling* 3, no. 3–4 (December 2009): 311–22, https://doi.org/10.1007/s12079-009-0068-0.

139 **Elevated OPN promotes scar tissue formation**

Minghua Wu et al., "Osteopontin in Systemic Sclerosis and Its Role in Dermal Fibrosis," *The Journal of Investigative Dermatology* 132, no. 6 (June 2012): 1605–14, https://doi.org/10.1038/jid.2012.32; Aggarwal et al., "Nephrolithiasis."

139 **loss of tissue integrity sets off uncontrolled scar tissue growth**

Hans-Joachim Anders and Liliana Schaefer, "Beyond Tissue Injury-Damage-Associated Molecular Patterns, Toll-like Receptors, and Inflammasomes Also Drive Regeneration and Fibrosis," *Journal of the American Society of Nephrology: JASN* 25, no. 7 (July 2014): 1387–1400, https://doi.org/10.1681/ASN.2014010117; N. Engin Aydin and Ufuk Usta, "Oxalate Deposition in Tissues," *Nephrology Dialysis Transplantation* 19, no. 5 (May 1, 2004): 1323–24, https://doi.org/10.1093/ndt/gfh086; D. J. Coltart and R. E. Hudson, "Primary Oxalosis of the Heart: A Cause of Heart Block," *British Heart Journal* 33, no. 2

(March 1971): 315–19; Thierry Derveaux et al., "Detailed Clinical Phenotyping of Oxalate Maculopathy in Primary Hyperoxaluria Type 1 and Review of the Literature," *Retina* (Philadelphia, PA), April 28, 2016, https://doi.org/10.1097/IAE.00000000 00001058.

139   the replacement of normal cells is impaired by oxalate damage

A. H. Campos and N. Schor, "Mechanisms Involved in Calcium Oxalate Endocytosis by Madin-Darby Canine Kidney Cells," *Brazilian Journal of Medical and Biological Research* 33, no. 1 (January 2000): 111–18, https://doi.org/10.1590/S0100 -879X2000000100015; J. C. Lieske and F. G. Toback, "Interaction of Urinary Crystals with Renal Epithelial Cells in the Pathogenesis of Nephrolithiasis," *Seminars in Nephrology* 16, no. 5 (September 1996): 458–73; M. A. Boogaerts et al., "Mechanisms of Vascular Damage in Gout and Oxalosis: Crystal Induced, Granulocyte Mediated, Endothelial Injury," *Thrombosis and Haemostasis* 50, no. 2 (August 30, 1983): 576–80.

139   normal cells diminish, but the scar tissue continues

Levin, Kantoff, and Jaffe, "Uremic Levels of Oxalic Acid Suppress Replication and Migration of Human Endothelial Cells."

139   fibrosis can occur in organs, joints

Levin, Kantoff, and Jaffe, "Uremic Levels of Oxalic Acid."

140   *non-resolving fibrosis* is a feature of many chronic

Michael Zeisberg and Raghu Kalluri, "Cellular Mechanisms of Tissue Fibrosis. 1. Common and Organ-Specific Mechanisms Associated with Tissue Fibrosis," *American Journal of Physiology - Cell Physiology* 304, no. 3 (February 1, 2013): 201, https://doi.org/ 10.1152/ajpcell.00328.2012.

140   Taking anti-inflammatory agents doesn't stop fibrosis

Hans-Joachim Anders and Daniel A. Muruve, "The Inflammasomes in Kidney Disease," *Journal of the American Society of Nephrology: JASN* 22, no. 6 (June 2011): 1007–18, https://doi.org/10.1681/ASN.2010080798.

140   "[e]limination of the inciting stimulus

Don C. Rockey, P. Darwin Bell, and Joseph A. Hill, "Fibrosis–a Common Pathway to Organ Injury and Failure," *The New England Journal of Medicine* 372, no. 12 (March 19, 2015): 1144, https://doi.org/10.1056/NEJMra1300575.

140   oxalate crystals cause fibrosis

Sunisa Yoodee et al., "Effects of Secretome Derived from Macrophages Exposed to Calcium Oxalate Crystals on Renal Fibroblast Activation," *Communications Biology* 4 (August 11, 2021): 959, https://doi.org/10.1038/s42003-021-02479-2.

140   when normal cells regain their ability to reproduce

A. Saxon et al., "Renal Transplantation in Primary Hyperoxaluria," *Archives of Internal Medicine* 133, no. 3 (March 1974): 464–67; I. Mandell, E. Krauss, and J. C. Millan, "Oxalate-Induced Acute Renal Failure in Crohn's Disease," *The American Journal of Medicine* 69, no. 4 (October 1980): 628–32; S. R. Khan et al., "Crystal Retention by Injured Urothelium of the Rat Urinary Bladder," *The Journal of Urology* 132, no. 1 (July 1984): 153–57.

140   Oxalate is a powerful *mast cell* activator

Ronald E. Bray and Paul P. VanArsdel, "In Vitro Histamine Release from Rat Mast Cells by Chemical and Physical Agents," *Proceedings of the Society for Experimental Biology*

and Medicine 106, no. 2 (February 1, 1961): 255–59, https://doi.org/10.3181/00379727
-106-26302.

141   mast cells secrete over 200 response chemicals

Theoharis C. Theoharides, Irene Tsilioni, and Huali Ren, "Recent Advances in Our
Understanding of Mast Cell Activation—or Should It Be Mast Cell Mediator
Disorders?," *Expert Review of Clinical Immunology* 15, no. 6 (June 2019): 639–56,
https://doi.org/10.1080/1744666X.2019.1596800.

141   associated with mast-cell activation

Lawrence B. Afrin, "Mast Cell Activation Disease and the Modern Epidemic of Chronic
Inflammatory Disease," *Translational Research: The Journal of Laboratory and Clinical
Medicine* 174 (2016): 33–59, https://doi.org/10.1016/j.trsl.2016.01.003; Lawrence B.
Afrin et al., "Diagnosis of Mast Cell Activation Syndrome: A Global 'Consensus-2,'"
Diagnosis (Berlin, Germany) 8, no. 2 (May 26, 2021): 137–52, https://doi.org/10.1515/
dx-2020-0005.

141   Symptoms are not the most reliable indicators

L. Boquist et al., "Primary Oxalosis," *The American Journal of Medicine* 54, no. 5 (May
1973): 673–81. "Physical findings are sparse . . . The clinical features most commonly
encountered are renal colic [. . .] hematuria, recurrent urinary tract infections[. . .]. Less
commonly encountered are joint manifestations, Raynaud's disease . . . secondary
hyperparathyroidism [. . .] nerve fiber degeneration and perineural fibrosis were
found . . . but vascular changes with impaired blood supply may have played a role."

142   Calcium deficiency, even when minimal, is bad

L. Böhn, S. Störsrud, and M. Simrén, "Nutrient Intake in Patients with Irritable Bowel
Syndrome Compared with the General Population," *Neurogastroenterology and Motility:
The Official Journal of the European Gastrointestinal Motility Society* 25, no. 1 (January
2013): 23-30.e1, https://doi.org/10.1111/nmo.12001; Tarek Mazzawi et al., "Effects of
Dietary Guidance on the Symptoms, Quality of Life and Habitual Dietary Intake of
Patients with Irritable Bowel Syndrome," *Molecular Medicine Reports* 8, no. 3 (September
2013): 845–52, https://doi.org/10.3892/mmr.2013.1565; Marion J. Torres et al., "Food
Consumption and Dietary Intakes in 36,448 Adults and Their Association with Irritable
Bowel Syndrome: Nutrinet-Santé Study," *Therapeutic Advances in Gastroenterology* 11
(2018): 1756283X17746625, https://doi.org/10.1177/1756283X17746625; Harold D.
Foster, *Health, Disease & the Environment* (London: Bellhaven Press, 1992); Ian J. Deary,
Alan E. Hendrickson, and Alistair Burns, "Serum Calcium Levels in Alzheimer's Disease:
A Finding and an Aetiological Hypothesis," *Personality and Individual Differences* 8, no. 1
(January 1, 1987): 75–80, https://doi.org/10.1016/0191-8869(87)90013-4; Nicholas J.
Talley, "What Causes Functional Gastrointestinal Disorders? A Proposed Disease Model,"
American Journal of Gastroenterology 115, no. 1 (January 2020): 41–48, https://doi.org/
10.14309/ajg.0000000000000485.

142   body maintains normal calcium and magnesium levels

M. Yasui, Y. Yase, and K. Ota, "Distribution of Calcium in Central Nervous System
Tissues and Bones of Rats Maintained on Calcium-Deficient Diets," *Journal of the
Neurological Sciences* 105, no. 2 (October 1991): 206–10, https://doi.org/10.1016/0022
-510x(91)90146-x; M. Yasui et al., "Distribution of Magnesium in Central Nervous
System Tissue, Trabecular and Cortical Bone in Rats Fed with Unbalanced Diets of
Minerals," *Journal of the Neurological Sciences* 99, no. 2–3 (November 1990): 177–83,
https://doi.org/10.1016/0022-510x(90)90154-f.

143 common first symptoms of primary hyperoxaluria

Eduardo Salido et al., "Primary Hyperoxalurias: Disorders of Glyoxylate Detoxification," *Biochimica Et Biophysica Acta* 1822, no. 9 (September 2012): 1453–64, https://doi.org/10.1016/j.bbadis.2012.03.004.

143 **people with IBS or depression also tend to suffer from rheumatoid arthritis**

Gardner and Boles, "Beyond the Serotonin Hypothesis"; Tobias Liebregts et al., "Immune Activation in Patients with Irritable Bowel Syndrome," *Gastroenterology* 132, no. 3 (March 2007): 913–20, https://doi.org/10.1053/j.gastro.2007.01.046.

143 **Persons with celiac disease or IBS are more likely to also develop osteoporosis**

D. J. Stobaugh, P. Deepak, and E. D. Ehrenpreis, "Increased Risk of Osteoporosis-Related Fractures in Patients with Irritable Bowel Syndrome," *Osteoporosis International: A Journal Established as Result of Cooperation between the European Foundation for Osteoporosis and the National Osteoporosis Foundation of the USA* 24, no. 4 (April 2013): 1169–75, https://doi.org/10.1007/s00198-012-2141-4; Katriina Heikkilä et al., "Celiac Disease and Bone Fractures: A Systematic Review and Meta-Analysis," *The Journal of Clinical Endocrinology & Metabolism* 100, no. 1 (January 1, 2015): 25–34, https://doi.org/10.1210/jc.2014-1858; Ardita Aliko et al., "Oral Mucosa Involvement in Rheumatoid Arthritis, Systemic Lupus Erythematosus and Systemic Sclerosis," *International Dental Journal* 60, no. 5 (October 2010): 353–58.

143 **oxalate crystals injected into only *one* back foot**

C. W. Denko and M. Petricevic, "Sympathetic or Reflex Footpad Swelling Due to Crystal-Induced Inflammation in the Opposite Foot," *Inflammation* 3, no. 1 (March 1978): 81–86.

147 **oxalate exposure can reduce nutrient uptake**

Zeynep Celebi Sözener et al., "Environmental Factors in Epithelial Barrier Dysfunction," *Journal of Allergy and Clinical Immunology* 145, no. 6 (June 1, 2020): 1517–28, https://doi.org/10.1016/j.jaci.2020.04.024.

147 **Oxalate has been associated with gut inflammation**

Samuel A. Brown and Alexander O. Gettler, "A Study of Oxalic-Acid Poisoning," *Proceedings of the Society for Experimental Biology and Medicine* 19, no. 5 (February 1, 1922): 204–8, https://doi.org/10.3181/00379727-19-95.

147 **those who suffered "from stomach and nervous complaints**

James Begbie, "On Stomach and Nervous Disorder, as Connected with the Oxalic Diathesis," *Monthly Journal of Medical Science* 9 (1849): 943.

147 **"excluding all those foodstuffs known to be rich in oxalates**

Anonymous, "Oxaluria," *Lancet*, March 28, 1925, 673.

147 **evidenced by the similar urinary patterns**

Michael E. Moran, "Associated Systemic Diseases," in *Urinary Stone Disease: The Practical Guide to Medical and Surgical Management*, ed. Marshall L. Stoller and Maxwell V. Meng, Current Clinical Urology (Totowa, NJ: Humana Press, 2007), 237–57, https://doi.org/10.1007/978-1-59259-972-1_12.

148 **Debra's speedy recovery from spastic bowel suggests**

The complete reversal of these symptoms over a few days implies a functional, rather than structural, impairment.

148   associations between gut problems and pain

Tryptophan deficiency can lead to lower serotonin levels. Michael Maes et al., "Serotonin-Immune Interactions in Major Depression: Lower Serum Tryptophan as a Marker of an Immune-Inflammatory Response," *European Archives of Psychiatry and Clinical Neuroscience* 247, no. 3 (June 1, 1997): 154–61, https://doi.org/10.1007/BF03033069.

149   **Hiccups are common with oxalate poisoning**

Chien-Liang Chen et al., "Neurotoxic Effects of Carambola in Rats: The Role of Oxalate," *Journal of the Formosan Medical Association = Taiwan Yi Zhi* 101, no. 5 (May 2002): 337–41.

149   **The neurological and psychiatric symptoms of oxalate poisoning**

Shang-Hang Chen et al., "Star Fruit Intoxication in a Patient with Moderate Renal Insufficiency Presents as a Posterior Reversible Encephalopathy Syndrome," *Acta Neurologica Taiwanica* 19, no. 4 (December 2010): 287–91.

150   **"Symptoms of neurological effects [of oxalate poisoning] can be**

R. Von Burg, "Oxalic Acid and Sodium Oxalate," *Journal of Applied Toxicology: JAT* 14, no. 3 (May 1, 1994): 233–37.

150   **Low energy and calcium imbalance are factors in age-related**

Urszula Wojda, Elzbieta Salinska, and Jacek Kuznicki, "Calcium Ions in Neuronal Degeneration," *IUBMB Life* 60, no. 9 (September 2008): 575–90, https://doi.org/10.1002/iub.91; Daniel Carleton Gajdusek, *Interference with Axonal Transport of Neurofilament as the Common Etiology and Pathogenesis of Neurofibrillary Tangles, Amyotrophic Lateral Sclerosis, Parkinsonism-Dementia, and Many Other Degenerations of the CNS: A Series of Hypotheses, Perspectives for Research* (US Department of Health and Human Services, National Institutes of Health, 1984).

150   **MS is a disease in which the energy-hungry insulating myelin sheath**

Sedel et al., "Targeting Demyelination and Virtual Hypoxia with High-Dose Biotin as a Treatment for Progressive Multiple Sclerosis"; Elizabeth A. Young et al., "Imaging Correlates of Decreased Axonal Na+/K+ ATPase in Chronic Multiple Sclerosis Lesions," *Annals of Neurology* 63, no. 4 (2008): 428–35, https://doi.org/10.1002/ana.21381.

150   **Energy metabolism problems in brain cells promote**

Gardner and Boles, "Beyond the Serotonin Hypothesis."

150   **elevated levels of oxalate may "starve" cells of sulfur ions**

Oxalate competes with sulfur for entry to cells; cells in need of sulfur may collect oxalate and frustrate the attempts to imbibe sulfur ions.

150   *neurosteroids*—**are hormones made in the brain**

Thomas Alec Lightning, Tarsis F. Gesteira, and Jonathan Wolf Mueller, "Steroid Disulfates - Sulfation Double Trouble," *Molecular and Cellular Endocrinology* 524 (March 15, 2021): 111161, https://doi.org/10.1016/j.mce.2021.111161; Mercedes M. Pérez-Jiménez et al., "Steroid Hormones Sulfatase Inactivation Extends Lifespan and Ameliorates Age-Related Diseases," *Nature Communications* 12, no. 1 (January 4, 2021): 49, https://doi.org/10.1038/s41467-020-20269-y.

150   **oxalate depletes their calcium or magnesium**

Abolfazl Avan et al., "Platinum-Induced Neurotoxicity and Preventive Strategies: Past, Present, and Future," *The Oncologist* 20, no. 4 (April 2015): 411–32, https://doi.org/10

.1634/theoncologist.2014-0044; Laurence Gamelin et al., "Predictive Factors of Oxaliplatin Neurotoxicity: The Involvement of the Oxalate Outcome Pathway," *Clinical Cancer Research: An Official Journal of the American Association for Cancer Research* 13, no. 21 (November 1, 2007): 6359–68, https://doi.org/10.1158/1078-0432.CCR-07-0660; Laurence Gamelin et al., "Prevention of Oxaliplatin-Related Neurotoxicity by Calcium and Magnesium Infusions: A Retrospective Study of 161 Patients Receiving Oxaliplatin Combined with 5-Fluorouracil and Leucovorin for Advanced Colorectal Cancer," *Clinical Cancer Research* 10, no. 12 (June 15, 2004): 4055–61, https://doi.org/10.1158/1078-0432.CCR-03-0666; F. Grolleau et al., "A Possible Explanation for a Neurotoxic Effect of the Anticancer Agent Oxaliplatin on Neuronal Voltage-Gated Sodium Channels," *Journal of Neurophysiology* 85, no. 5 (May 2001): 2293–97.

150   Another way oxalate produces pain is by triggering inflammatory "storms"

J. E. Fantasia et al., "Calcium Oxalate Deposition in the Periodontium Secondary to Chronic Renal Failure," *Oral Surgery, Oral Medicine, and Oral Pathology* 53, no. 3 (March 1982): 273–79; Aydin and Usta, "Oxalate Deposition in Tissues."

151   Being mast-cell activators, nerve toxins, and connective tissue destabilizers

Lawrence B. Afrin and Gerhard J. Molderings, "A Concise, Practical Guide to Diagnostic Assessment for Mast Cell Activation Disease," *World Journal of Hematology* 3, no. 1 (2014): 1–17; Afrin, "Mast Cell Activation Disease and the Modern Epidemic of Chronic Inflammatory Disease."

151   Effects on intestinal neurons help explain the anxiety, fatigue

Talley, "What Causes Functional Gastrointestinal Disorders?"; Liebregts et al., "Immune Activation in Patients with Irritable Bowel Syndrome."

151   Migraines tend to cluster with other oxalate-related symptoms

"Common migraine comorbidities affect multiple organ systems in addition to the [brain]. These include Raynaud's phenomenon, hypertension, interstitial cystitis/bladder pain syndrome (IC/BPS), allergy and asthma, irritable bowel syndrome (IBS), osteo- and rheumatoid arthritis, anxiety, tremor, and depression. The molecular underpinnings common to and connecting these disorders are not known, but may include . . . signaling events that activate pain, inflammation, or oxidative pathways." Andrea I. Loewendorf et al., "Roads Less Traveled: Sexual Dimorphism and Mast Cell Contributions to Migraine Pathology," *Frontiers in Immunology* 7 (2016): 2, https://doi.org/10.3389/fimmu.2016.00140.

151   Oxalate-related damage, metabolic stress, and inflammation also contribute

As Ermer et al. (2016) put it, "[H]igh plasma oxalate levels . . . launch a vicious cycle of inflammasome-mediated systemic inflammation . . . In particular, the cardiovascular implications of high oxalate levels in the circulation are of great concern."

T. Ermer et al., "Oxalate, Inflammasome, and Progression of Kidney Disease," *Current Opinion Nephrol Hypertens* 25, no. 4 (July 2016): 363–71.

Barbara A. Gilchrest, John W. Rowe, and Martin C. Mihm, "Clinical and Histological Skin Changes in Chronic Renal Failure: Evidence for a Dialysis-Resistant, Transplant-Responsive Microangiopathy," *The Lancet*, Originally published as Volume 2, Issue 8207, 316, no. 8207 (December 13, 1980): 1271–75, https://doi.org/10.1016/S0140-6736(80)92337-5; Miroslav Mydlík and Katarína Derzsiová, "Oxalic Acid as a Uremic Toxin," *Journal of Renal Nutrition: The Official Journal of the Council on Renal Nutrition of the National Kidney Foundation* 18, no. 1 (January 2008): 33–39, https://doi

.org/10.1053/j.jrn.2007.10.008; J. S. Yudkin et al., "Inflammation, Obesity, Stress and Coronary Heart Disease: Is Interleukin-6 the Link?," *Atherosclerosis* 148, no. 2 (February 2000): 209–14, https://doi.org/10.1016/s0021-9150(99)00463-3; J. Danesh et al., "Low Grade Inflammation and Coronary Heart Disease: Prospective Study and Updated Meta-Analyses," *BMJ (Clinical Research Ed.)* 321, no. 7255 (July 22, 2000): 199–204, https://doi.org/10.1136/bmj.321.7255.199; Wolfgang Koenig, "Inflammation and Coronary Heart Disease: An Overview," *Cardiology in Review* 9, no. 1 (February 2001): 31–35.

151 **Elevated levels of oxalate inhibit normal endothelial cell function**

Phoebe A. Recht et al., "Oxalic Acid Alters Intracellular Calcium in Endothelial Cells," *Atherosclerosis* 173, no. 2 (April 2004): 321–28, https://doi.org/10.1016/j.atherosclerosis .2003.11.023.

151 **cells can't replace themselves at a fast enough rate**

Levin, Kantoff, and Jaffe, "Uremic Levels of Oxalic Acid Suppress Replication and Migration of Human Endothelial Cells."

151 **Endothelial dysfunction in turn promotes a pro-inflammatory environment**

Boogaerts et al., "Mechanisms of Vascular Damage in Gout and Oxalosis"; Georg Schlieper et al., "Vascular Calcification in Chronic Kidney Disease: An Update," *Nephrology Dialysis Transplantation* 31, no. 1 (January 1, 2016): 31–39, https://doi.org/ 10.1093/ndt/gfv111.

151 **Vascular inflammation, or *vasculitis*, is an immune response**

"Giant Cell Arteritis," *Johns Hopkins Vasculitis Center* (blog), accessed July 1, 2020, https://www.hopkinsvasculitis.org/types-vasculitis/giant-cell-arteritis/.

151 **to problems in the arteries and veins**

G. S. Arbus and S. Sniderman, "Oxalosis with Peripheral Gangrene," *Archives of Pathology* 97, no. 2 (February 1974): 107–10.

152 **This is an aspect of a condition called vasospastic angina**

Hongtao Sun et al., "Coronary Microvascular Spasm Causes Myocardial Ischemia in Patients with Vasospastic Angina," *Journal of the American College of Cardiology* 39, no. 5 (March 6, 2002): 847–51, https://doi.org/10.1016/s0735-1097(02)01690-x.

152 **Oxalate-instigated calcium dysregulation is linked to abnormal blood pressure**

Hawa N. Siti, Y. Kamisah, and J. Kamsiah, "The Role of Oxidative Stress, Antioxidants and Vascular Inflammation in Cardiovascular Disease (a Review)," *Vascular Pharmacology* 71 (August 2015): 40–56, https://doi.org/10.1016/j.vph.2015.03.005; Carl E. Burkland, "Etiology and Prevention of Oxalate Calculi in the Urinary Tract: A Plan of Therapy," *The Journal of Urology* 46, no. 1 (1941): 82–88.

152 **calcium deficiency can cause vascular calcification and hypertension**

L. M. Resnick, "Calcium Metabolism in Hypertension and Allied Metabolic Disorders," *Diabetes Care* 14, no. 6 (June 1991): 505–20, https://doi.org/10.2337/diacare.14.6.505; Maoqing Wang et al., "Calcium-Deficiency Assessment and Biomarker Identification by an Integrated Urinary Metabonomics Analysis," *BMC Medicine* 11 (March 28, 2013): 86, https://doi.org/10.1186/1741-7015-11-86; Schlieper et al., "Vascular Calcification in Chronic Kidney Disease."

152   calcification-promoting proteins (including osteopontin)

Andrew P. Sage et al., "Hyperphosphatemia-Induced Nanocrystals Upregulate the Expression of Bone Morphogenetic Protein-2 and Osteopontin Genes in Mouse Smooth Muscle Cells in Vitro," *Kidney International* 79, no. 4 (February 2, 2011): 414–22, https://doi.org/10.1038/ki.2010.390; Johan M. Lorenzen et al., "Osteopontin in the Development of Systemic Sclerosis–Relation to Disease Activity and Organ Manifestation," *Rheumatology* (Oxford, England) 49, no. 10 (October 2010): 1989–91, https://doi.org/10.1093/rheumatology/keq223.

152   vascular smooth muscle cells with disturbed calcium metabolism

Nonanzit Pérez-Hernández et al., "Vascular Calcification: Current Genetics Underlying This Complex Phenomenon," *Chinese Medical Journal* 130, no. 9 (May 5, 2017): 1113–21, https://doi.org/10.4103/0366-6999.204931; Rukshana C. Shroff et al., "Chronic Mineral Dysregulation Promotes Vascular Smooth Muscle Cell Adaptation and Extracellular Matrix Calcification," *Journal of the American Society of Nephrology: JASN* 21, no. 1 (January 2010): 103–12, https://doi.org/10.1681/ASN.2009060640.

152   vessels directly collect calcium oxalate deposits in the cells

Levin, Kantoff, and Jaffe, "Uremic Levels of Oxalic Acid Suppress Replication and Migration of Human Endothelial Cells"; Gilchrest, Rowe, and Mihm, "Clinical and Histological Skin Changes in Chronic Renal Failure"; Mydlík and Derzsiová, "Oxalic Acid as a Uremic Toxin"; W. R. Salyer and D. Keren, "Oxalosis as a Complication of Chronic Renal Failure," *Kidney International* 4, no. 1 (July 1973): 61–66. There is generalized vasospastic tendency in these cells that increases their susceptibility.

152   Vascular damage and related inflammation increase the crystal deposition

Fantasia et al., "Calcium Oxalate Deposition in the Periodontium Secondary to Chronic Renal Failure"; Gerald F. Falasca et al., "Superoxide Anion Production and Phagocytosis of Crystals by Cultured Endothelial Cells," *Arthritis & Rheumatism* 36, no. 1 (January 1, 1993): 105–16, https://doi.org/10.1002/art.1780360118.

152   "high plasma oxalate levels . . . launch a vicious cycle

Ermer et al., "Oxalate, Inflammasome, and Progression of Kidney Disease."

153   oxalate causes "vascular obliteration" and poor blood flow

Antonio J. Reginato, "Calcium Oxalate and Other Crystals or Particles Associated with Arthritis," in *Arthritis and Allied Conditions*, ed. William J. Koopman, 14th ed., vol. 2, 2 vols. (Philadelphia: Lippincott, Williams & Wilkins, 2001); Irama Maldonado, Vineet Prasad, and Antonio J. Reginato, "Oxalate Crystal Deposition Disease," *Current Rheumatology Reports* 4, no. 3 (May 1, 2002): 257–64, https://doi.org/10.1007/s11926 -002-0074-1; Joseph A. Blackmon et al., "Oxalosis Involving the Skin: Case Report and Literature Review," *Archives of Dermatology* 147, no. 11 (November 2011): 1302–5, https://doi.org/10.1001/archdermatol.2011.182; E. Jorquera-Barquero et al., "Oxalosis and Livedo Reticularis," *Actas Dermo-Sifiliográficas* 104, no. 9 (November 2013): 815–18, https://doi.org/10.1016/j.ad.2012.04.019.

153   leading to sudden death

W. R. Salyer and G. M. Hutchins, "Cardiac Lesions in Secondary Oxalosis," *Archives of Internal Medicine* 134, no. 2 (August 1974): 250–52: "oxalate-induced fibrosis contributed significantly to the congestive heart failure of these patients [with chronic renal insufficiency," 251.

153   symptoms (seen in PH patients) are shortness of breath, chest pain

Farouk Mookadam et al., "Cardiac Abnormalities in Primary Hyperoxaluria," *Circulation Journal: Official Journal of the Japanese Circulation Society* 74, no. 11 (November 2010): 2403–9.

153   with other oxalate-related autoimmune conditions

Kevin G. Moder, Todd D. Miller, and Henry D. Tazelaar, "Cardiac Involvement in Systemic Lupus Erythematosus," *Mayo Clinic Proceedings* 74, no. 3 (March 1, 1999): 275–84, https://doi.org/10.4065/74.3.275; Maurizio Turiel et al., "The Heart in Rheumatoid Arthritis," *Autoimmunity Reviews* 9, no. 6 (April 1, 2010): 414–18, https://doi.org/10.1016/j.autrev.2009.11.002; William P. Follansbee, Tony R. Zerbe, and Thomas A. Medsger, "Cardiac and Skeletal Muscle Disease in Systemic Sclerosis (Scleroderma): A High Risk Association," *American Heart Journal* 125, no. 1 (January 1, 1993): 194–203, https://doi.org/10.1016/0002-8703(93)90075-K.

153   Elevated serum oxalate is a risk factor for cardiovascular events

Anja Pfau et al., "High Oxalate Concentrations Correlate with Increased Risk for Sudden Cardiac Death in Dialysis Patients," *Journal of the American Society of Nephrology: JASN* 32, no. 9 (September 2021): 2375–85, https://doi.org/10.1681/ASN.2020121793.

153   elevated blood oxalate levels and heart attacks is so strong

Natalia Stepanova et al., "Plasma Oxalic Acid and Cardiovascular Risk in End-Stage Renal Disease Patients: A Prospective, Observational Cohort Pilot Study," *Korean J. Intern. Med* 10 (2020): 1–20, https://doi.org/10.3904/kjim.2020.561.

154   pre-dialysis blood oxalate levels can be 10 to 100 times higher

Levin, Kantoff, and Jaffe, "Uremic Levels of Oxalic Acid Suppress Replication and Migration of Human Endothelial Cells."

154   Also, although red blood cells contain oxalate

Sven Oehlschläger et al., "Role of Cellular Oxalate in Oxalate Clearance of Patients with Calcium Oxalate Monohydrate Stone Formation and Normal Controls," *Urology* 73, no. 3 (March 2009): 480–83, https://doi.org/10.1016/j.urology.2008.11.028.

154   Oxalate overload is associated with unstable or degenerating connective tissues

Serpil Ünver Saraydin, Dursun Saraydin, and Zeynep Deniz Şahin İnan, "A Digital Image Analysis Study on the Disintegration Kinetics of Reticular Fibers in the Ethylene Glycol-Induced Rat Liver Tissue," *Microscopy Research and Technique* 83, no. 12 (2020): 1585–93, https://doi.org/10.1002/jemt.23554; Muhammad Abdul Mabood Khalil et al., "Scleroderma Renal Crisis in a Newly Diagnosed Mixed Connective Tissue Disease Resulting in Dialysis-Dependent Chronic Kidney Disease despite Angiotensin-Converting Enzyme Inhibition," *CEN Case Reports* 2, no. 1 (May 2013): 41–45, https://doi.org/10.1007/s13730-012-0036-z.

154   extensive degeneration of the skeletal muscles

The pathologist also found dead cells in her brain and spinal cord, small bleeds in her pelvis, and immune cell reactions in her heart. I. Dvořáčková, "Tödliche Vergiftung nach intravenöser Verabreichung von Natriumoxalat," *Archiv für Toxikologie* 22, no. 2 (March 1, 1966): 63–67, https://doi.org/10.1007/BF01342653.

154 Fibromyalgia sufferers have a lower density of mitochondria

A. Bengtsson, "The Muscle in Fibromyalgia," *Rheumatology* (Oxford, England) 41, no. 7 (July 2002): 721–24, https://doi.org/10.1093/rheumatology/41.7.721.

154 these factors interfere with energy production

Thomas J. Romano and John W. Stiller, "Magnesium Deficiency in Fibromyalgia Syndrome," *Journal of Nutritional Medicine* 4, no. 2 (January 1, 1994): 165–67, https://doi.org/10.3109/13590849409034552; Paul Le Goff, "Is Fibromyalgia a Muscle Disorder?," *Joint Bone Spine* 73, no. 3 (May 2006): 239–42, https://doi.org/10.1016/j.jbspin.2005.03.022. Compensations for compromised energy metabolism and insufficient blood supply include increased numbers and uneven distribution of mitochondria in muscles. Biopsies from muscle pain patients show ragged red fibers, which are damaged and inflamed muscle fibers that have mitochondrial disease. Ragged red fibers in muscles increase with "normal" aging, a reflection of progressive damage to mitochondrial energy metabolism in muscles with age. Given that symptoms of fibromyalgia eventually abate on the low-oxalate diet, oxalates' muscle-damaging (mitochondria-killing) potential is perhaps part of the explanation. Bengtsson, "The Muscle in Fibromyalgia"; Z. Rifai et al., "Ragged Red Fibers in Normal Aging and Inflammatory Myopathy," *Annals of Neurology* 37, no. 1 (January 1995): 24–29, https://doi.org/10.1002/ana.410370107.

155 Patients on dialysis

A. J. Reginato et al., "Arthropathy and Cutaneous Calcinosis in Hemodialysis Oxalosis," *Arthritis and Rheumatism* 29, no. 11 (November 1986): 1387–96; A. J. Reginato and B. Kurnik, "Calcium Oxalate and Other Crystals Associated with Kidney Diseases and Arthritis," *Seminars in Arthritis and Rheumatism* 18, no. 3 (February 1989): 198–224; Reginato, "Calcium Oxalate and Other Crystals or Particles Associated with Arthritis"; Elisabeth B. Matson and Anthony M. Reginato, "Calcium-Containing Crystal-Associated Arthropathies in the Elderly Population," 2011; A. Coral, M. van Holsbeeck, and C. Hegg, "Case Report 599: Secondary Oxalosis Complicating Chronic Renal Failure (Oxalate Gout)," *Skeletal Radiology* 19, no. 2 (1990): 147–49.

155 Oxalate arthritis typically occurs in previously damaged joints

A. Rosenthal, L. M. Ryan, and D. J. McCarty, "Arthritis Associated with Calcium Oxalate Crystals in an Anephric Patient Treated with Peritoneal Dialysis," *JAMA* 260, no. 9 (September 2, 1988): 1280–82, https://doi.org/10.1001/jama.1988.03410090112041; P. Hasselbacher et al., "Stimulation of Secretion of Collagenase and Prostaglandin E2 by Synovial Fibroblasts in Response to Crystals of Monosodium Urate Monohydrate: A Model for Joint Destruction in Gout," *Transactions of the Association of American Physicians* 94 (1981): 243–52; G. S. Hoffman et al., "Calcium Oxalate Microcrystalline-Associated Arthritis in End-Stage Renal Disease," *Annals of Internal Medicine* 97, no. 1 (July 1982): 36–42.

155 Immune reactions to the oxalate crystals

Erick Prado de Oliveira and Roberto Carlos Burini, "High Plasma Uric Acid Concentration: Causes and Consequences," *Diabetology & Metabolic Syndrome* 4 (April 4, 2012): 12, https://doi.org/10.1186/1758-5996-4-12; Hoffman et al., "Calcium Oxalate Microcrystalline-Associated Arthritis in End-Stage Renal Disease"; Fabio Martinon et al., "Gout-Associated Uric Acid Crystals Activate the NALP3 Inflammasome," *Nature* 440, no. 7081 (March 9, 2006): 237–41, https://doi.org/10.1038/nature04516; H. S. Cheung and D. J. McCarty, "Mechanisms of Connective Tissue Damage by Crystals Containing Calcium," *Rheumatic Diseases Clinics of North America* 14, no. 2 (August 1988): 365–76.

155   pains flared after eating high-oxalate foods

Hoffman et al., "Calcium Oxalate Microcrystalline-Associated Arthritis in End-Stage Renal Disease," citing Lueper M. 1932 Rhumatisme chronique et oxalemie. *Nutr Tome II Ann Clin Biol Ther.*

155   gouty arthritis results from any of five types of crystals

P. A. Simkin, "Articular Oxalate Crystals and the Taxonomy of Gout," *JAMA* 260, no. 9 (September 2, 1988): 1285–86.

155   arthritis, bursitis, and tendinitis can be due to

P. A. Simkin, "Towards a Coherent Terminology of Gout," *Annals of the Rheumatic Diseases* 52, no. 9 (September 1993): 693–94.

156   bones become harder and denser, yet more porous

Renata Caudarella, "Citrate and Mineral Metabolism: Kidney Stones and Bone Disease," *Frontiers in Bioscience: A Journal and Virtual Library* 8 (September 1, 2003): s1084-1106; Reginato and Kurnik, "Calcium Oxalate and Other Crystals Associated with Kidney Diseases and Arthritis."

156   may lead to spinal stenosis and other bone deformities

R. Q. Knight et al., "Oxalosis: Cause of Degenerative Spinal Stenosis. A Case Report and Review of the Literature," *Orthopedics* 11, no. 6 (June 1988): 955–58.

156   crystal deposits promote bone loss

G. Gherardi et al., "Bone Oxalosis and Renal Osteodystrophy," *Archives of Pathology & Laboratory Medicine* 104, no. 2 (February 1980): 105–11.

156   immune reactions to crystals is even more destructive

D. Brancaccio et al., "Bone Changes in End-Stage Oxalosis," *AJR. American Journal of Roentgenology* 136, no. 5 (May 1981): 935–39, https://doi.org/10.2214/ajr.136.5.935; C. L. Benhamou et al., "Primary Bone Oxalosis: The Roles of Oxalate Deposits and Renal Osteodystrophy," *Bone* 8, no. 2 (1987): 59–64; C. L. Benhamou et al., "[Bone involvement in primary oxalosis. Study of 20 cases]," *Revue du Rhumatisme et des Maladies Ostéo-Articulaires* 58, no. 11 (November 30, 1991): 763–69.

156   (*osteoclasts*, a type of immune cell) issue acid and enzymes

S. L. Teitelbaum, "Bone Resorption by Osteoclasts," *Science* (New York, NY) 289, no. 5484 (September 1, 2000): 1504–8, https://doi.org/10.1126/science.289.5484.1504.

156   oxalate deposits may become shockingly severe

Leila Benmoussa, Marion Renoux, and Loredana Radoï, "Oral Manifestations of Chronic Renal Failure Complicating a Systemic Genetic Disease: Diagnostic Dilemma. Case Report and Literature Review," *Journal of Oral and Maxillofacial Surgery: Official Journal of the American Association of Oral and Maxillofacial Surgeons* 73, no. 11 (November 2015): 2142–48, https://doi.org/10.1016/j.joms.2015.05.029; B. S. Moskow, "Periodontal Manifestations of Hyperoxaluria and Oxalosis," *Journal of Periodontology* 60, no. 5 (May 1989): 271–78, https://doi.org/10.1902/jop.1989.60.5.271.

156   oxalate problems occurring in the wake of ileojejunal bypass surgery

H. J. Lapointe and R. Listrom, "Oral Manifestations of Oxalosis Secondary to Ileojejunal Intestinal Bypass," *Oral Surgery, Oral Medicine, and Oral Pathology* 65, no. 1 (January 1988): 76–80.

157   *oxalate toxicity always sits at the root cause of hearing loss*

Liam Boehm, Liam Stops Tinnitus, personal communication.

157   Anemia can result from oxalate

Gustavo Tapia, José-Tomas Navarro, and Maruja Navarro, "Leukoerythroblastic Anemia Due to Oxalosis with Extensive Bone Marrow Involvement," *American Journal of Hematology* 83, no. 6 (June 2008): 515–16, https://doi.org/10.1002/ajh.20935; Nasir A. Bakshi and Hazzaa Al-Zahrani, "Bone Marrow Oxalosis," *Blood* 120, no. 1 (July 5, 2012): 8, https://doi.org/10.1182/blood-2011-12-400192; Karolina M. Stepien et al., "Acute Renal Failure, Microangiopathic Haemolytic Anemia, and Secondary Oxalosis in a Young Female Patient," *International Journal of Nephrology* 2011 (July 19, 2011), https://doi.org/10.4061/2011/679160; H. A. Buc et al., "The Metabolic Effects of Oxalate on Intact Red Blood Cells," *Biochimica et Biophysica Acta* 628, no. 2 (March 3, 1980): 136–44, https://doi.org/10.1016/0304-4165(80)90360-8.

158   (interstitial cystitis) and urinary control problems

Mauro Cervigni and Franca Natale, "Gynecological Disorders in Bladder Pain Syndrome/Interstitial Cystitis Patients," *International Journal of Urology: Official Journal of the Japanese Urological Association* 21, Suppl 1 (April 2014): 85–88, https://doi.org/10.1111/iju.12379.

158   immune activation leading to chronic or episodic bladder pain

Jennifer Yonaitis Fariello and Robert M. Moldwin, "Similarities between Interstitial Cystitis/Bladder Pain Syndrome and Vulvodynia: Implications for Patient Management," *Translational Andrology and Urology* 4, no. 6 (December 2015): 643–52, https://doi.org/10.3978/j.issn.2223-4683.2015.10.09; Cervigni and Natale, "Gynecological Disorders in Bladder Pain Syndrome/Interstitial Cystitis Patients."

158   Oxalate crystals cause acute kidney injury

Mulay et al., "Cytotoxicity of Crystals Involves RIPK3-MLKL-Mediated Necroptosis"; Andrea Matson and Burt Faibisoff, "Gluteal Black Market Silicone–Induced Renal Failure: A Case Report and Literature Review," *Plastic and Reconstructive Surgery Global Open* 5, no. 11 (November 20, 2017), https://doi.org/10.1097/GOX .0000000000001578.

158   oxalate crystal deposits in the kidney cause tissue damage

Ermanila Dhana, Isis Ludwig-Portugall, and Christian Kurts, "Role of Immune Cells in Crystal-Induced Kidney Fibrosis," *Matrix Biology*, SI: Fibrosis—Mechanisms and Translational Aspects, 68–69 (August 1, 2018): 280–92, https://doi.org/10.1016/j.matbio .2017.11.013.

158   stones are predominately oxalate crystal aggregates

D. T. D. Hughes, "The Clinical and Pathological Background of Two Cases of Oxalosis," *Journal of Clinical Pathology*, no. 12 (1959): 498; N. D. Adams et al., "Calcium-Oxalate-Crystal-Induced Bone Disease," *American Journal of Kidney Diseases: The Official Journal of the National Kidney Foundation* 1, no. 5 (March 1982): 294–99; Boogaerts et al., "Mechanisms of Vascular Damage in Gout and Oxalosis."

158   after meals cause cellular distress

John C. Lieske, F. Gary Toback, and Sergio Deganello, "Direct Nucleation of Calcium Oxalate Dihydrate Crystals onto the Surface of Living Renal Epithelial Cells in Culture," *Kidney International* 54, no. 3 (September 1998): 796–803, https://doi.org/10.1046/j.1523-1755.1998.00058.x; Lakhmir S. Chawla et al., "Acute Kidney Injury and Chronic Kidney Disease as Interconnected Syndromes," *The New England Journal of Medicine* 371, no. 1 (July 3, 2014): 58–66, https://doi.org/10.1056/NEJMra1214243.

"An increase in either GI oxalate absorption or hepatic oxalate production increases plasma oxalate and thus urinary oxalate, and contributes to the risk of stone formation and other adverse kidney outcomes, such as nephrocalcinosis. Enteric hyperoxaluria can result from increased bioavailability of dietary oxalate or increased GI oxalate permeability. Decreased intestinal secretion of oxalate into the gut lumen has also been associated with hyperoxaluria in animal models. The bioavailability of dietary oxalate is, in part, determined by the calcium content of ingested food . . ." Celeste Witting et al., "Pathophysiology and Treatment of Enteric Hyperoxaluria," *Clinical Journal of the American Society of Nephrology: CJASN*, September 8, 2020, https://doi.org/10.2215/CJN.08000520.

158   **high urine oxalate leads to crystal clumping**

R. L. Hackett, P. N. Shevock, and S. R. Khan, "Cell Injury Associated Calcium Oxalate Crystalluria," *The Journal of Urology* 144, no. 6 (December 1990): 1535–38; S. R. Khan et al., "Crystal-Cell Interaction and Apoptosis in Oxalate-Associated Injury of Renal Epithelial Cells," *Journal of the American Society of Nephrology: JASN* 10, no. Suppl 14 (1999): 457–63; J. M. Fasano and S. R. Khan, "Intratubular Crystallization of Calcium Oxalate in the Presence of Membrane Vesicles: An in Vitro Study," *Kidney International* 59, no. 1 (January 2001): 169–78, https://doi.org/10.1046/j.1523-1755.2001.00477.x.

159   **"a common biology underlies calcium stone formation**

Eric N. Taylor, "Stones, Bones, and Cardiovascular Groans," *Clinical Journal of the American Society of Nephrology: CJASN* 10, no. 2 (February 6, 2015): 175, https://doi .org/10.2215/CJN.12311214.

159   **The baffling and disparate symptoms of oxalate overload**

Alessio Fasano, "Zonulin, Regulation of Tight Junctions, and Autoimmune Diseases," *Annals of the New York Academy of Sciences* 1258, no. 1 (July 2012): 25–33, https://doi .org/10.1111/j.1749-6632.2012.06538.x.

Chapter 11

160   **Many assume that in the absence**

Stephen J. Genuis and Kasie L. Kelln, "Toxicant Exposure and Bioaccumulation: A Common and Potentially Reversible Cause of Cognitive Dysfunction and Dementia," *Behavioural Neurology* 2015 (2015): 620143, https://doi.org/10.1155/2015/620143.

162   **Immune cells perceive the damaging oxalates**

P. Matzinger, "Tolerance, Danger, and the Extended Family," *Annual Review of Immunology* 12 (1994): 991–1045, https://doi.org/10.1146/annurev.iy.12.040194.005015.

165   **fibrotic kidneys loaded with calcium oxalate crystals**

A. Allen et al., "Enteric Hyperoxaluria and Renal Failure Associated with Lymphangiectasia.," *Nephrology Dialysis Transplantation* 12, no. 4 (April 1, 1997): 802–6, https://doi.org/10.1093/ndt/12.4.802.

165   **"No specific treatment was initiated at this point"**

Allen et al., "Enteric Hyperoxaluria and Renal Failure," 802.

168   **Urea (the principal source of ammonia smells) has antioxidant effects**

B. Finlayson, R. Roth, and L. Dubois, "Perturbation of Calcium Ion Activity by Urea," *Investigative Urology* 10, no. 2 (September 1972): 138–40; Jaroslav Streit, Lan-Chi

Tran-Ho, and Erich Königsberger, "Solubility of the Three Calcium Oxalate Hydrates in Sodium Chloride Solutions and Urine-Like Liquors," *Monatshefte Für Chemie / Chemical Monthly* 129, no. 12 (December 1, 1998): 1225–36, https://doi.org/10.1007/PL00010134.

Chapter 12

173 **The best treatment**

Elizabeth C. Lorenz et al., "Update on Oxalate Crystal Disease," *Current Rheumatology Reports* 15, no. 7 (July 2013): 340, https://doi.org/10.1007/s11926-013-0340-4.

Chapter 13

181 **[T]he significant can only be**

Nassim Nicholas Taleb, *Antifragile: Things That Gain from Disorder* (New York: Random House, 2012).

Chapter 14

196 **There has been, of late years**

Sarah Josepha Buell Hale, *Early American Cookery: "The Good Housekeeper,"* 1841 (Mineola, N.Y.: Dover Publications, 1996).

214 **greater intake of animal protein**

John Knight et al., "Increased Protein Intake on Controlled Oxalate Diets Does Not Increase Urinary Oxalate Excretion," *Urological Research* 37, no. 2 (April 2009): 63–68, https://doi.org/10.1007/s00240-009-0170-z.

215 **toxic giant snails**

The snail *Limicolaria aurora* is used as a food in Nigeria (381mg/100g). S. C. Noonan and G. P. Savage, "Oxalate Content of Foods and Its Effect on Humans," *Asia Pacific Journal of Clinical Nutrition* 8, no. 1 (March 1999): 64–74. Citing Anthony P. Udoh, Edet O. Akpanyung, and Ironge E. Igiran, "Nutrients and Anti-Nutrients in Small Snails (*Limicolaria aurora*)," *Food Chemistry* 53, no. 3 (January 1, 1995): 239–41, https://doi.org/10.1016/0308-8146(95)93927-J., and the dogwhelk, which contains a whopping 1686mg/100g (A. P. Udoh, R. I. Effiong, and D. O. Edem, "Nutrient Composition of Dogwhelk (*Thais cattifera*), a Protein Source for Humans," *Tropical Science* (United Kingdom), 1995.

215 **meat from other animals (pigs and poultry)**

Food oxalate content for all cited foods appears with references in the data tables available via my website, www.sallyknorton.com.

221 **boiling fresh broccoli for 12 minutes will reduce the oxalate**

Weiwen Chai and Michael Liebman, "Effect of Different Cooking Methods on Vegetable Oxalate Content," *Journal of Agricultural and Food Chemistry* 53, no. 8 (April 1, 2005): 3027–30, https://doi.org/10.1021/jf048128d.

221 **after six days of fermentation**

A. Jagannath, Manoranjan Kumar, and P. S. Raju, "The recalcitrance of oxalate, nitrate and nitrites during the controlled lactic fermentation of commonly consumed green leafy vegetables," NFS *Nutrition & Food Science* 45, no. 2 (2015): 336–46.

221 **A traditional Hawaiian food called** *poi*

Amy C. Brown and Ana Valiere, "The Medicinal Uses of Poi," *Nutrition in Clinical Care: An Official Publication of Tufts University* 7, no. 2 (2004): 69–74.

Chapter 15

225 **Oxalate in the body**

A. Bergstrand et al., "Oxalosis in Renal Transplants Following Methoxyflurane Anaesthesia," *British Journal of Anaesthesia* 44, no. 6 (June 1972): 569–74.

229 **Using a sauna can improve blood pressure**

Jari A. Laukkanen, Tanjaniina Laukkanen, and Setor K. Kunutsor, "Cardiovascular and Other Health Benefits of Sauna Bathing: A Review of the Evidence," *Mayo Clinic Proceedings* 93, no. 8 (August 2018): 1111–21, https://doi.org/10.1016/j.mayocp.2018.04.008.

229 **"a lazy person's exercise with regard to health improvement"**

Martin L. Pall, "Do Sauna Therapy and Exercise Act by Raising the Availability of Tetrahydrobiopterin?," *Medical Hypotheses* 73, no. 4 (October 2009): 610–13, https://doi.org/10.1016/j.mehy.2009.03.058.

230 **Cold showers, or even cold-water immersion, deliver**

Nikolai A. Shevchuk, "Adapted Cold Shower as a Potential Treatment for Depression," *Medical Hypotheses* 70, no. 5 (January 1, 2008): 995–1001, https://doi.org/10.1016/j.mehy.2007.04.052.

231 **Sun exposure is frequently viewed as "all bad"**

Richard B. Weller, "Sunlight Has Cardiovascular Benefits Independently of Vitamin D," *Blood Purification* 41, no. 1–3 (2016): 130–34, https://doi.org/10.1159/000441266; Marianne Berwick et al., "Sun Exposure and Mortality from Melanoma," *Journal of the National Cancer Institute* 97, no. 3 (February 2, 2005): 195–99, https://doi.org/10.1093/jnci/dji019; Graham Holliman et al., "Ultraviolet Radiation-Induced Production of Nitric Oxide:A Multi-Cell and Multi-Donor Analysis," *Scientific Reports* 7, no. 1 (September 11, 2017): 11105, https://doi.org/10.1038/s41598-017-11567-5; Prue H. Hart et al., "Exposure to Ultraviolet Radiation in the Modulation of Human Diseases," *Annual Review of Pathology* 14 (January 24, 2019): 55–81, https://doi.org/10.1146/annurev-pathmechdis-012418-012809.

231 **the regular consumption of seed oils**

V. E. Reeve, M. Bosnic, and C. Boehm-Wilcox, "Dependence of Photocarcinogenesis and Photoimmunosuppression in the Hairless Mouse on Dietary Polyunsaturated Fat," *Cancer Letters* 108, no. 2 (November 29, 1996): 271–79, https://doi.org/10.1016/s0304-3835(96)04460-6.

231 **Grain-fed chicken is another source**

Khaled Kanakri et al., "The Effect of Different Dietary Fats on the Fatty Acid Composition of Several Tissues in Broiler Chickens," *European Journal of Lipid Science and Technology* 120, no. 1 (2018): 1700237, https://doi.org/10.1002/ejlt.201700237.

232 **omega-3 fats provided by seafoods are skin protective**

Suzanne M. Pilkington et al., "Omega-3 Polyunsaturated Fatty Acids: Photoprotective Macronutrients," *Experimental Dermatology* 20, no. 7 (July 2011): 537–43, https://doi.org/10.1111/j.1600-0625.2011.01294.x.

232 **tannin-rich foods act as co-carcinogens**

King-Thom Chung, Cheng-I Wei, and Michael G. Johnson, "Are Tannins a Double-Edged Sword in Biology and Health?," *Trends in Food Science & Technology* 9, no. 4 (April 1, 1998): 168–75, https://doi.org/10.1016/S0924-2244(98)00028-4.

Recall that tannins are polyphenols associated not only with skin cancer, but also esophageal, stomach, lung, and kidney cancers.

232 **direct toxic effects of sunscreen lotions**

Germaine M. Buck Louis et al., "Urinary Concentrations of Benzophenone-Type Ultraviolet Radiation Filters and Couples' Fecundity," *American Journal of Epidemiology* 180, no. 12 (December 15, 2014): 1168–75, https://doi.org/10.1093/aje/kwu285.

233 **Not many foods are particularly good sources of calcium beyond milk**

Jean A. Thompson Pennington and Judith Spungen, *Bowes & Church's Food Values of Portions Commonly Used* (Philadelphia: Lippincott, Williams & Wilkins, 2010).

236 **Adequate calcium intake also helps to prevent kidney stones**

Ita P. Heilberg and David S. Goldfarb, "Optimum Nutrition for Kidney Stone Disease," *Advances in Chronic Kidney Disease* 20, no. 2 (March 2013): 165–74, https://doi.org/10.1053/j.ackd.2012.12.001.

236 **calcium supplement–takers have a lower risk of death**

N. C. Harvey et al., "The Role of Calcium Supplementation in Healthy Musculoskeletal Ageing : An Expert Consensus Meeting of the European Society for Clinical and Economic Aspects of Osteoporosis, Osteoarthritis and Musculoskeletal Diseases (ESCEO) and the International Foundation for Osteoporosis (IOF)," *Osteoporosis International: A Journal Established as Result of Cooperation between the European Foundation for Osteoporosis and the National Osteoporosis Foundation of the USA* 28, no. 2 (February 2017): 447–62, https://doi.org/10.1007/s00198-016-3773-6.

236 **cardiovascular benefits from calcium supplements**

Gabriela Cormick et al., "Calcium Supplementation for Prevention of Primary Hypertension," *The Cochrane Database of Systematic Reviews*, no. 6 (June 30, 2015): CD010037, https://doi.org/10.1002/14651858.CD010037.pub2.

237 **considered by some to be the optimum calcium supplement**

C. Y. Pak, "Citrate and Renal Calculi: An Update," *Mineral and Electrolyte Metabolism* 20, no. 6 (1994): 371–77; Andrea Palermo et al., "Calcium Citrate: From Biochemistry and Physiology to Clinical Applications," *Reviews in Endocrine & Metabolic Disorders* 20, no. 3 (2019): 353–64, https://doi.org/10.1007/s11154-019-09520-0.

239   magnesium helps oxalate get out without crystallizing

Jaroslav Streit, Lan-Chi Tran-Ho, and Erich Königsberger, "Solubility of the Three
Calcium Oxalate Hydrates in Sodium Chloride Solutions and Urine-Like Liquors,"
Monatshefte Für Chemie / Chemical Monthly 129, no. 12 (December 1, 1998):
1225–36, https://doi.org/10.1007/PL00010134; Bryan G. Alamani and Jeffrey D. Rimer,
"Molecular Modifiers of Kidney Stones," *Current Opinion in Nephrology and
Hypertension* 26, no. 4 (2017): 256–65, https://doi.org/10.1097/
MNH.0000000000000330; P. O. Schwille et al., "Magnesium, Citrate, Magnesium
Citrate and Magnesium-Alkali Citrate as Modulators of Calcium Oxalate Crystallization
in Urine: Observations in Patients with Recurrent Idiopathic Calcium Urolithiasis,"
Urological Research 27, no. 2 (April 1999): 117–26; Jürgen Vormann, "Magnesium and
Kidney Health—More on the 'Forgotten Electrolyte,'" *American Journal of Nephrology*
44, no. 5 (2016): 379–80, https://doi.org/10.1159/000450863.

239   foods can't begin to make up for magnesium deficiency

Jürgen Vormann, "Magnesium," in *Biochemical, Physiological, and Molecular Aspects of
Human Nutrition*, ed. Martha H. Stipanuk and Marie A. Caudill, Third (St. Louis:
Elsevier, 2013), 747–58.

239   low magnesium may be contributing

Ryu Yamanaka, Yutaka Shindo, and Kotaro Oka, "Magnesium Is a Key Player in
Neuronal Maturation and Neuropathology," *International Journal of Molecular Sciences*
20, no. 14 (July 12, 2019), https://doi.org/10.3390/ijms20143439; Uwe Gröber, Joachim
Schmidt, and Klaus Kisters, "Magnesium in Prevention and Therapy," *Nutrients* 7, no. 9
(September 23, 2015): 8199–8226, https://doi.org/10.3390/nu7095388.

239   Without adequate magnesium, recovery from oxalate toxicity is difficult

Mildred S. Seelig, *Magnesium Deficiency in the Pathogenesis of Disease: Early Roots of
Cardiovascular, Skeletal, and Renal Abnormalities* (Springer Science & Business Media,
2012); Faruk Turgut et al., "Magnesium Supplementation Helps to Improve Carotid
Intima Media Thickness in Patients on Hemodialysis," *International Urology and
Nephrology* 40, no. 4 (2008): 1075–82, https://doi.org/10.1007/s11255-008-9410-3.

239   L-threonate has increased ability to cross into the brain

Jia-Liang Chen et al., "Normalization of Magnesium Deficiency Attenuated Mechanical
Allodynia, Depressive-like Behaviors, and Memory Deficits Associated with
Cyclophosphamide-Induced Cystitis by Inhibiting TNF-α/NF-ΚB Signaling in Female
Rats," *Journal of Neuroinflammation* 17, no. 1 (April 2, 2020): 99, https://doi.org/10.1186/
s12974-020-01786-5.

240   The Recommended Dietary Allowance (RDA) is 4,700 mg

M. K. Hoy and J. D. Goldman, "Potassium Intake of the U.S. Population: What We Eat
In America, NHANES 2009- 2010. Food Surveys Research Group Dietary Data Brief,"
September 2012, http://ars.usda.gov/Services/docs.htm?docid=19476.

241   to rebuilding demineralized bones and the prevention of bone loss

F. J. He and G. A. MacGregor, "Potassium: More Beneficial Effects," *Climacteric: The
Journal of the International Menopause Society* 6, Suppl 3 (October 2003): 36–48.

241   High potassium intake prevents fibrosis and kidney-stone formation

Pietro Manuel Ferraro et al., "Dietary Protein and Potassium, Diet–Dependent Net Acid
Load, and Risk of Incident Kidney Stones," *Clinical Journal of the American Society of
Nephrology* 11, no. 10 (October 7, 2016): 1834–44, https://doi.org/10.2215/

CJN.01520216; Kuang-Yu Wei et al., "Dietary Potassium and the Kidney: Lifesaving Physiology," *Clinical Kidney Journal* 13, no. 6 (September 2, 2020): 952–68, https://doi .org/10.1093/ckj/sfaa157.

241　**directly inhibiting free radical formation**

R. D. McCabe et al., "Potassium Inhibits Free Radical Formation," *Hypertension* 24, no. 1 (July 1994): 77–82.

243　**half the dose used in clinical trials**

F. J. He et al., "Effects of Potassium Chloride and Potassium Bicarbonate on Endothelial Function, Cardiovascular Risk Factors, and Bone Turnover in Mild Hypertensives," *Hypertension* 55, no. 3 (2010): 681–88.

244　**turns on the sodium-retaining hormones**

Olena Andrukhova et al., "FGF23 Regulates Renal Sodium Handling and Blood Pressure," *EMBO Molecular Medicine* 6, no. 6 (June 2014): 744–59, https://doi.org/ 10.1002/emmm.201303716.

248　**deficiency of the sulfur amino acids**

Stephen Parcell, "Sulfur in Human Nutrition and Applications in Medicine," *Alternative Medicine Review: A Journal of Clinical Therapeutic* 7, no. 1 (February 2002): 22–44.

248　**MSM is also good for the skin, vascular system, and stomach lining**

Keyvan Amirshahrokhi and Ali-Reza Khalili, "Methylsulfonylmethane Is Effective against Gastric Mucosal Injury," *European Journal of Pharmacology* 811 (September 15, 2017): 240–48, https://doi.org/10.1016/j.ejphar.2017.06.034; Huijeong Ahn et al., "Methylsulfonylmethane Inhibits NLRP3 Inflammasome Activation," *Cytokine* 71, no. 2 (February 2015): 223–31, https://doi.org/10.1016/j.cyto.2014.11.001; Matthew Butawan, Rodney L. Benjamin, and Richard J. Bloomer, "Methylsulfonylmethane: Applications and Safety of a Novel Dietary Supplement," *Nutrients* 9, no. 3 (March 16, 2017): E290, https://doi.org/10.3390/nu9030290.

248　**repair and regeneration of bones and teeth**

Hanan Dakhil Aljohani, "Methylsulfonylmethane: Possible Role in Bone Remodeling" (Doctoral Dissertation, Baltimore, University of Maryland, 2020), https://www.proquest .com/openview/5903727aea3a869514ca09d36f7280f1/1?pq-origsite=gscholar&cbl=51922 &diss=y.

248　**help with fibromyalgia, arthritis, interstitial cystitis**

Parcell, "Sulfur in Human Nutrition and Applications in Medicine."

249　**if well tolerated, gradually increase**

Thomas A. Pagonis et al., "The Effect of Methylsulfonylmethane on Osteoarthritic Large Joints and Mobility," *International Journal of Orthopaedics* 1, no. 1 (June 23, 2014): 19–24, https://doi.org/10.6051/ijo.v1i1.745.

249　**breathing silica crystals is toxic**

Werner Götz et al., "Effects of Silicon Compounds on Biomineralization, Osteogenesis, and Hard Tissue Formation," *Pharmaceutics* 11, no. 3 (March 12, 2019), https://doi.org/ 10.3390/pharmaceutics11030117.

249　**Silicon can be more effective than collagen for connective tissue health**

H. Rico et al., "Effect of Silicon Supplement on Osteopenia Induced by Ovariectomy in Rats," *Calcified Tissue International* 66, no. 1 (January 2000): 53–55, https://doi.org/ 10.1007/s002230050010; Charles T. Price, Kenneth J. Koval, and Joshua R. Langford,

"Silicon: A Review of Its Potential Role in the Prevention and Treatment of Postmenopausal Osteoporosis," *International Journal of Endocrinology* 2013 (2013): 316783, https://doi.org/10.1155/2013/316783.

250 **Tap water may contain not only toxic metals but also many other additives**

Malwina Diduch, Zaneta Polkowska, and Jacek Namieśnik, "Chemical Quality of Bottled Waters: A Review," *Journal of Food Science* 76, no. 9 (December 2011): R178-196, https://doi.org/10.1111/j.1750-3841.2011.02386.x.

250 **water contains plastic residues picked up from its packaging**

Diduch, Polkowska, and Namieśnik, "Chemical Quality of Bottled Waters"; Arnold F. Dijkstra and Ana Maria de Roda Husman, "Chapter 14 — Bottled and Drinking Water," in *Food Safety Management*, ed. Yasmine Motarjemi and Huub Lelieveld (San Diego: Academic Press, 2014), 347–77, https://doi.org/10.1016/B978-0-12-381504-0.00014-7.

251 **water is an important source of minerals**

Zhiqun Qiu et al., "Multi-Generational Drinking of Bottled Low Mineral Water Impairs Bone Quality in Female Rats," *PloS One* 10, no. 3 (2015): e0121995, https://doi.org/10.1371/journal.pone.0121995.

251 **de-ionized water filters restore trace amounts**

Monique H. Vingerhoeds et al., "Sensory Quality of Drinking Water Produced by Reverse Osmosis Membrane Filtration Followed by Remineralisation," *Water Research* 94 (February 19, 2016): 42–51, https://doi.org/10.1016/j.watres.2016.02.043.

254 **Citric acid (or citrate) in the urine and elsewhere**

Palermo et al., "Calcium Citrate."

254 **well-established, highly effective, and well-tolerated treatment**

Renata Caudarella, "Citrate and Mineral Metabolism: Kidney Stones and Bone Disease," *Frontiers in Bioscience: A Journal and Virtual Library* 8 (September 1, 2003): s1084-1106.

254 **increases the protective effects of other anti-clumping molecules**

Ehud Ohana et al., "SLC26A6 and NaDC-1 Transporters Interact to Regulate Oxalate and Citrate Homeostasis," *Journal of the American Society of Nephrology* 24, no. 10 (October 1, 2013): 1617–26, https://doi.org/10.1681/ASN.2013010080.

254 **it also reduces osteopontin levels**

Renata Caudarella and Fabio Vescini, "Urinary Citrate and Renal Stone Disease: The Preventive Role of Alkali Citrate Treatment," *Archivio Italiano Di Urologia, Andrologia: Organo Ufficiale [Di] Società Italiana Di Ecografia Urologica E Nefrologica / Associazione Ricerche in Urologia* 81, no. 3 (September 2009): 182–87; Karen Byer and Saeed R. Khan, "Citrate Provides Protection against Oxalate and Calcium Oxalate Crystal Induced Oxidative Damage to Renal Epithelium," *The Journal of Urology* 173, no. 2 (February 2005): 640–46, https://doi.org/10.1097/01.ju.0000143190.49888.c7; D. P. Simpson, "Citrate Excretion: A Window on Renal Metabolism," *The American Journal of Physiology* 244, no. 3 (March 1983): F223-234; Leslie C. Costello and Renty B. Franklin, "Plasma Citrate Homeostasis: How It Is Regulated; And Its Physiological and Clinical Implications. An Important, But Neglected, Relationship in Medicine," *HSOA Journal of Human Endocrinology* 1, no. 1 (2016): 1–18.

254　Citrate also promotes strong bones and teeth

Changyu Shao et al., "Citrate Improves Collagen Mineralization via Interface Wetting: A Physicochemical Understanding of Biomineralization Control," *Advanced Materials* 30, no. 8 (February 2018), https://doi.org/10.1002/adma.201704876. p.6 of 7. Citing: a) F. Dickens, *Biochem. J.* 1941, 35, 1011; b) R. L. Hartles, in *Advances in Oral Biology*, Vol. 1 (Ed.: H. S. Peter), Elsevier, Amsterdam, The Netherlands, 1964.

254　reverse the loss of bone

Caudarella and Vescini, "Urinary Citrate and Renal Stone Disease."

254　can lower urinary citrate

J. G. Pattaras and R. G. Moore, "Citrate in the Management of Urolithiasis," *Journal of Endourology* 13, no. 9 (November 1999): 687–92, https://doi.org/10.1089/end.1999.13.687.

254　Bicarbonate can also reduce tissue acidity

Vivian Barbosa Pinheiro et al., "The Effect of Sodium Bicarbonate upon Urinary Citrate Excretion in Calcium Stone Formers," *Urology* 82, no. 1 (July 2013): 33–37, https://doi.org/10.1016/j.urology.2013.03.002; David P. Simpson, "Tissue Citrate Levels and Citrate Utilization after Sodium Bicarbonate Administration," *Proceedings of the Society for Experimental Biology and Medicine* 114, no. 2 (November 1, 1963): 263–65, https://doi.org/10.3181/00379727-114-28647.

256　a lesser-known citrate called hydroxycitrate

Jihae Chung et al., "Molecular Modifiers Reveal a Mechanism of Pathological Crystal Growth Inhibition," *Nature* 536, no. 7617 (August 25, 2016): 446–50, https://doi.org/10.1038/nature19062; Doyoung Kim, Jeffrey D. Rimer, and John R. Asplin, "Hydroxycitrate: A Potential New Therapy for Calcium Urolithiasis," *Urolithiasis* 47, no. 4 (August 2019): 311–20, https://doi.org/10.1007/s00240-019-01125-1.

256　repeated ingestion of manufactured citric acid may elicit

Iliana E. Sweis and Bryan C. Cressey, "Potential Role of the Common Food Additive Manufactured Citric Acid in Eliciting Significant Inflammatory Reactions Contributing to Serious Disease States: A Series of Four Case Reports," *Toxicology Reports* 5 (August 9, 2018): 808–12, https://doi.org/10.1016/j.toxrep.2018.08.002.

257　extracellular acid that goes with inflammation and oxalate illness

Ione de Brito-Ashurst et al., "Bicarbonate Supplementation Slows Progression of CKD and Improves Nutritional Status," *Journal of the American Society of Nephrology: JASN* 20, no. 9 (September 2009): 2075–84, https://doi.org/10.1681/ASN.2008111205.

257　alkalizing effects and that can help raise citrate in the urine

Roshan M. Patel et al., "Coconut Water: An Unexpected Source of Urinary Citrate," *BioMed Research International* 2018 (2018): 3061742, https://doi.org/10.1155/2018/3061742.

259　vitamin B$_1$, activates other B vitamins and is important

H. Sidhu et al., "Oxalate Metabolism in Thiamine-Deficient Rats," *Annals of Nutrition & Metabolism* 31, no. 6 (1987): 354–61, https://doi.org/10.1159/000177294; Saori Nishijima et al., "Effect of Vitamin B$_6$ Deficiency on Glyoxylate Metabolism in Rats with or without Glyoxylate Overload," *Biomedical Research* 27, no. 3 (2006): 93–98, https://doi.org/10.2220/biomedres.27.93; Wen-Ching Huang et al., "The Effects of

Thiamine Tetrahydrofurfuryl Disulfide on Physiological Adaption and Exercise Performance Improvement," *Nutrients* 10, no. 7 (June 29, 2018), https://doi.org/10.3390/nu10070851.

259   **thiamin is effective in alleviating a wide variety of chronic conditions**

Flore Depeint et al., "Mitochondrial Function and Toxicity: Role of the B Vitamin Family on Mitochondrial Energy Metabolism," *Chemico-Biological Interactions* 163, no. 1–2 (October 27, 2006): 94–112, https://doi.org/10.1016/j.cbi.2006.04.014.

259   **foods contain factors that destroy thiamin**

Laura L. Frank, "Thiamin in Clinical Practice," *JPEN. Journal of Parenteral and Enteral Nutrition* 39, no. 5 (July 2015): 503–20, https://doi.org/10.1177/0148607114565245; K. Rungruangsak et al., "Chemical Interactions between Thiamin and Tannic Acid. I. Kinetics, Oxygen Dependence and Inhibition by Ascorbic Acid," *The American Journal of Clinical Nutrition* 30, no. 10 (October 1977): 1680–85, https://doi.org/10.1093/ajcn/30.10.1680.

259   **low thiamin causes a variety of issues with neurological health**

Depeint et al., "Mitochondrial Function and Toxicity."

259   **for any condition involving depleted or damaged mitochondria**

Derrick Lonsdale and Chandler Marrs, *Thiamine Deficiency Disease, Dysautonomia, and High Calorie Malnutrition* (London: Academic Press, 2017).

259   **doses greater than 400 mg a day**

Antonio Costantini et al., "High-Dose Thiamine Improves the Symptoms of Fibromyalgia," BMJ Case Reports 2013 (May 20, 2013), https://doi.org/10.1136/bcr-2013-009019; Ann M. Manzardo et al., "Change in Psychiatric Symptomatology after Benfotiamine Treatment in Males Is Related to Lifetime Alcoholism Severity," Drug and Alcohol Dependence 152 (July 1, 2015): 257–63, https://doi.org/10.1016/j.drugalcdep.2015.03.032.

259   **Fatigue may be relieved more quickly**

Antonio Costantini et al., "High-Dose Thiamine Improves Fatigue after Stroke: A Report of Three Cases," *Journal of Alternative and Complementary Medicine* (New York, NY) 20, no. 9 (September 2014): 683–85, https://doi.org/10.1089/acm.2013.0461.

260   **Inflammation consumes B$_6$**

En-Pei Chiang et al., "Inflammation Causes Tissue-Specific Depletion of Vitamin B$_6$," *Arthritis Research & Therapy* 7, no. 6 (2005): R1254-1262, https://doi.org/10.1186/ar1821; Valentina Lotto, Sang-Woon Choi, and Simonetta Friso, "Vitamin B$_6$: A Challenging Link between Nutrition and Inflammation in CVD," *The British Journal of Nutrition* 106, no. 2 (July 2011): 183–95, https://doi.org/10.1017/S0007114511000407.

260   **B$_6$ deficiency can (1) increase oxalate absorption**

S. Farooqui et al., "Effect of Pyridoxine Deficiency on Intestinal Absorption of Calcium and Oxalate: Chemical Composition of Brush Border Membranes in Rats," *Biochemical Medicine* 32, no. 1 (August 1984): 34–42.

260   **(2) elevate glycine levels**

Nishijima et al., "Effect of Vitamin B$_6$ Deficiency on Glyoxylate Metabolism in Rats with or without Glyoxylate Overload."

260 (3) lower citrate levels in the urine

Nishijima et al., "Effect of Vitamin B$_6$ Deficiency."

260 low plasma P-5-P increases the risk of cardiovascular disease

Per Magne Ueland et al., "Inflammation, Vitamin B$_6$ and Related Pathways," *Molecular Aspects of Medicine* 53 (2017): 10–27, https://doi.org/10.1016/j.mam.2016.08.001.

260 problems with production of the heme molecule

Evonne Teresa Nicole Ruegg, "Investigating the Porphyrias through Analysis of Biochemical Pathways" (master's thesis, University of Canterbury, 2014).

260 When vitamin B$_6$ levels are deficient, increasing your vitamin B$_6$ intake

Ueland et al., "Inflammation, Vitamin B$_6$ and Related Pathways," 20.

260 *pyridoxine HCl, is a form that the body cannot use*

Mary Rose Sweeney, Joseph McPartlin, and John Scott, "Folic Acid Fortification and Public Health: Report on Threshold Doses above Which Unmetabolised Folic Acid Appear in Serum," BMC *Public Health* 7 (March 22, 2007): 41, https://doi.org/10.1186/1471-2458-7-41.

261 *"even at relatively low dose, vitamin B$_6$ supplementation*

Misha F. Vrolijk et al., "The Vitamin B$_6$ Paradox: Supplementation with High Concentrations of Pyridoxine Leads to Decreased Vitamin B$_6$ Function," *Toxicology in Vitro: An International Journal Published in Association with BIBRA* 44 (October 2017): 206–12, https://doi.org/10.1016/j.tiv.2017.07.009.

261 The symptoms of a vitamin B$_6$ deficiency

B. E. Caffery, "Influence of Diet on Tear Function," *Optometry and Vision Science: Official Publication of the American Academy of Optometry* 68, no. 1 (January 1991): 58–72.

261 B$_6$ deficiency is associated with dry eyes

Caffery, "Influence of Diet on Tear Function."

261 neurological complaints occurring after taking 50 mg of pyridoxine

Vrolijk et al., "The Vitamin B$_6$ Paradox."

261 using P-5-P supplements for arthritis provide 100 mg doses

S. C. Huang et al., "Vitamin B(6) Supplementation Improves pro-Inflammatory Responses in Patients with Rheumatoid Arthritis," *European Journal of Clinical Nutrition* 64, no. 9 (September 2010): 1007–13, https://doi.org/10.1038/ejcn.2010.107.

262 Suboptimal biotin levels also occur

Hamid M. Said, "Intestinal Absorption of Water-Soluble Vitamins in Health and Disease," *The Biochemical Journal* 437, no. 3 (August 1, 2011): 357–72, https://doi.org/10.1042/BJ20110326.

262 biotin deficiency in pregnancy

Pregnancy needs for biotin are >2–3 times the USDA Adequate Intake level of 30 mcg. Donald M. Mock, "Biotin: From Nutrition to Therapeutics," *The Journal of Nutrition* 147, no. 8 (August 1, 2017): 1487–92, https://doi.org/10.3945/jn.116.238956.

262 **linked to blood sugar problems, increased inflammation**

Depeint et al., "Mitochondrial Function and Toxicity." citing C. Fernandez-Mejia, "Pharmacological Effects of Biotin," *J. Nutr. Biochem.* 16 , no. 7 (2005): 424–27. https:// doi.org/10.1016/j.jnutbio.2005.03.018.

262 **shown to help enzymes work better**

Anne-Laure Tardy et al., "Vitamins and Minerals for Energy, Fatigue and Cognition: A Narrative Review of the Biochemical and Clinical Evidence," *Nutrients* 12, no. 1 (January 16, 2020): 228, https://doi.org/10.3390/nu12010228.

262 **over 90 percent of the patients**

Frédéric Sedel et al., "Targeting Demyelination and Virtual Hypoxia with High-Dose Biotin as a Treatment for Progressive Multiple Sclerosis," *Neuropharmacology* 110, no. Pt B (November 2016): 644–53, https://doi.org/10.1016/j.neuropharm.2015.08.028.

263 **unmetabolized folic acid from fortified foods**

Joel B. Mason et al., "A Temporal Association between Folic Acid Fortification and an Increase in Colorectal Cancer Rates May Be Illuminating Important Biological Principles: A Hypothesis," *Cancer Epidemiology, Biomarkers & Prevention: A Publication of the American Association for Cancer Research, Cosponsored by the American Society of Preventive Oncology* 16, no. 7 (July 2007): 1325–29, https://doi.org/10.1158/1055-9965 .EPI-07-0329; A. David Smith, Young-In Kim, and Helga Refsum, "Is Folic Acid Good for Everyone?," *The American Journal of Clinical Nutrition* 87, no. 3 (March 2008): 517–33, https://doi.org/10.1093/ajcn/87.3.517.

263 **is seen as a safety-net precaution**

Hans K. Biesalski and Jana Tinz, "Multivitamin/Mineral Supplements: Rationale and Safety," *Nutrition* 36 (April 1, 2017): 60–66, https://doi.org/10.1016/j.nut.2016.06.003.

264 *"Vitamin C should not be viewed as a benign*

S. Mashour, J. F. Turner, and R. Merrell, "Acute Renal Failure, Oxalosis, and Vitamin C Supplementation—A Case Report and Review of the Literature," *Chest* 118, no. 2 (August 2000): 561–63, https://doi.org/10.1378/chest.118.2.561.

266 **most probiotic products are ineffective**

Niv Zmora et al., "Personalized Gut Mucosal Colonization Resistance to Empiric Probiotics Is Associated with Unique Host and Microbiome Features," *Cell* 174, no. 6 (September 2018): 1388-1405.e21, https://doi.org/10.1016/j.cell.2018.08.041; Jotham Suez et al., "Post-Antibiotic Gut Mucosal Microbiome Reconstitution Is Impaired by Probiotics and Improved by Autologous FMT," *Cell* 174, no. 6 (September 6, 2018): 1406-1423.e16, https://doi.org/10.1016/j.cell.2018.08.047; Aaron Lerner, Yehuda Shoenfeld, and Torsten Matthias. "Probiotics: If It Does Not Help It Does Not Do Any Harm. Really?" *Microorganisms* 7, no. 4 (April 11, 2019): 104. https://doi.org/10.3390/ microorganisms7040104.

266 **oxalate-eating gut bacteria do help**

M. Hatch et al., "*Oxalobacter* Sp. Reduces Urinary Oxalate Excretion by Promoting Enteric Oxalate Secretion," *Kidney International* 69, no. 4 (February 2006): 691–98, https://doi.org/10.1038/sj.ki.5000162; Donna Arvans et al., "*Oxalobacter formigenes*– Derived Bioactive Factors Stimulate Oxalate Transport by Intestinal Epithelial Cells," *Journal of the American Society of Nephrology*, October 13, 2016, ASN.2016020132, https://doi.org/10.1681/ASN.2016020132; Siddharth Siva et al., "A Critical Analysis of the Role of Gut *Oxalobacter formigenes* in Oxalate Stone Disease," *BJU International* 103, no. 1 (January 1, 2009): 18–21, https://doi.org/10.1111/j.1464-410X.2008.08122.x.

266   ***Oxalobacter formigenes* cannot be reestablished**

John C. Lieske, "Probiotics for Prevention of Urinary Stones," *Annals of Translational Medicine* 5, no. 2 (January 2017): 29, https://doi.org/10.21037/atm.2016.11.86; Dawn Milliner, Bernd Hoppe, and Jaap Groothoff, "A Randomised Phase II/III Study to Evaluate the Efficacy and Safety of Orally Administered *Oxalobacter formigenes* to Treat Primary Hyperoxaluria," *Urolithiasis* 46, no. 4 (2018): 313–23, https://doi.org/10.1007/s00240-017-0998-6; Paulina Wigner, Michał Bijak, and Joanna Saluk-Bijak, "Probiotics in the Prevention of the Calcium Oxalate Urolithiasis," *Cells* 11, no. 2 (January 14, 2022): 284, https://doi.org/10.3390/cells11020284.

266   **long-term use of vitamin E and vitamin C supplements**

Goran Bjelakovic et al., "Antioxidant Supplements for Prevention of Mortality in Healthy Participants and Patients with Various Diseases," *Cochrane Database of Systematic Reviews*, no. 3 (2012), https://doi.org/10.1002/14651858.CD007176.pub2; David R Thomas, "Vitamins in Aging, Health, and Longevity," *Clinical Interventions in Aging* 1, no. 1 (March 2006): 81–91.

267   **antioxidant supplements can inhibit the normal adaptive response**

Sergio Di Meo and Paola Venditti, "Evolution of the Knowledge of Free Radicals and Other Oxidants," *Oxidative Medicine and Cellular Longevity* 2020 (2020): 9829176, https://doi.org/10.1155/2020/9829176.

267   **Familiar and universally available**

Chris Centeno, "Are You an NSAID Addict? What Can You Do?," Regenexx, March 12, 2015, https://www.regenexx.com/nsaid-addict-can/.

267   **more than 30 million people worldwide were using these drugs**

Carlos Sostres, Carla J Gargallo, and Angel Lanas, "Nonsteroidal Anti-Inflammatory Drugs and Upper and Lower Gastrointestinal Mucosal Damage," *Arthritis Research & Therapy* 15, no. Suppl 3 (2013): S3, https://doi.org/10.1186/ar4175.

267   **Anti-inflammatories may even shorten life**

Di Meo and Venditti, "Evolution of the Knowledge of Free Radicals and Other Oxidants."

267   **NSAIDs are ineffective for oxalate-related arthritis**

A. J. Reginato et al., "Arthropathy and Cutaneous Calcinosis in Hemodialysis Oxalosis," *Arthritis and Rheumatism* 29, no. 11 (November 1986): 1387–96.

Chapter 16

270   **No written law**

Carrie Chapman Catt, " 'Why We Ask for the Submission of an Amendment'," (US Senate Hearing on woman's suffrage, Washington, DC, February 13, 1900).

Index

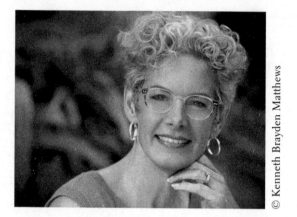

ABOUT THE AUTHOR

Sally K. Norton, MPH, received her bachelor's degree in nutritional science from Cornell University and her master's degree in public health from the University of North Carolina, Chapel Hill.